New, Old, and F[orgotten]

Remedies: Papers ~~by~~ ~~Many~~

Writers

Various

Alpha Editions

This edition published in 2022

ISBN: 9789356712713

Design and Setting By

Alpha Editions

a www.alphaedis.com

Email - info@alphaedis.com

Contents

PREFACE.

During the many years that the compiler has had the management of the publishing department of Messrs. Boericke & Tafel—long to look back over, yet short to live—so many inquiries came in for "literature," or, in the form, "where can I find something about" this, that, or the other, remedy, that finally I became convinced that there might be a niche in the great world's already over-crowded library for a book containing, in part, at least, the information desired by my numerous correspondents. This determined, and the great publishing house willing to back the enterprise, came the task of collecting the material. The work once begun, it was soon found that it is much easier to plan such a volume than to carry out the plan, for it involved no inconsiderable amount of delving in dusty piles of old journals to discover the sought for matter, which, when brought to light, had to be scanned closely to determine whether it was of a nature to justify this literary resurrection. However, in the odd hours of time that could be bestowed the work was finally completed and—the result is before you, kindly reader.

That this collection of papers has many gems is, I believe, not to be questioned; that some better papers on the remedies than those herein presented may exist is also probable; that it may contain some that are of doubtful value is not to be denied, and even some that have no right in such a book may have crept in. But what it is, it is; take the good and, in the current phrase of the hour, "forget" the rest.

The part born by the editor, beyond delving for and selecting the remedies, will be found scattered through the book in[Pg iv] bracketed small type, and consists simply in announcing who the writer of the paper was and where it may be found; no attempt has been made at editing any of the papers, or commenting on them, beyond a little cutting out of a little verbosity here and there, or of matter not bearing on the use of the remedy.

The material was drawn from journals of all "schools," wherever a paper could be found that seemed to contain something not to be found in medical-book literature, and to be honestly written.

The new remedies of the laboratory have been purposely ignored because they do not come in the scheme of this book, they having a literature of their own that, not infrequently, may be had "free on request" to the laboratories. Only remedies (with a few exceptions) such as nature gives us are included in this work.

And now the task completed naught remains but for the compiler to subscribe himself,

EDWARD POLLOCK ANSHUTZ.

1011 Arch St., Philadelphia, January 2, 1900.

ACALYPHA INDICA.

NAT. ORD., Euphorbiaceæ.
COMMON NAME, Indian Acalypha, Indian Nettle.
PREPARATION.—The fresh plant is macerated with two parts by weight of alcohol.

(Dr. Tonnère, of Calcutta, India, seems to have been the first to call attention to this plant as a remedy. In a small work, *Additions to the Homœopathic Materia Medica*, collected and arranged by Henry Thomas, M. D., and published in London in the year 1858, appears the following credited to that physician.)

Tincture of the *Acalypha Indica*, prepared and administered in the sixth decimal dilution, is specific in hæmorrhage from the lungs. In three cases in which I have employed it, the persons were affected with phthisis. In one case there was a tuberculous affection of the upper portion of the left lung, of some two years' standing. Hæmoptysis had been going on for three months; the expectoration had been in the morning pure blood; in the evening dark lumps of clotted blood, and the fits of coughing were very violent at night. In this case all homœopathic remedies had been tried unsuccessfully, when I accidentally discovered the virtues of the *Acalypha Indica*, that remedy having been given me by a native for jaundice. I prepared the mother tincture upon the homœopathic principle, and took 10 drops, which brought on a severe fit of dry cough, followed by spitting of blood. Having noted all the symptoms experienced by myself, and finding that they were nearly all similar to those of my patients, I gave six drops 6th [decimal] dilution in half a tumbler of water, a spoonful to be taken every half hour, beginning immediately (9 A.M.). At 6 P.M., the blood stopped. I continued this for eight days, and the blood has never reappeared (now three months since). The patient is improving, and auscultation proves the disease has decreased, and I am in hopes to affect a cure, yet one month since I have been giving them the medicine they have not spit any blood, although previously one of them never passed a day without spitting a great quantity. *Calcarea carb.* is an antidote to the *Acalypha*.

Another transatlantic medical friend writes:—"I hope you obtained some of the *Acalypha Indica* while you were here. I have found it perfectly successful in arresting hæmoptysis in three cases of consumption in the last stage; I could not perceive any other effect from its use, but the cessation of the hemorrhagic sputa was, I think, a great advantage."

Its use in my hands has been very satisfactory, but I have only tried it in similar cases to those already cited. The first instance of my using it—in a hopeless case of phthisis—a continued and wearisome hæmoptysis succumbed to its exhibition, and quiet sleep succeeded its use—the patient eventually died of pulmonary paralysis.

In a case of passive hæmorrhage from the lungs, after *Arnica* was used with little benefit, *Acalypha* benefited, and then failed; after which the use of *Arnica* entirely stayed the hæmorrhagic flow. (Perhaps *Hamamelis* would have at once cured, but it was not at hand.)[A]

K., a phthisical patient, had hæmoptysis to a considerable extent; in a short time his voice failed him; he took half-drop doses of 7th [decimal] dilution of *Acalypha* in water every half hour, and in a few hours the blood spitting left him entirely.

(In 1885 Dr. Peter Cooper, of Wilmington, Delaware, read a paper on the drug *Acalypha Indica* of which the following is an abstract:)

Professor Jones recapitulates as follows: "*Time.* Hæmorrhage occurs in morning. *Blood.* Bright-red and not profuse in morning; dark and clotted in afternoon. *Pulse.* Neither quickened nor hard; rather soft and easily compressible. *Cough.* Violent and in fits at night; patient has a played-out feeling in the morning and gains in strength as the day advances.

N. B.—Worthy of trial in all pathological hæmorrhages having notedly a morning exacerbation."

Such is an outline presentation of the drug given us by so eminent an authority as Professor Jones, of the University of Michigan. It was his "N. B.," his suggestion that *Acalypha* was worthy of trial in all pathological hæmorrhages from any source, providing the morning aggravation was present, that fixed my attention upon the drug especially. At the time I had a case of hæmorrhage per rectum that had baffled me for several months. No remedy had aided the case in the least, so far as I could see, unless it was Pond's Extract used locally in the form of injection; and I finally came to the conclusion that the relief apparently due to the *Hamamelis* was merely a coincidence. I had given all the hæmorrhagic remedies I knew of or could hear of. Still the bleeding came just as often, with increasing severity. Each time the patient was sure she would "bleed to death," and I was not positive she would be disappointed. In fact, I was so hopeless that I used to delay the answer to her summons as long as possible, so that the bleeding might have time to exhaust itself. She became reduced in flesh and the hæmorrhagic drugs became reduced in number, until like the nine little Indians sitting on a gate the last one tumbled off and then there was none. As soon as I read Dr. Jones' monograph on *Acalypha Indica*, I determined to try it. She had all the symptoms—bright-red blood in the morning; dark and clotted in the afternoon and evening; weak and languid in the forenoon, stronger during the afternoon—except one, *i.e.*, instead of the blood coming from the lungs it came from within the portals of the anus. I procured the 6x dil. and served it in water. It gave speedy, almost immediate relief. Each subsequent attack came less profuse and at longer intervals. She has not had a hæmorrhage now for two months, while before she was having from seven to one (continuous) a week. She is gaining in flesh, is in every way improved, and keeps *Acalypha Indica* constantly by her.

FOOTNOTES:

[A] Homœopathic Review, vol. 1, p. 256.

ACIDUM LACTICUM.

COMMON NAME, Lactic acid.

ORIGIN.—Lactic acid is obtained from sour milk, resulting from the fermentation of the sugar of milk under the influence of casein.

PREPARATION *for Homœopathic Use.*—One part by weight of pure lactic acid is dissolved in 99 parts by weight of alcohol.

(A very complete proving of this remedy will be found in Allen's *Encyclopædia of Pure Materia Medica*, but little use seems to have been made of it, though the following by Dr. Tybel-Aschersleben, *Allgemeine Hom. Zeitung*, March 13, 1890, seems to show that it is very efficient in certain forms of rheumatism).

We are by no means rich in remedies against arthritic rheumatism, and those which we do use lack the reputation of being reliable. A new and a valuable remedy will therefore be a welcome addition to this list. I say reliable, inasmuch as this remedy is truly homœopathically indicated for, according to Foster, of Leitz, Niemeyer's Pathology, 10th edition, 2d vol., pp. 561: "*Lactic acid in large doses and used for a long time will produce symptoms entirely analogous to arthritic rheumatism.*" We also find mention elsewhere that the use of lactic acid occasioned rheumatic pains in the thigh.

CLINICAL CASES.

1. A young girl æt. 15 was afflicted with acute arthritic rheumatism, she received *Acid Lacticum* 2x dil., a dose every 2 or 3 hours, and was so much improved in two weeks that the pain had subsided, and for her remaining weakness *China off.* sufficed.

2. A nine-year-old girl was confined to her bed for three weeks with acute arthritic rheumatism. *Acid Lacticum 2* speedily cured her.

3. A miner, B., had been afflicted over six weeks with acute arthritic rheumatism. The first dose of *Acid Lactic 2* gave relief and a second dose cured the man.

4. In a case with swollen and very painful joints one dose of *Acidum Lactic 2* sufficed to overcome the pain and the swelling. Against the remaining weakness *China* proved efficacious.

5. Arthritic rheumatism of the wrist vanished slowly after using *Acid Lactic 2* from two to three weeks.

6. A patient afflicted with arthritic rheumatism for four weeks, accompanied by copious perspiration, soon mended under the use of *Acid Lactic 2* and was entirely cured within two weeks.

7. Even in a case of chronic arthritis with inflation of the Epiphyses of Metacarpal bones and consequent partial displacement of the fingers, *Lactic Acid 2* produced such a decided amelioration that two months later the report said: all pains are gone even the anchylosis has disappeared.

(It has also been successfully employed in cases where the digestive powers are weak and is said to be preferable to other acids in such cases. It has also been successfully employed in cases of dyspepsia.)

ÆTHIOPS ANTIMONIALIS.

(This remedy is prepared by triturating together equal parts of *Æthiops mineralis* and *Antimonium crudum*; we may add that the first named consists of a trituration of equal parts of *Mercurius viv.* and washed flowers of sulphur. Therefore *Æthiops antimon.* consists of mercury, crude antimony and sulphur.

The following clinical cases illustrating the use of the preparation is by Dr. H. Goullon and was published in Vol. II of the *Zeitschrift fuer Homœopathie*.)

The following case was cured in a few days by *Æthiops antimonalis* after having been treated by a homœopath who strictly followed Hahnemann's rules, but failed to make an impression beyond a certain point.

Miss A. inherited from her father, who was reported to have suffered from laryngitis, a distinct disposition to scrofulosis and tuberculosis. This was proved two years ago by a bloody cough caused by lung catarrh. After the lung was affected she suffered from profuse sweats, especially down the back, but of special interest was the appearance of a "quince colored" swelling of the size of a pea at the extreme corner of the left eye with suppuration which threatened the bulbus. A skilled specialist removed by operation this pus-hearth, which no doubt acted as a fontanel. The immediate result was a large furuncle under the arm and the affliction for which I was consulted. A patient presented herself to me whose appearance was shocking. Numerous parts of her face were literally covered with thick, elevated fissured scabs. A scrofulent liquid was oozing out, and the worst were those parts on the side of the lower lip, the nostrils and the root of the nose. On the whole, a certain symmetry could be observed in the arrangements of these frightful diseased products.

This eruption, which according to its nature must be called herpetic-eczematous, had existed for five months. The patient, who has red hair, and is between 20 and 30 years old, contracted this disease at the sight of a fainting sister. This kind of genesis is an established fact. I remember of reading in Stark's "General Pathology" of an instance where a mother was affected with eczema of the lips immediately on seeing her child fall on a knife.

Our patient, however, lost the above mentioned sweats, which proves that the fright had a metastatic effect. I learned that at first there appeared very small spots which developed into pustules, infecting half of the forehead. Scratching aggravated the condition, so that some places assumed a cup-like appearance, somewhat as favus.

When patient came to me the face was oozing so terribly that the pillow was thoroughly soaked in the morning, and she suffered greatly. When asked the nature of the pains she said that they were sometimes itching, sometimes tensive, and often indescribable, suddenly appearing and disappearing.

What should be done? Certainly no strictly homœopathic indication presented itself since one might think of *Sulphur*, another of *Arsenicum*, *Silicea*, *Hepar sulphur*, *Causticum*, *Mezereum*, etc. In such case I have laid down, as a rule for my guidance, never to experiment at the cost of the patient (and my own as well as Hahnemann's), but to employ a so-called empirical remedy. I know *Æthiops antimonialis* as a very effective remedy through its recommendation (by the Berlin Society of Homœopathic Physicians) in ophthalmia scrofulosa of the worst kind, a fact which I proved myself to be correct. In this case, also, we find the deepest and most stubborn disturbance of the organic juices and a subject with every indication of the worst form of scrofula, ending in lethal cancer—dyscrasia or tuberculosis.

The patient received the remedy in doses of the 1st centesimal trituration, every evening and morning, as much as a point of a knife blade would hold. There was no attempt at external removal of the eruption, a method so much favored by the allopaths, and yet the simple internal effort was magical, since after a few days the scabs were dried up, had fallen off, and the terrible oozing as well as the pain had ceased. The happy patient presented herself again on Friday, after having taken the medicine for the first time on Sunday evening. Very great changes could, indeed, be noticed which justified the hope for a speedy and total cure.

I again ask all my colleagues which was the principle of healing in this case? We may soonest think of Schüssler's therapeutic maxim, the biochemic principle. The definition that this preparation acts as a blood purifier is not sufficient, and yet it may be accepted as the most intelligent.

Schoeman triturates the *Æthiops antimonalis* with *Æthiops mercurialis* (or *mineralis*), which last consists of equal parts of quicksilver and sulphur, and says of the product: "It acts analogous to *Æthiops mercurialis*, but stronger, and is therefore preferred to it in scrofulous eruptions of the skin, scald, milk-scab, scrofulosis conjunctivitis, keratitis, blepharitis glandulosa, otorrhœa and swellings of the glands. It is especially valuable for children as a mild but nevertheless effective remedy."

AGAVE AMERICANA.

NAT. ORD., Amaryllidaceæ.
COMMON NAMES, American Aloe, Maguey, Century Plant.
PREPARATION.—The fresh leaves are pounded to a pulp and macerated
with two parts by weight of alcohol.

(We find the following concerning this little known remedy in Volume I,
1851, of the *North American Journal of Homœopathy*.)

1. *Agave Americana or Maguey.*—[Dr. Perin, U. S. A., stationed at Fort
McIntosh, in Texas, having many cases of scurvy to treat, and finding the
usual allopathic routine ineffectual, was led to make inquiry as to the
domestic remedies in use among the natives. Among others, his attention
was called to the *Agave Americana* or *American Aloe*, and he reports to the
Surgeon General the following cases in which it was the drug relied on. We
extract from the *N. Y. Jour. Med.*:]

Private Turby, of Company "G," 1st U. S. Infantry, was admitted into
hospital March 25th, in the following state: Countenance pale and dejected;
gums swollen and bleeding; left leg, from ankle joint to groin, covered with
dark purple blotches; leg swollen, painful, and of stony hardness; pulse
small, feeble; appetite poor; bowels constipated.

He was placed upon lime juice, diluted and sweetened, so as to make an
agreeable drink, in as large quantities as his stomach would bear; diet
generous as could be procured, consisting of fresh meat, milk, eggs, etc.;
vegetables could not be procured.

April 11th. His condition was but slightly improved; he was then placed
upon the expressed juice of the maguey, in doses of f. ʒij. three times daily;
same diet continued.

April 17th. Countenance no longer dejected, but bright and cheerful;
purple spots almost entirely disappeared; arose from his bed and walked
across the hospital unassisted; medicine continued.

May 4th. So much improved so as to be able to return to his company
quarters, where he is accordingly sent; medicine continued.

May 7th. Almost entirely well; continued medicine.

Private Hood, "G" Company, 1st U. S. Infantry, was admitted into
hospital April 10th. His general condition did not differ much from Private
Turby's. He had been on the sick report for eight days; had been taking
citric acid drinks, but grew gradually worse up to the time of his admission,

when he was placed upon lime-juice until the 13th, at which time no perceptible change had taken place. On that date he commenced the use of the expressed juice of the maguey; same diet as the case above described.

April 21st. General state so much improved that he was sent to his company quarters.

May 22d. Well; returned to duty.

Eleven cases, all milder in form than the two just related, were continued upon the lime-juice; diet the same. On the 21st of April they exhibited evidences of improvement, but it was nothing when compared with the cases under the use of the maguey.

Seven cases were under treatment during the same time, making use of citric acid. On the 21st of April no one had improved, and three were growing worse.

At this time so convinced was I of the great superiority of the maguey over either of the other remedies employed that I determined to place all the patients upon that medicine. The result has proved exceedingly gratifying; every case has improved rapidly from that date. The countenance, so universally dejected and despairing in the patients affected with scurvy, is brightened up by contentment and hope in two days from the time of its introduction; the most marked evidences of improvement were observable at every successive visit. From observing the effects of the maguey in the cases which have occurred in this command, I am compelled to place it far above that remedy which, till now, has stood above every other—the lime-juice.

This no doubt will appear strong language, but further experience will verify it.

The juice of the maguey contains a large amount of vegetable and saccharine matter, and of itself is sufficiently nutritious to sustain a patient for days.

This succulent plant grows indigenous in most parts of the State, and, if I am correctly informed, in New Mexico and California. In Mexico it is well-known as the plant from which they manufacture their favorite drink, the "Pulque," and grows in great abundance. As it delights in a dry sandy soil, it can be cultivated where nothing but the cactus will grow; for this reason, it will be found invaluable to the army at many of the western posts, where vegetables cannot be procured.

The manner in which it is used is as follows, viz.:—The leaves are cut off close to the root, they are placed in hot ashes until thoroughly cooked, when they are removed, and the juice expressed from them. The expressed juice is then strained, and may be used thus, or may be sweetened. It may be given in doses of f. ℥ij. to f. ℥iij. three times daily.

It is not disagreeable to take, and in every instance it has proved to agree well with the stomach and bowels.

After the leaves have been cooked, the cortical portion near the root may be removed, and the white internal portion may be eaten; it appears to be a wholesome and nutritious food. I have seen muleteers use it in this way, and they seem to be very fond of it. I have been informed, upon good authority, that several tribes of Indians in New Mexico make use of it in the same manner. The use of the leaf in this way, I believe, will ward off most effectually incipient scorbutus.

(In El Siglo Medico, 1890, Dr. Fernandez Avila reports the case of a boy, æt. 8, who had been bitten by a supposedly mad dog on Feb. 18. The wound healed up, but on July 7th the boy developed all the symptoms of rabies and on the 17th was so violent that he had to be tied and had not tasted food for seventy-two hours as all remedies failed to produce any effect, the doctor, having read that *Agave Americana* was efficacious in such cases, and having none of the tincture at hand, gave the boy a piece of the plant itself which he greedily ate; it was given to him as long as he would take it. On the 25th his symptoms had all abated and he was dismissed cured.)

AMBROSIA ARTEMISIFOLIA.

NAT. ORD., Compositæ.
COMMON NAMES, Rag Weed, Hog Weed.
PREPARATION.—The fresh leaves and flowers are pounded to a pulp and macerated with two parts by weight of alcohol.

(The following concerning this little used remedy was contributed to the HOMŒOPATHIC RECORDER, 1889, by Dr. C. F. Millspaugh, at that time the editor):

Of late years much attention has been called to the species of the genus Ambrosia (the Rag Weeds) as being, through the agency of their pollen, the cause of hay fever. Many people afflicted with this troublesome complaint lay the charge directly at its doors, while others claim that, in all probability, it is the direct cause, as their sufferings always commence during the anthesis of the plant. The general impression, however, both among the laity and the medical fraternity, has been that the effect was a purely mechanical one, the nasal mucous membranes being directly irritated by the pollen dust in substance. If this were true, would not every one suffer from hay fever? Impressed with the above report, I had the pleasure of curing two attacks while writing my work upon "American Medicinal Plants," in which the above species figures. Since the publication of the work, all the cases I have had of the disease (four) have yielded beautifully to the 3d centesimal potency of the drug.

The four cases, Mr. B——, Mrs. I——, Mr. C—— and Miss P——, presented the following generic symptoms: Inflammation of the mucous membranes of the nose, adventing yearly in the autumn. At first dryness, then watery discharges, finally involving the frontal sinuses and the conjunctival membrane. In Mr. B. and Miss P. the irritation extended to the trachea and bronchial tubes, in Mr. B. amounting to severe asthmatic attacks. In all cases the coryza was very severe, and in previous years lasted, in spite of all treatment, from four to eight weeks. Mr. B. has found relief from *Ambrosia* 3₁, three times a day, in from four to six days, for three successive years, with no return of the trouble in the same year; Mrs. I. has been relieved in from two to four days for two years; Mr. C. gets immediate relief in twenty-four hours (three seasons); Miss P., in this her first experience with *Ambrosia*, found entire relief from six doses.

AMYGDALUS PERSICA.

NAT. ORD., Rosaceæ. Amygdaleæ.
SYNONYM, Persica vulgaris.
COMMON NAME, Peach.
PREPARATION.—The tincture is made by pjounding to a pulp the fresh bark of the twigs and macerating in two parts by weight of alcohol. The infusion is made by taking of the bark one part and of boiling Distilled Water ten parts. Infuse in a covered vessel for one hour and strain.

(Outside the old herbalists the virtues of the bark and leaves of the peach tree have received little attention. The following contributed by Dr. C. C. Edson in the *Chicago Medical Times*, 1890, however, aroused some attention):

Some ten years ago I had a little patient whose principle difficulty seemed to be an inability to retain anything whatever upon its stomach. It would vomit up promptly everything I gave it, and I had given it everything I had ever heard of and also had eminent council, but it was no go; I was literally at my rope's end. At this juncture an elderly lady neighbor, one of "the good old mothers," timidly suggested an infusion of peach bark. Well, as it was any port in storm, I started to find the coveted bark, which I was fortunate enough to procure after a long tramp through the country and two feet of snow. I prepared an infusion, gave the little patient a few swallows, and presto! the deed was done, the child cured. * * It fills all the indications of the leaves and many more. It fills the indications of hydrocyanic acid, ingluvin, ipecac or any other anti-emetic. It will more frequently allay the vomiting of pregnancy than any remedy I have ever tried. And nearly every case of retching or vomiting (except it be reflex) will promptly yield under its use. * * * For an adult the dose is five drops, and in urgent cases repeat every five to ten minutes until the symptoms subside, after which give it at intervals of one to four hours as indicated. After ten years' use I am thoroughly convinced that any physician once giving it a thorough trial will never again be without it. Of course it is not a specific for all "upheavals of the inner man," but will I think meet more indications than any other known remedy of its class.

(This brought out the following from Dr. Kirkpatrick in the same journal):

I must say that I feel a little plagued after reading what Dr. Edson says about *Amygdalus*; he has taken the wind out of my sails, but I must give my experience. Quite a number of years since a good friend in the profession called on me, and asked me to visit one of his patients, honestly stating that he thought she would die. I went a few miles in the country to see her. She had been vomiting blood for two or three days, and, notwithstanding she had had oxalate of cerium, bismuth, pepsin, ingluvin and other good remedies, everything she swallowed would come up, so that she looked more like a corpse than a living being. I ordered them to go out and get me some of the young switches of the last year's growth from the peach tree; I had them pound them to loosen the bark; I then nearly filled a tumbler with this bark, then covered it with water. I ordered her a teaspoonful to be taken after each time she vomited, one dose being given then, and one every hour after the vomiting stopped. The result was, she vomited no more and made a good recovery.

* * * In recent cases I have very rarely had to give the second prescription to relieve morning sickness. I was visiting a doctor in Quincy; while there he told me he was afraid he would have either to make a lady abort or let her die, from the fact that he had failed to stop her vomiting. I happened to have a sample of the medicine with me; I gave it to him, he took it to the lady and in a few days he reported her well. I may say, like Dr. Edson, it is a standard remedy with me. I have found it very useful in hæmorrhage from the bladder. Some of my lady patients find it very good in nervous headache. I have used the tincture prepared from the leaves, but it is far inferior to that prepared from the bark of the young shoots. A medical friend was going to see a lady who had morning sickness; he told me he had thought of advising her to use popcorn; I handed him a small bottle of my *Amygdalus* and told him to take a couple of ears of corn in his pocket and try both. The next time I met him he said my medicine had done the work.

(Dr. Oliver S. Haines, of Philadelphia, also contributed the following experience):

Apropos of the remarks made by Dr. C. C. Edson upon the efficacy of infusion of peach *bark* in the gastric irritability of children, we might mention the following authentic case:

An infant, during its second summer, had been much reduced by acute dyspeptic diarrhœa. A marked feature of this case was the persistent vomiting of all food. The stomach would tolerate no form of baby food with or without milk. The child's parents had consulted some eminent physicians of our city. The child had been treated homœopathically. None of the remedies chosen seemed to produce the desired effect. After a consultation it was deemed best to send the infant to the mountains. The change aggravated its condition. While the parents hourly expected their baby would die, it was suggested that they send for an old practitioner living in the mountains near at hand. This man had a local reputation as a saver of dying babies. His prescription was as follows: Two or three fresh peach *leaves* were to be put in a cup of boiling water, the infant to receive a "drink" of this infusion at frequent intervals. The effects of this remedy were as remarkable in this case as in the case narrated by Dr. Edson. Our child soon retained food and eventually recovered.

It seems this ancient disciple of Esculapius had long used peach leaves and regarded them as possessing specific virtues.

ANAGALIS ARVENSIS.

NAT. ORD., Primulaceæ.

COMMON NAMES, Scarlet Pimpernel. Poor Man's Weather-Glass.

PREPARATION.—The fresh plant, of the scarlet-flowered variety, gathered before the development of the flowers, is pounded to a pulp and subjected to pressure. The expressed juice is mingled with an equal part by weight of alcohol.

(This paper was arranged from the provings by Dr. W. H. A. Fitz for the Organon and Materia Medica Society of Philadelphia, and published in the *Medical Advance*, 1891)

We think of this remedy for the following clinical indications: Hypochondriasis, mania, epilepsy. Amblyopia, cataract, spots on the cornea. Syphilis, hepatitis and indurated liver, visceral obstruction, inflammation of rectum (horses), hemorrhoids, inflammation of kidneys, gleet, copious urination (horses), gravel, syphilis with deranged mind, nosebleed, pain in small of back, gonorrhœa, amenorrhœa, cancer of mammea, sterility (cows), consumption, lumbago, itching, gout, bloody sweat (murrain of calves), dropsy, ill-conditioned ulcers, snake bites and hydrophobia, promotes the expulsion of splinters, inflammation of stomach (horses).

It is characterized by great tickling and itching. We find tickling and pricking in the urethra, in left ear; on tip of nose; at soft palate as from something cold; in symphysis pubis; as from a brush against epiglottis (with hoarseness); pain in right leg and at os illium; itching on vertex and occiput; of eyelids; in left ear; on cheek bones; itching and tickling stitches on left corner of mouth and upper lip; in rectum; at anus after evacuation of bowels; on left side of chest, principally on nipple; on neck and scapula; on inside of upper arm, just above elbow joint; on back of right hand; tetter on hands and fingers. In fact, great itching all over the skin.

HEADACHE just over supra-orbital ridges, with eructations and rumbling in bowels; spasmodic lancination in temples, extending to eyes; pressive aching in forehead and occiput from a current of air blowing on him; intense headache and nausea, with pains throughout the body. Occiput: dull or tearing pains and inclination to vomit; violent headache, with hard, knotty stools; knocking pains in left side; dull pain all night.

PAINS: Teeth pain as from cold.

STITCHES: In scalp, over left ear and on occiput; in eyeballs; in temples; in left corner of mouth; in right ear; in left side, region of fourth and fifth ribs; in left tibia, when sitting, when moving leg or foot; disturb sleep.

NEURALGIC PAINS: In right cheek bones.

Rheumatic, gouty pains.

TEARING PAINS: In occiput; in right cheek bone; in upper molars; in spermatic cords; in muscles of left leg; disturb sleep.

DRAWING PAINS: In right testicle and cord; tensive drawing in left shoulder to neck, returns when lifting or stretching arms; in muscles of upper arm; especially when moving hands or arm in writing; in right carpal and metacarpal bones (sometimes left), returning at regular intervals; also tearing; in muscles of left leg.

PRESSING PAINS: In forehead and occiput; with stitching in eyeballs; in eyes; on lungs; in sacrum.

DULL PAIN: In occiput; in hollow tooth, with trembling of heart; in upper molars; in gums, accompanied by hard stools.

CRAMPS: In right thenar; ceasing there as it goes to the left.

VIOLENT PAIN: As if caused by external pressure on occiput, behind the left ear; in sacrum when lifting, they take her breath; in muscles of forearm, inside near elbow joint; in carpal and metacarpal bones, extending to shoulder; in palm of right hand, extending between thumb and forefinger, as if a pin were thrust through.

SENSATION: In lungs as if struck by a cushion full of pins; anxiety in chest; skin of forehead feels too tight; tension in bend of left knee, as if swollen or sore. Cold or chilly sensation on right frontal protuberance; in teeth, as if something cold were placed on tongue; at soft palate, as from touch of something cold; chilly, trembling; scratching in throat after eating; when reading aloud.

Soreness on chest.

Burning in urethra.

Heat rising to head.

Dryness in throat.

Things seem to float to and fro; he cannot write.

PAIN: In right ear, as if meatus auditorius were obstructed; in facial muscles, in lungs, in the front and the back up to the scapulæ; in right side of back, followed by violent sneezing; in upper arm, outside, near the shoulder; pain and twitching in the left thumb; in bend of left knee; in upper part of metatarsus of right foot; in great and little toe of left foot in morning; in sole of left foot.

Hence we find under—

LOCALITY AND DIRECTION—below upwards.

Pains in upper limbs.

RIGHT: Chilly sensation in frontal protuberance; pain in the eyeball; in palm of hand; in about knee and tibia; in foot; pain and stitches in ear; tickling pains in leg and os ilii; drawing in testes and cord; pressure on lungs; itching on scapula; weak, lame feeling in leg.

LEFT: Knocking inside of occiput; pain in knee and posterior muscles of leg; in tibia; in foot; glittering before eye; stitches over ear; in corner of mouth (and itching); tensive drawing from shoulder; drawing in muscles of leg; itching in ear; on side of chest; tight feeling in bend of knee.

MOTION: In bed: trembling of heart with toothache; chilliness.

POSITION: Sitting with legs crossed; pain in and about right knee; stretching arm; tensive drawing from left shoulder up to neck; lifting; tensive drawing in left shoulder; pain in sacrum.

REST: Walking: pressure on right lung; motion: of leg or foot < stitches in and left tibia.

TIME: Night: dull pain in occiput; neuralgia in cheek; tickling at palate; erections.

Morning: burning in urethra when urinating; pain in feet.

Towards evening: spells of chilliness.

Evening: glittering before left eye; trembling, anxious feeling in chest; toothache.

AGGRAVATIONS: Pain right eyeball < from touching lids; burning in urethra when urinating, mostly in mornings; violent pain in sacrum when lifting a slight load; tensive drawing, ascending from left shoulder to nape of neck; < raising and extending arm; pain in right eyeball < from touch.

AMELIORATIONS: Coffee relieves headache; burning in urethra before and during erection, *ceases* during coition.

CAUSES: Mental work causes great prostration (*Picric acid*); when cutting with shears, cramps in ball of thumb; pressure on right lung after eating, or when walking; pressing in eyes after headache; obstruction and pain in right ear after pressure in eyes.

MENTAL STATE: Exhilarated, mind very active; everything gives pleasure.

NOSE: Nosebleed, violent sneezing, expelling lumps of yellow phlegm; running of water from nose; copious secretion of yellow phlegm.

MOUTH: Viscid saliva in mouth, raised by coughing; water in mouth with tearing pains in molars.

ABDOMEN: Distended with wind; weak feeling in abdomen.

STOOLS: Piles; passes offensive flatus; stools soft and pappy; watery diarrhœa; stools hard, like stone, knotty.

URINE: Dark, straw-colored; orifice seems agglutinated; presses to urinate; urine escapes in divided streams.

SKIN: Rough, dry; dry, bran-like tetter in rings; groups of small vesicles, smarting and itching, oozing a yellowish-brown lymph, which soon turns into a scurf, new vesicles appearing beneath.

ULCERS and swelling on joints; promotes expulsion of splinters (*Hepar*).

RELATIONSHIP: Collateral relation. *Cyclamen*. Similar to *Coffee* (joyous, excited); *Picric acid* (prostration after mental exertion); *Cyclamen* (sneezing); *Lithia carb.* (rough skin, ringworm); *Sepia, Tellur.* (ringworm); *Pulsatilla* (chilliness; catarrhs); smelling of *Rhus*, and, an hour later, taking *Col.*, relieved sacral pains. *Rhus* relieved swollen gums.

- 21 -

ARSENICUM BROMATUM.

COMMON NAMES, Arsenous or Arsenious Bromide; Arsenic Tribromide. PREPARATION.—Add one drachm each Arsenious acid, Carbonate of Potassium and Tartar to eight ounces of Distilled Water; boil until entirely dissolved; after cooling add sufficient water to make eight ounces. Then add two drachms of pure Bromine. *Clemens.*

(The following paper was translated, 1888, from the German (*Deutsche Clinic*, March, 1859) of Dr. Th. Clemens, by the late Dr. Samuel Lilienthal):

Arsenious acid, Arsenic blanc, Arsenic oxide, Flowers of Arsenic (AsO_3) is commonly used as the only preparation in which it could be assimilated. In the Solutio Fowleri we find a combination with Kali carbonicum e Tartaro, a combination which allows to the Arsenious acid its full destructive power. Now comes Spiritus Angelicæ comp. and the pure chemical preparation smells like Theriac, but it ought hardly ever be allowed to add something to a pure chemical preparation in order to give it taste, color, and use. This Spir. Angel. comp. is made up of Anglica, Siordium, Juniper berries, Valerian, Camphor, and Alcohol, and Solutio Fowleri is prepared even to this day in the same manner, and ought therefore be expelled from every pharmacopœia, especially as it is sure to spoil in the pharmacies if kept too long on the shelves. Looking, therefore, for a better preparation, I prescribe now for the last decade: **R**. Arsen. albi. depurat. pulv., Kali carb. e Tartar. āā ʒj., coque cum Aqua destill. lb 1/2 ad perfect. solutionem, refriger., adde aqua destil. q. s. ut fiat solutio ʒxii., Dein adde Brom. pur. ʒii. This solution, which during first eight days is frequently shaken, becomes colorless in the fourth week, and is then ready for use. It must be kept in a dark, cool place.

I will now give my reason for choosing Bromine as a combination. The study of mineral waters is an old pet of mine; many of them contain Arsenic in combination with Bromine, and are all well known for their roborating and alterating qualities. I begun, therefore, my experiments with minute doses of *Brom. arsen.*; gradually these were increased, and I felt astonished what large doses were well borne, and how long I could use this preparation without injurious consequences. After a few drops of my solution I could prove Arsenic in all secretions, an experiment easily made by Marsh's test. Experiments on animals with toxic doses of either solution (Clemens and Fowler) showed that the same quantity *Arsenicum brom.* is less poisonous (one has to be careful with the selection of animals, as many of them, especially ruminants, bear very large doses of Arsenic without injury).

My preparation gives a rapid, not destructive, but roborating action on every part of the body.

In doses of two to four drops daily, always to be taken in a full glass of water, it always shows its specific action as an antipsoricum. Herpetic eruptions and syphilitic excrescences or exanthemata dry up and heal up, while simultaneously the relaxed and thoroughly infected body steadily increases in turgor vitals. Glandular tumors and indurations of dyscrasic origin, where any other treatment has failed, are scattered by the long-continued use of my preparation. I have in suitable cases given it for years without noticing any hurtful sequelæ, and after my patients were cured I kept them under observation for years afterwards, and know, therefore, that nothing injurious followed. This cannot be said of the usual arsenical preparations, and old Heim, a great admirer of Arsenic, opposed a lengthy use of it; he rather preferred larger doses, which is rather a dangerous procedure. Given for a long time for carcinoma, it stops the rapid progress of this fearful disease, and though at the same time Chloride of arsenic was used externally, a real cure remained an impossibility. My best successes were in obstinate cases of lues inveterata, in the first stages of tabes dorsalis (ataxie locomotrice), in the reconvalescence from exhausting acute diseases, in gastric suppurations, inactivity of bowels, tardy digestion, constipation. In cases where *Chininum sulph.* failed in intermittent fevers, I prescribe *Brom. arsen.* twice daily, four drops, each time in a full glass of water, gradually diminishing it to one daily dose, and in four weeks even the most obstinate cases yielded to this treatment. The patient feels encouraged by his increasing vigor, the fever-cakes disappear, the bowels move regularly, and appetite leaves nothing to be desired. Those mean obstinate cases of intermittens larvata, often appearing in the form of unbearable neuralgiæ, yield more rapidly to it than to the Quinine. It is often quite astonishing what good results can be obtained by the daily use of only one drop of this solution, kept up for a very long time in dyscrasic constitutions, who spent a fortune to regain their health and failed with every other treatment. Its full solubility and rapid assimilation are the reason that it can be used without injury, but it must be taken largely diluted. Let me give you a few cases for elucidation.

St., 46 years old, contracted syphilis several years ago and was relieved of it by mercurial treatment and Zittman's decoction. About six years ago he felt out of sorts, and a papular eruption appeared on forehead, temples, and especially at the root of the nose. Though treatment was immediately instituted, still in a few weeks the face of the patient was covered by an ugly, foul-smelling crust. Cod-liver oil was now taken internally, and applied externally till the scuffs fell off and the eruption concentrated on three points. For six months that treatment was kept up, but after being omitted for a few weeks, the eruption spread again to its former extent. Every treatment was tried in rotation without the least benefit. In the spring 1856 he entered my clinic. In the centre of the forehead, at the root of the nose, on both eyebrows, on the temples and right cheek there are moist herpetic eruptions covered with crusts, exuding on least pressure an acrid ichor and easily bleeding. Around these eruptions the skin is injected, reddened, interspersed with a large network of veins. Cough and expectoration hint to a beginning of tuberculosis, an heirloom in the family. Little appetite, disturbed digestion, tardy defecation, and evening fever. He is ordered Solutio arsen. brom. twice a day, four drops in a glass of water, and already after two weeks the eruption begins to dry up, appetite returns, and bowels are regular. A generous diet and fresh meat several times a day are accessories to an arsenical cure. After two months two crusts fall off and the skin under them is soft, shining, somewhat red. About July all eruption had gone, and the cough greatly improved. A few months ago I saw the patient again, and I feel sure that the disease is eradicated.

Miss W., 42 years old, passed her childhood in the West Indies, and brought from there a peculiar skin disease. When I saw her for the first time her features looked old for her age, skin gray and sallow, hair gray, rough, full of dandruff, and moisture oozing from the ears and forehead. The scalp feels hard and thickened. The cervical glands are indurated all around the neck. On the left chest an herpetic eruption of the size of a dollar, and on the mamma a hard tumor of the size of a fist. For a year past this tumor began to be painful and sensitive to pressure, and my advice was sought for relief of all her ailments, especially as her hands were also in a fearful state, where the eruption looked as if she had the itch. The nails were discolored, knobby, easily bleeding and covered with a gluey eruption. She had to wear and to change gloves every day. For nine years she never entered society, as the exhalation from her body disgusted even herself, and was hardly bearable, though sponging the whole body and daily renewal of linen was strictly adhered to. In such an obstinate chronic psoric case treatment with small doses is at first necessary, and *Arsen. brom.*, two drops twice daily, ordered, and her cold bath continued. After four weeks the dose was doubled, and after nine weeks the first glimmer of improvement could be seen. The tumor in the mamma was smaller and painless, and where before it was so sensitive as to be covered with oil-silk she could bear now the pressure of her clothing. After four months steady continuation of four drops twice daily, she was able to go without gloves. The scalp also was cleaner, less hard, and the ears more dry. But with the return of spring the eruption gained new vigor. The head and hands became covered with suppurating nodules and small exuding herpetic spots, which became confluent and itched terribly, a most classic picture of the herpes of the ancients. Though for years she had been accustomed to an aggravation in the spring, she never witnessed it in such severity. I now omitted the drug and ordered head and hands frequently washed with cold water. After eight days the storm calmed down, and it was remarkable to witness the steady decrease of the induration in the cervical glands and mamma. After four weeks the old treatment was renewed. During the summer months she took regularly her four drops twice daily, and in the beginning of autumn the dose was reduced to two drops, and so continued during the whole winter. The following spring crisis was the mildest one she ever experienced. During the summer she took her four drops, during fall and winter two drops. The third spring aggravation came with full severity, but lasted only three days, when desquamation followed. Another year of the same treatment and the fourth spring eruption showed itself slightly only in small papules behind the ears and between the fingers, and were hardly worth noticing. She now felt a slight weakness in right arm, which from childhood up was rather weaker than the other one. After the disappearance of the induration in the mamma the arm seemed to regain its former strength and the patient felt therefore rather astonished at the reappearance of the weakness when its cause seemed removed, but it yielded readily to a mild constant current applied a few times, and some faradic shocks each time from the shoulder through the arm, and in September she went to Nizza in order to use sea-bathing, with the advice to take for a whole year one drop daily of her solution. She considered herself now well, but still her skin was flabby, especially on the hands where the epidermis often desquamated, and the nails remained hard, brittle and without lustre.

I may here remark that I found repeatedly Arsenic in the urine of such patients. A case of obstinate intermittens larvata, characterized by vomiting of chyme, also yielded to *Arsen. brom.* One case more must suffice. A young man went to America but failed in his trade, and became barkeeper on a Mississippi steamer, which place he had to give up on account of intermittent fever. We find him then as hostler in Chicago where he was laid up with an attack of cholera, and as he did not fully recover his strength he returned to the old home again. When I saw him for the first time the diagnosis seemed to be first stage of Bright's disease. Anamnesis, ætiology, and present state, albumen in the urine, justified the diagnosis. Patient is pale, bloated, œdema pedum, no appetite, white tongue, thin feverish pulse, swollen spleen, watery diarrhœa alternating with constipation. Every drug produced vomiting, and he perfectly abhorred the old Quinine powders. I ordered four drops *Arsen. brom.* and a full meat diet. Improvement followed with the continuance of the treatment. After three weeks the spleen was reduced in size, his face showed better color, hardly any œdema. To strengthen the skin he was advised to take pineneedle baths, and after three months' treatment he could be discharged, a well man. He was advised to take for a few months one drop daily of his solution, and to take often an airing in the pineries which abound around Frankfort. Though he returned to America the latest reports from him are that he feels again as well as ever, but he keeps his drops about him.

Arsen. brom. is also a powerful remedy in diabetes mellitus and insipidus, for I cured cases with it where the patient had already been reduced from 138 pounds to 98, and where the urine could be condensed, by boiling, into syrupy consistency. Mixed diet may be allowed, though I insist upon large quantities of fresh meat during treatment with *Bromide of arsenic*. Let the patient take three drops thrice daily in a glass of water, and after a week the insatiable burning thirst will be quenched, and these doses must be continued till the quantity of sugar in the urine is reduced, when the drug might be taken twice a day and continued for a long time. A diabetic patient needs fresh pure air if he wishes to get well; confinement in a room or in the office prevents the action of any treatment, for it needs ozone to reduce the sugar of the blood into carbonic acid and water.

ASPIDOSPERMINE.[B]

PREPARATION.—Trituration of the alkaloid.

(Dr. Edwin M. Hale communicated the following concerning this alkaloid to the *Homœopathic Recorder* for 1889):

Dyspnœa.—This alkaloid is from the South American tree—*Quebracho.* The maximum dose, according to Merck, is 1/10th grain. I use the 1/500th trituration, which I find most efficient in doses of 2 to 5 grains.

CASE I.—A boy of ten. The attacks of spasmodic dyspnœa were a sequel of hay fever. The aggravation was at night, when lying down, or sleep was impossible. I tried *Ipecac* and *Arsenic,* but with no effect. *Aralia,* also. (I never had any curative or palliative effects from *Aralia.*)

Prescribed *Aspidospermine,* 1/500th trituration, 2 grains every two hours, all day. The night was comfortable, could lie down and sleep. Continued the remedy for four days, when he was so much better that the medicine was suspended.

CASE II.—Cardiac dyspnœa in a man of 60. Valvular disease, hypertrophy with dilatation. Distressing difficulty of breathing from the slightest exertion; had to sit upright day and night. Face livid from venous stasis. *Strophanthus* regulated and strengthened the heart's action, but only slightly benefited the dyspnœa. Five grains of *Aspidospermine,* 1/500th trituration, every two hours effected a marvellous change. He could walk about the house and out to his carriage with but little discomfort. He has now continued it three weeks. Observes no unpleasant symptoms. Can lie on his back and right side and is very grateful for the relief. It seems to act as well as an aid to *Digitalis,* or *Strophanthus,* in cardiac dyspnœa.

FOOTNOTES:

[B] *Aspidospermine* or *Quebrachine* is derived from the Chilian "white Quebracho" (*Aspidospermia Quebracho*). At Santigo de Chile the bark is used as a substitute for Cinchona as a febrifuge. The alkaloid forms salts with Citric, Hydrochloric and Sulphuric acids.

AURUM MURIATICUM NATRONATUM.

COMMON NAME.—Chloride of Gold and Sodium.
PREPARATION.—A mixture composed of equal parts of dry chloride of Gold and chloride of Sodium, triturated in the usual way.

(The following is an extract from a paper by Dr. H. Goullon in the *Allg. Hom. Zeit.*, bd. 114, No. 12, on the therapeutics of this remedy):

Never have I observed gold so startling in its action as in the following case: The patient is a type of the scrofulous habit; reddish hair, pasty complexion, thick nose, coarse features. About thirty years of age. He has had the misfortune of being infected by syphilis, and the still greater ill-luck of being treated by mercurial inunctions and iodine to excess. All these circumstances conjoined helped to produce a complication of morbid conditions which would put medical art to a severe test. Let us recall the region in which gold makes such brilliant cures, and we find it especially suitable in an uncommon swelling of the left testicle. In this case I do not exaggerate, when I say that the scrotum was as large as a gourd of moderate size and the tumor was four or five times larger in circumference than the right testicle, which was also swollen. The entire mass simulated an oblong, heavy weight, like those one meets with in old-fashioned clocks, and could hardly find space in the capacious suspensory.

The skin was also involved. On the elbow was a wide-spread herpetic eruption; on different parts of the body were gummy indurations; the ear discharged; in short, the many characteristic manifestations of the syphilitic poison were to be seen throughout the cutaneous and mucous systems. There were also ulcerous formations in the oral cavity and on the sides of the tongue.

After about four weeks the patient again set foot upon the floor, saying: 'The drops have done wonders.' And indeed the influence upon the testicles was so striking that now the right, which was formerly the smaller, seemed the larger, without having actually at all increased in size. Not the less remarkable had been the action of gold on the general condition. The patient, formerly irritable and uneasy, is cheerful and comfortable; enjoys sound sleep, whereas before he was disturbed with morbid dreams; has lost his previous debility and disgust for everything; and says that his digestive power is quite a different thing. He assimilates articles of diet which he did not formerly dare to take, unless he wished to suffer with flatulence, gastric acidity and vomiting. Among other things punch, which he 'could not even smell,' agrees well.

But, evidently, the mode of administering gold in such cases is not a matter of indifference. And although I have only recently published a cure with high potencies (in which I subsequently corrected the mistake of the 100th *Dec.* for the *Centes.*, which was what I used of the *Natrum muriaticum*), I cannot commit myself to high potencies in syphilitic complications. Experience in these cases is always in favor of substantial doses. But, as we shall soon see, these proportionally massive and heavy doses are always quite out of the allopathic posological range, and even on this ground one must set boundaries, and seek for the conversion of the traditional school. By two or three clinical experiences of this sort many a Saul would become a Paul in spite of all former prejudices, *vis inertia*, and most tormenting skepticism. One-half grain *Aurum muriaticum natronatum* was dissolved in 6 grms. Spiritus vini, but of this first 6 drops are again put into a wineglass of water, of which the patient takes a teaspoonful thrice daily.

(Dr. Tritschler, of the Gynæcological Clinic of Tübingen, furnishes the following on the use of this remedy in diseases of women. From *Allg. Hom. Zeit.*, bd. 94. Nos. 17. 18, 19):

Permit me now to specify some practical instances of the curative powers of *Aurum*, and especially of *Aurum muriaticum natronatum*, in reference to gynæcology.

CHRONIC METRITIS.

The first case is that of a woman with chronic metritis and prolapsus uteri. Hydrarg. chlorat. mit. was given at first, which acted favorably on the inflammation, but whose further use was prevented by its giving rise to salivation. The intumescence of the uterus continued about the same. Chloride of gold entirely reduced the chronic inflammation, and restored the uterus to its natural position without external means.

INDURATION OF UTERUS.

The second case was an unmarried woman at the climacteric, the vaginal portion of whose uterus showed an induration which disappeared during the administration of chloride of gold.

HYSTERICAL SPASMS.

The third case was a woman with periodical attacks of hysterical spasms, which involved the entire body, with unconsciousness lasting several hours, asthma, palpitation, etc., beginning with a sense of coldness, ascending from the abdomen, and perceptible even to the bystanders. Sometimes the attack began with pulsation through the occiput. Examination showed an inflamed uterus, filling not only the true pelvis, and interfering with urination and defecation, but the enlarged uterus perceptible through the thick abdominal walls above the pubes. At the end of seven months, *Aur. mur. nat.* had entirely reduced the swelling. The woman has enjoyed good health for several years, quite free from the so-called hysteria.

INDURATION OF CERVIX.

It happened that a woman presented an induration of the cervix, together with a remarkable softening in the posterior uterine wall. The result of treatment with chloride of gold was, that in proportion to the decrease of the induration there was an increase in the consistency of the softened posterior wall. The woman, who had been married for three years and childless, became pregnant for the first time and has since borne several children. With this experience, the Gold-chloride was also given for a softening of the atrophied cervical canal, in one case until it was curved at right angles to the body of the uterus; also in a diffused softening of the uterine tissues, with the result that the hitherto sterile woman, after toning up the uterine tissue, attained the joy of motherhood. * * * * *

Habitual abortion and premature labor recurring at about the same month of pregnancy generally depended upon induration in some portion of the uterus, which, preventing its natural expansion during gestation, gives rise to premature expulsion of the fœtus. By the use of *Aur. mur. nat.* before and during pregnancy, the absorption of this induration will conduce to the proper termination of parturition.

A swelling of the ovary, reaching as far as the umbilicus, I have cured with *Aur. mur. nat.*, and have improved others of considerable extent very decidedly. Martini has cured five cases of ovarian dropsy in the greatest possible degree with the same remedy.

Ulcers of the os and the vaginal portion, which had resulted from inflammation and induration, some as large as a dollar, and of a gangrenous character, were healed by the use of gold, without any topical applications.

The profession considers ulceration and induration of the uterus incurable. This dogma of theirs is based on the fact that the usual change, the disturbance of nutrition, can neither be remedied nor hindered in its advance. Now since ulcers are generally found only in an advanced stage of softening and induration, it is conceivable why the school—seeking a cure solely in the use of local means—turns away almost entirely from the employment of internal remedies. According to the opinions of the specialists the use of different remedies, partly insoluble, partly soluble, pure or in combination, permanent or transient, is indicated. Others apply ointments on sponges to the surface of the ulcers, keeping them in contact with it by tampons. Others again prescribe injections, and with these expect to attain the end. Finally, glowing-hot iron, the galvano-cautery, or the knife and scissors remove partially or entirely the vaginal portion.

Now, if the malady continues to thrive on the wounds made by these procedures, if old cicatrices break out again, if too a permanent cure is out of the question, there is ground for supposing that the *product* of illness, the ulcer, may be cauterized, burnt and cut away, but that the cause, the diathesis, the tendency to it, can only be removed by internal medication. *
* * * *

CHRONIC METRITIS.

One day an official in Dresden brought his wife to me, who was 41 years of age. The couple, all of whose children had died soon after birth, longed once more for children. The woman had aborted several times, and both were intelligent enough to see that everything could not be right with the sexual organs, and even begged for a gynæcological examination. The result was in a few words: inflammation of both lips of the uterus, a thickening of the cervical canal with a swelling of the posterior uterine wall as hard as cartilage, and retroversio uteri. Menstruation too early, dysmenorrhœa, blood dark, tarry, passing in clots. Yellowish, fetid leucorrhœa. Stools retained, appetite changeable; pains in the broad ligaments on both sides during rest as well as on exertion. The so-called "facies uterina"—weeps much. Frequent exclamations on the distastefulness of life since the death of all her children, and on account of her present childlessness. Should I register in my journal in the beginning of a scirrhus? I wrote simply: metritis chronica; intumescentia labiorum orificii et colli uteri.

Prognosis, not unfavorable as far as regards the swelling, after my already well-tested experience with *Aur. mur. nat.* But how about the removal of sterility acquired in her 41st year. I was more cautious about this. The cure took six months, and was not only accompanied by absorption of the affected parts, but the woman became pregnant in good time and gave birth to a boy with comparative comfort. Thus would the wishes of the worthy couple have been fulfilled, if their joy had not been banished once more by the death of the child in four weeks from an attack of eclampsia.

ANTEVERSION WITH PROLAPSUS.

I now come in conclusion to a gratifying case, which I relate partly because we make ourselves guilty of sins of omission in certain instances through neglect of the needful investigation. A woman in her twentieth year, quite healthy, had been delivered with forceps for the first time two years before, nominally on account of deficient labor pains. There was nothing unusual about the confinement. Immediately after the first getting up, she began to have constant pain in the right side of the uterine region, and soon a feeling "as if something would fall out of the parts." The family physician paid no attention to these persistent complaints for a whole year, until finally a constantly increasing leucorrhœa demanded an examination. He now expressed himself as unable to make a diagnosis alone, and the lady was referred to a celebrated gynæcologist in Leipsic. Cauterizations were now undergone at the professor's house at short intervals, and further treatment of a similar character was to be carried out at the patient's own house, which was, however, discontinued when the patient was referred to me. Examination showed: metritis following upon sub-involution of the uterus, anteversion with prolapsus of the whole organ. Both uterine lips were swollen, and on examination with the speculum a greenish-yellow discharge was seen to flow from the uterus. All local treatment was discontinued, the woman received for the first time in April, 1876, *Aur. mur. nat.*, and in June, 1876, again became pregnant; the treatment with gold was continued until the 8th month of pregnancy, in consequence of which the uterus was found in its normal position on examination twelve days after her safe confinement on March 30th. The menses, which up to this time had been very painful, returned for the first time on the 25th of April, and were quite free from suffering.

But now let us ask, whether we have in the salts of gold a simile for the diseases of the female sexual organs under the comprehensive name of chronic metritis. We find in the homœopathic proving, inflammatory affections of the internal organs; fainting depression and emaciation; great anxiety, sadness, dizziness, whimsical mood, weariness of life, morbid desires, and headache; nausea, vomiting; pressure in the gastric region; cardialgia, contractive, drawing pains in the abdomen. *Stitches in the left hypochondrium, pinching and burning in the right*, the abdomen sensitive to touch, with distension; dull pains in the abdomen; drawing and stinging in the whole abdomen; eruption of small papules above the pubes; *decreased excretion of urine*, pressure on urinating, burning on urinating; redness, burning, swelling and moisture of the labia, *discharge of yellow mucus*, menstruation too soon and lasts too long; amenorrhœa; labor-like pains, as if the menses would appear; symptoms which certainly correspond to the whole picture of chronic metritis and its results.

The mode of administration which I have used for *Aur. mur. nat.* is in trituration. Generally I have had the patient herself divide into three parts a 10 gr. powder of the 3d trit., and take one of these dry just one hour after each meal. But I have also used the 1st and 2d trituration. The effect cannot be seen before four weeks, hence I seldom make a further examination before that time. Many women notice a remarkable increase of the appetite during the use of gold. After the administration of the 1st trit. I have observed frequent, dark stools. An increase in the urine with a thick, gray sediment is often seen. * * *

UTERINE DISEASES.

Uterine diseases, according to my experience of many years, make more marriages unfruitful than all the other known or fancied hindrances to child-bearing. They can exist many years even with a blooming appearance, without apparently disturbing the general health, and on that account are often overlooked and mistaken by physicians themselves, who are not concerned about gynæcological examinations, or else make only superficial investigations, not having their eyes at the ends of their fingers. I beg, therefore, if this communication should give rise to a more extensive use of *Aur. mur. nat.*, above all things, a thorough gynæcological examination, not leaving this to the so-called surgeons and midwives. If women complain of gastric troubles, dizziness, pain in the loins and back, disturbances of urination or defecation, with a more or less pronounced hysterical appearance, and withal purposely or unwittingly deceive themselves and the physician; if, added to these, leucorrhœa and a sensation as if everything would drop out of the abdominal cavity, one may say of the patient that her uterus is diseased, and may base upon that his proposal for an examination, which will give the correct information of the nature of the malady. As a rule, every deep-seated, morbid alteration in the uterine tissues entails suffering upon the nervous system, which, being in such close relation with the uterus, not seldom apparently suffers the most.

HYSTERIA.

Because the uterus receives its nerves from the sympathetic system, which governs nutrition, circulation, respiration with distribution of animal heat, gestation, etc., these functions being out of sight, it is difficult to get at the root of the matter as regards the uterus in a suffering woman. Her sensations and fancies offer, according to her education, organization, etc., a wide field in which to make her a burden to herself and others. Her mind is generally out of order, she knows not why. In the more advanced stages of disease, the functions of the higher nervous system, the organs of sense, and even the mental activities are disordered. Then appears that chameleon of diseases, which goes by the name of *hysteria*, suitable in so far as hysteria almost without exception takes root in the "hystera" or uterus. I shall certainly not deny the possibility of primary or purely nervous diseases of the uterus, hysteria sine materia; I am nevertheless convinced that in at least nine cases out of ten, hysteria depends upon objective, sensible, perceptible changes in the uterus. It is these whose existence I ascertain by a thorough examination, and according to these that I regulate my treatment; they give me in every case a more certain starting point than a lengthy account of true and imaginary suffering. If I find, however, no palpable abnormality in the tissue to remove, and prescribe *Aur. mur. nat.* simply as an excellent nervine, following Niemeyer, it occasionally does good, but generally leaves me in the lurch.

AVENA SATIVA.

NAT. ORD., Graminaceæ.

COMMON NAME, Oats.

PREPARATION.—The fresh green plant, gathered in August, is pounded to a pulp and macerated with two parts by weight of alcohol.

(Comparatively little has been written concerning this remedy, the tincture of oats. It acquired a bad reputation somewhere in the "eighties" by being advertised as a proprietary remedy making wonderful cures, but analysis showed the advertised "avena" to contain opium. The following outline of the drug is by Dr. E. H. Russell, in *North American Journal of Homœopathy*):

Avena sativa is pre-eminently an anti-neurotic, quieting the nervous system to a remarkable degree. Its special sphere of action seems to be upon the male sexual organs, regulating the functional irregularities of these parts perhaps as much as any drug can. It is a most useful remedy in all cases of nervous exhaustion, general debility, nervous palpitation of the heart, insomnia, inability to keep the mind fixed upon any one subject, etc., more especially when any or all of these troubles is apparently due to nocturnal emissions, masturbation, over sexual intercourse, and the like. For these disorders it is truly specific. It is one of the most valuable means for overcoming the bad effects of the morphine habit. In most cases in which the habitue has not used more than four grains daily the opiate may be abruptly discontinued, and even substituted, without any serious results. If a larger quantity than this amount has been taken for some time, it is better to gradually reduce the daily dose of morphine, in the usual manner, simply prescribing the *Avena* in addition. The latter should be given in the same dose, as a rule, regardless of the amount of morphine taken. In other words, it is not necessary to increase the *Avena* as the opiate is withdrawn. When the quantity of morphine has not exceeded four grains daily it should be stopped at once, as stated above, and *Avena* given in its stead in fifteen-drop doses, four times a day, in a wineglassful of hot water. By this method the disagreeable after-effects will be much less than though the dose of morphine is gradually reduced, and the patient will find life quite bearable, as a rule, at the end of a week.

Avena sativa should always be given in appreciable doses of the tincture. Fifteen drops three or four times a day, well diluted, will usually meet the case. It may be given in doses of from five to sixty drops in rare instances. It should, however, never be given in larger quantities than twenty minims unless the patient is thoroughly accustomed to the remedy, and has found the usual dose insufficient. Otherwise there is danger of getting the physiological effect of the drug, which is *pain at the base of the brain*. When this symptom makes its appearance the medicine should be discontinued for a day or two, and then given in reduced doses. There seems to be no danger whatever of forming the habit of taking this drug, as it can be suddenly abandoned at any time without evil consequences, even when given in large quantities. In one case it was prescribed by the writer in sixty-drop doses, night and morning, *for one year*, and then abruptly stopped, nothing being substituted therefore, without bad effects.

Whenever a quick action is desired, and in all cases where *Avena* is given to overcome the morphine habit, it should be prepared in hot water. It is also a good plan to prescribe it in this fashion wherever indigestion complicates the case.

The writer has employed this drug in his private practice for a number of years with the most gratifying results. He has very rarely found it to fail when indicated, and on account of his high opinion of the remedy he has taken great pleasure in thus bringing it prominently to the attention of the medical profession.

———————————————————————

AZADIRACHTA INDICA.

PREPARATION.—The fresh bark is pounded to a pulp and macerated in two parts by weight of alcohol.

(The following synopsis of *Azadirachta Ind.*, is contributed by P. C. Majumdar, M. D., of Calcutta, India):

Azadirachta Indica. Syn.: Sanskrit, Nimba; Bengala and Hindi, Nim. Belongs to the natural order Meliaeæ. It is a large tree. Bark is used for making tinctures from which provings were instituted. The leaves, bark, wood, roots and fruits, in short, every part of this tree, is intensely bitter. According to Ayurveda (Hindu System of Medicine) the different parts of this tree possess different medicinal properties. Bhava Misra, Charak, Susratha and several other Sanskrit authors agree that its bark, though very disagreeable in taste, is generally used with success in cases of lassitude, thirst, cough, fever, loss of appetite, helmenthiasis, boils, bilious derangements, catarrh, vomiting, cutaneous diseases, hiccough, gonorrhœa, etc.; its leaves are used in some forms of ophthalmic disease, helmenthiasis and disorders brought on by deranged bile or use of poisonous things. A decoction of fresh leaves is used as a favorite wash to cure old ulcers of long standing. It removes within a short time the sloughs and promotes the healing. The fruit is purgative, demulcent, and is used in some forms of cutaneous affections. A kind of oil is produced from the seed of ripe fruits, and this oil is said to cure lepra, eczema and some other obstinate skin diseases.

Nim is also praised by some of the Allopathic physicians for its tonic, antiseptic, astringent and anti-periodic properties. Its febrifuge action is well-known in our country. Kanirages (native physicians) use Nim as the principal substance in their febrifuge medicines. The vast range of its action is chiefly due to azaderine, margocine and katechin, the three active principles found in this tree. Nim was proved by me and one of my students, U. C. Bagchi. A full report of the proving was published in the *Indian Homœopathic Review*, Vol. iii, No. 1. Here I give the most reliable and peculiar symptoms obtained in its proving.

Mind: Depressed and forgetful, mistakes in writing and spelling words, weak and dull, full of anxiety, inactive, could not think or remember names of persons very familiar, or what has been done in the previous day. No desire to go out or walk out. Loss of memory.

Head: Giddiness, as if the head were moving to and fro, especially when rising from a sitting posture; headache, pressure in the head, by moving it;

headache, throbbing in the temporal arteries, especially of the right side, with a little vertigo; aching, drawing and throbbing in the whole head; headache, by wet compress, with much pain in the right eyeball; headache, on moving; headache on the right side with much pain. Frontal headache, especially on the right side, in the open air. Throbbing in the vertex, by stooping; scalp is painful and sensitive to touch, even the hair is painful. Vertigo at 10 A.M.; intense headache, pain in the whole head; on walking pain is felt in the back part of the head.

Eyes: Burning in the eyes; burning of the eyes continued throughout even the next day; burning, dull and heavy. Pain in the eye, by slightest pressure; red, congested and burning with slight coryza; sense of pressure in the right eye; eyes red and sunken; pressive pain in the right eyeball.

Ears: Buzzing in the ears; a peculiar cracking sound is heard in the ear like tickling with a feather, which is increased on opening the mouth.

Nose: Running of watery fluid from the nose.

Face: Flushings of the face; flushing and heat in the face; face pale.

Mouth: No thirst but mouth is clammy, water has relish; taste good, but mouth is clammy and bitter. On the sides and surface of the tongue a painful burning sensation is felt as if scalded; papillæ seem to be enlarged and prominent. Putrid taste in the mouth. Saliva coming out which tastes salty. Slight difficulty in deglutition, especially water and meat.

Throat: Bitter taste in the throat; left-sided sore throat.

Stomach: No thirst; appetite very acute and keen; very great thirst for large quantity of cold water; very great thirst at long interval. Heart-burn and water-brash. Uneasy sensation in the thorax.

Abdomen: Great uneasiness in the abdomen with flatulent rumbling in the bowels; twisting pain in the epigastric region; no tenderness in the abdomen; clutching pain in the umbilical region, obliging to bend forwards, which affords some relief; abdomen a little distended, passing of offensive flatus; painful tension in the hypochondriac region.

Stools: Insufficient; bowels very much constipated; stools hard, small and knotty; stools hard, but natural; stools copious, soft, semi-solid. Diarrhœa, no satisfaction after stool.

Genito-urinary organs: Great excitement of sexual organ (in male); sexual desire a little diminished. Urine scanty and high-colored, and scalding; urine white, clear and copious; urine of strong odor (once with purple sediment).

Respiratory organs: Very troublesome cough after bathing at 1 P.M. Sputa white in small lumps expelled with much difficulty. Sighing, breathing at intervals. Slight hoarseness. Cough with greyish expectoration; cough with thick sputa; short, dry cough in the afternoon; very troublesome cough with white sputa and tasteless. Deep breathing at long intervals; breathing very rapid and hot.

Chest and throat: Aching in the lower part of the right chest, below the nipple. Stitches in the chest. Crampy pains in the lower part of chest. Transitory stitches in the chest, especially in the right side.

Pulse, quick and hard, feeble.

Neck and back: Pain and debility in the nape of the neck.

Extremities: Numbness of the limbs, as if the limbs are paralyzed. Gnawing in the legs. Strength of the hand diminished. Burning of the hands and soles of the feet. Numbness of the hands only, especially the right hand. Rheumatic pains in the lower extremities.

Sleep and dreams: Sleeplessness and tossing in bed; dreamy and interrupted sleep at night. Dreams of quarrels and beating in the latter part of night.

Fever: Fever commences with very slight chill or without chill from 4:30 P.M., and abates from 7:30 P.M.; afternoon fever. Glowing heat and burning, especially in the face, eyes, palms of the hands and soles of the feet, in open air.

Copious sweat, especially on the forehead, neck and upper part of the body; sweating commences on the forehead, gradually extending towards the trunk; no sweat in the lower part of the body.

Skin: Itching of various parts of the body, without the appearance of any eruption; itching of the body. Sudamina on the back.

BACILLINUM, TUBERCULINUM AND AVIAIRE, THE VIRUSES OF TUBERCULOSIS.

PREPARATION.—Triturate in the usual way.

(The literature on these several preparations is so extensive that we must confine ourselves to the paper read by Dr. Francois Cartier, Physician to the Hospital St. Jacques, Paris, at the International Homœopathic Congress, 1896, it covering the ground more completely than any other. For fuller information on *Bacillinum* the reader is referred to Dr. J. Compton Burnett's book, the *New Cure for Consumption*.)

I must disclaim any intention of traversing afresh the pathogenesy of *Tuberculin*, or of instituting an examination into the various treatises put forth on the subject of the virus of tuberculosis by the allopathic as well as by the homœopathic school.

The materia medica of *Tuberculin* takes its rise in the complex result of the use of Koch's lymph, in experiments upon animals, and in certain symptoms observed by those who have experimented upon themselves with different products of tuberculous nature. I shall therefore indicate the published sources, and I specially desire to place before the Homœopathic Congress of London the tuberculous virus under certain aspects which are perhaps new; and if my conclusions seem somewhat paradoxical I am content to accept, with a good grace, the criticisms of my colleagues.

Fourteen years anterior to the researches of Koch, Hering, Swan and Biegler availed themselves, as a homœopathic remedy, of the maceration of tuberculous lungs, and of the sputa of tuberculous subjects.

Dr. J. Compton Burnett in his book, "A Cure for Consumption," several years before Koch's experiments, noticed symptoms resulting from taking the preparation which he calls *Bacillinum*.

Drs. de Keghel[C] and J. H. Clarke[D] instituted an inquiry into the symptoms produced by the employment of Koch's lymph in the case of tuberculous and non-tuberculous patients.

Dr. Mersch[E] published a pathogenesy, based to a large extent upon that of Dr. de Keghel; it is an excellent work.

Dr. d'Abzen,[F] of Lisbon, sent to the Tuberculosis Congress of 1895, at Coimbra, a study of the works of Koch and Pasteur, and an enumeration of the treatises published by homœopathists.

We must notice also an English translation of Dr. Mersch's pathogenesy, by Dr. Arnulphy, of Chicago, in which special attention is paid to the symptoms observed in healthy and non-tuberculous persons, with some original remarks about *Tuberculin*. It is published in the *Clinique* for this year (February, 1896).

Nor must we overlook a series of writers who have published isolated observations of the cases of persons cured with *Tuberculin*. Such are Drs. Lambreghts, Joussett, Zoppritz, Horace Holmes, Richardson, Young, Clarke, Pinart, Youman, U. H. Merson, Snow, Lamb, Clarke, Ebersole, W. James, Kunkel, A. Zoppritz, Steinhauf, Van den Berghe, &c.

Finally, for my own part, in my articles in *L'Art Médical*, published three years ago, and in the *Hahnemannian Monthly* (July, 1894), I have insisted on homœopathic action of the viruses of tuberculosis.

In certain of the pathogenesies of *Tuberculin* we find thrown pell-mell together symptoms appertaining to Koch's lymph, as well as others which belong to the product baptized by several names, such as *Bacillinum* and *Tuberculin*, in the recommendation of which Hering and Swan, and Dr. J. Compton Burnett, in England, have made themselves conspicuous.

Bacillinum—since it must be distinguished from Koch's *Tuberculin*—is a maceration of a typical tuberculous lung.[G] Koch's lymph is an extract in glycerine of dead tuberculous bacilli. The former is compound natural infection; the latter is a product of laboratory experiment. In the one, various bacteriological species are associated which give, clinically, an appearance of cachexia and of hectic fever; from the other we may sometimes observe vascular, cardiac, renal changes having no connection with the clinical "syndrome" of pulmonary tuberculosis. To place these products together in the same pathogenesy gives an absolutely wrong sense, and the fact that both contain Koch's bacillus gives no excuse for confounding them. In my opinion there are, from a homœopathic point of view, distinct differences between *Bacillinum* and the Koch's lymph.

Experimentally Koch's bacillus, like many other microbes, does not reproduce a clinical symptom-group; and we homœopaths must have an assemblage of clearly-defined symptoms before prescribing a poison on homœopathic principles. Such is unfortunately the case with many other microbes in pure culture. The experimental diphtheria does not resemble clinical diphtheria. The pneumococcus, pathogenetic of pneumonia, is met with in many other diseases, such as pleurisy, salpingitis, meningitis, etc. Koch's bacillus, too, sometimes remarkably mild in its effects, and seeming to meet with no reaction in the system, evolves aside as in the verrucous tuberculosis; while at other times nothing is able to arrest the action of this terrible microbe, and the world still waits in vain for the man who shall find the means of combatting it. The toxins of tuberculosis are far from reproducing clinical tuberculosis; yet even here we find a curious aspect sometimes assumed by certain poisons drawn from the pure cultivation of microbes. We cannot produce with *Tuberculin* symptoms analogous to those of real tuberculosis—as it is possible, for instance, to produce tetanus with the toxine alone, *Tetanin*.

As a general rule, in the case of a healthy man, Koch's lymph would not develop any reaction, its effects manifesting themselves in a febrile congestion, which betrays the presence of tubercles. In our pathogeneses (those of Mersch-Arnulphy), we note the following symptoms—"catarrhal pneumonia with soft hepatisation, and tendency to abscess formation; at post-mortems it is not a gelatinous or fibrinous exudation which oozes out from the alveoli, but an opaque and watery fluid; 'never,' so says Virchow, 'is there found the characteristic lesion of croupous pneumonia.'" A pneumonia from which issues an aqueous and opaque liquid! I confess I do not understand it.

Experimentally this same lymph of Koch gives symptoms of inflammation of the arteries which are not found in clinical tuberculosis.

Animals inoculated with progressive doses of *Avian tuberculin*, or with serum of tuberculous animals, undergo wasting and loss of appetite, and other general symptoms. They may die of cachexia, or may develop an isolated abscess; but they do not present characteristic symptoms as they would under the action of *Cantharis*, of *Phosphorus*, or of *Lead*.

Finally, inoculation with dead bacilli may produce real tuberculosis.

In the pathogenesy put forth by homœopathists, pulmonary symptoms do not occupy a prominent place. Dr. Burnett, who has experimented on himself with *Bacillinum*, notes at the end of his symptoms, after the headache, a slight and almost insignificant cough.

In explaining the clinical forms of infectious complaints, we are frequently forced to admit the increasingly preponderant part played by association of microbes—as it is the frequent case in diphtheria—and especially the modifications which depend directly on the disposition of the organ attacked, and not upon the action of the microbe itself.

An examination of the above considerations leads me to the following conclusions:

1. That the importance of the materia medica of the tubercular virtues ought not to be exaggerated. There are few characteristic symptoms to take off; it is more wise to guide oneself in the homœopathic application of the therapeutics by the clinical symptoms of the evolution of the various

tuberculosis, rather than by the intoxication produced by their active products, the *Tuberculins*.

2. Koch's lymph, *Bacillinum* and *Avian tuberculin* must be studied separately, clinically as well as experimentally. *Bacillinum* presents symptoms very different from those of *Avian tuberculin*, and especially from those of Koch's lymph; and I intend to divide my remarks into three parts, corresponding to these three substances, which have actually become homœopathic remedies.

————————————

At the time of the introduction of the ever-memorable Koch's lymph, there were included under the head of poisonings by this drug vascular lesions, as I have mentioned above, acute arteritis, arterio-sclerosis, changes in the vessels of the heart and the kidneys, and acute nephritis. Apropos of acute nephritis, the supposition was that the kidney became congested because of the presence in that part of certain tubercular islets, and that the kidney responded, like the tuberculous lung, under the influence of the *Tuberculin*, by acute congestion.

However this might be, these vascular lesions drew attention to the homœopathicity of Koch's lymph in nephritis. Dr. Jousset has experimented in it with encouraging results, using homœopathic dilutions, in Bright's disease; and at the meeting of the Société Homœopathique Francaise on April 18, 1895, Drs. Tessier, Silva and Jousset, father and son, mentioned the diminution of albumen in cases of chronic and incurable nephritis, and the appearance of that substance in acute cases.

Dr. Arnulphy, in a series of articles in the Chicago *Clinique*, which I have read attentively, speaks favorably of Koch's lymph in homœopathic dilutions in cases of tuberculosis. Personally I have not used it, and I am loth to pass judgment on observations recorded in every good faith. I would merely remark to my honorable colleague that Koch's lymph was used in our school in all the homœopathic dilutions possible at the moment of its far-resounding discovery—a fact which he should know as well as myself. To mention only one instance—Drs. Simon, V. L. Simon Boyer and Chancerel used the drug at the Hahnemann Hospital in Paris at the time of the arrival in France of the first consignment of lymph from Germany; and I am nearly certain that there is not at this time a single country where homœopathists have not used this remedy in all the infinitesimal dilutions. Homœopaths and allopaths have actually taken pretty much the same side as regards the primitive formula put forward by Koch (I am not now speaking of trials of new tuberculins); and Dr. Arnulphy would be fortunate enough were he able to revive its credit after its several years' oblivion as a cure of tuberculosis.

Clinically this lymph of Koch has led to wonderful cures in lobular pneumonia, for it produces pneumonia, broncho pneumonia, and congestion of the lungs in the tuberculous patient. Its homœopathic action would thus appear more trustworthy than its isopathic, and Dr. Arnulphy makes this remark: "I make bold to state that no single remedy in our materia medica, not excepting *Ipecac*, *Iodine*, *Tartar emetic*, and even *Phosphorus*, approaches the singular efficacy of *Tuberculin* in well-authenticated cases of that affection (broncho pneumonia, be it) in the child, the adult, or the aged. Its rapidity of action in some cases is little short of wonderful, and all who have used it in this line are unanimous in their unbounded praise of its working."

The four cases quoted by Dr. Mersch (*Journal Belge d' Homéopathie*, November, 1894, January and May, 1895) are very instructive:

The first is that of a member of the Dutch Parliament who had contracted a pneumonia which reached a chronic stage. While undergoing a relapse his expectoration assumed a rusty-red color, which color disappeared completely in three days on treatment with *Tuberculin* 30th.

The second case is that of a person who was seized, after an attack of measles, with broncho-pneumonia. On the fifth day Dr. Mersch prescribed *Tuberculin* 6th. In a day or two the condition of the chest was completely altered.

In the third case an old lady was likewise attacked with broncho-pneumonia, together with digestive troubles, and was for a long time in a serious state. After the lapse of a single night, which was a rather distressing one, under the action of the remedy the amelioration was great, and it was with difficulty that Dr. Mersch found a touch of bronchitis in the very place where the day before he had heard nothing but the tubular *souffle*. The prescription ran: *Tuberculin* 6th, eight packets of ten globules each, one to be taken every two hours.

Finally, in a fourth case, the patient was a lady of vigorous physique, and twenty-five years of age, who had capillary bronchitis, combined with the symptoms of angina pectoris. Dr. Mersch had once more had an opportunity of viewing with astonishment the rapidity with which the therapeutic action of *Tuberculin* may be manifested in such cases.

Bacillinum deserves study from two points of view, isopathically in the treatment of tuberculosis, homœopathically in the treatment of affections of the respiratory organs without tuberculosis. To fully understand its action it is necessary to know with exactness its composition. Dr. J. Compton Burnett has christened it *Bacillinum*, because he recognized in its lower dilutions the presence of Koch's bacilli. As a matter of fact, *Bacillinum* contains in its elements everything that a cavity of a tuberculous lung is capable of containing; that is to say, many other things besides Koch's bacillus. The bacillus of Koch is feebly pyogenetic, and the purulent contents of the cavities include pyogenetic staphylococci and streptococci, to say nothing of the organic products which play a large part in the production of the hectic fever of tuberculosis. It is a combination of toxins, then, which constitutes *Bacillinum*, and especially of toxins of a purulent nature. I lay stress upon this last fact, as it goes to sustain the opinion that I hold on the action of *Bacillinum*.

The infinitesimal dose of Homœopathy is in no way inimical to the entrance of all the elements constituting a substance into its materia medica. The salts of potassium owe their effect to their base as well as to their acid; *Graphites* is analogous to *Carbo* and *Ferrum*, because it contains both carbon and iron; *Hepar sulphuris calcareum* acts by reason of its sulphur as well as of its lime. *Bacillinum*, then, combines in its action all its constituent products, owing its efficacy to its suppurative microbes as well as its inclusion of Koch's bacillus.

This method of viewing the matter, which is peculiar to myself, permits me to include in one and the same category the action of *Bacillinum* in consumption and its action in non-tuberculous bronchitis.

I have studied conscientiously the action of *Bacillinum* in tuberculosis, and I must confess that I am looking out still for an authentic case of cure by this remedy. Nevertheless, in the midst of the paucity of drugs for the treatment of tuberculosis, I am happy to state that *Bacillinum* has produced in my hands considerable amelioration of the symptoms of this disease. Perhaps in certain cases it produces what Bernheim would call "la treve tuberculeuse." But sooner or later the drug, after ameliorating the symptoms, loses its effect, and the disease again gets the upper hand. I wish I could be as optimistic as Dr. J. Compton Burnett in his interesting book, "A New Cure for Consumption;" but that is impossible.

In looking over my observations I find that the symptom which has always undergone the greatest mitigation has been the *expectoration*. When *Bacillinum* acts on tuberculosis the sputum is less abundant, less purulent, less green, and more aërated. It is this which has always struck me most in the action of *Bacillinum*. It is rarely that a patient satisfied with the remedy fails to remark, "I expectorate less." In cases of dry cough at the beginning of tuberculosis I have noticed that the drug evidently arrests the tubercular process.

I would most severely criticise, as well for myself as for others, cases of so-called "cure of tuberculosis." There certainly are persons in whom the disease does not develop. These may have been accidentally infected, and their phagocytes may have struggled against their microbe foe. But in the case of an individual in whom the tubercle finds a suitable field for development, it is the merest chance that he entirely recovers without ulterior relapse; mostly it is a seeming cure, caused by a time of pause in the microbian pullulation.

Last year I had under my care, at the Hospital St. Jacques, a truly extraordinary case. It has been followed out by Dr. Jousset, by Dr. Cesar, head of the hospital laboratory, and by the house-physicians. It was that of a woman who entered the hospital suffering from influenza, and who, a few days after a slight amelioration of her symptoms, was attacked with a pulmonary congestion, clearly localized in the top of the left lung, and accompanied by all the clinical symptoms of tuberculosis—râles and moist crepitation, dulness, exaggeration of the thoracic vibration, nummular expectoration, fever, perspiration, spitting of blood—everything was there. Examination of the sputa showed distinctly the presence of Koch's bacilli. Everyone at the hospital diagnosed tuberculosis, myself the first. I gave her *Avian tuberculin* and in three weeks all the symptoms had disappeared. That woman left the hospital completely cured, and *a year afterwards* her health was still perfect. In my opinion this patient never had consumption; she was attacked with pseudo-phymic bronchitis, a complication which is very often found with influenza, and which may very easily be mistaken for tuberculosis; and in spite of the presence in the sputa of Koch's bacillus I would not register it as a case of tuberculosis, because, in contradistinction to that single case, I could mention twenty cases of tuberculosis whose symptoms neither *Avian tuberculin* nor any other such drug has cured.

There is absolutely no connection between the clinical evolution of real tuberculosis and observations based on the autopsies of old persons whose lungs contain cavities, but whose death was not due to tuberculosis. To admit, with Professor Brouardel, that three-fourths of those who have died a violent death are possessed of tuberculous lesions, whose existence was not suspected while the subject was living, would be running absolutely counter to clinical experience. The time is probably at hand when the different kinds of tuberculosis will be distinguished and separated, as we distinguish and separate the varieties of serious pleurisy and purulent pleurisy, of broncho-pneumonia arising from the presence of pneumococci, of streptococci, or of staphylococci. Malassez has already described cases of pseudo-tuberculosis, or zoogleic-tuberculosis, whose existence has only been acknowledged of late years. Courmont has discovered a pseudo-bacillosis of a bovine origin. We have a pseudo-bacillosis of a strepto bacillar origin, not to mention the "professional" tuberculoses, such as that to which persons are exposed who have to breathe the fumes of charcoal.

To return to *Bacillinum*, I consider this remedy as a powerful moderator of the muco-purulent secretion of consumption. While diminishing the secretion it modifies the auscultation; there is less thick sputum, the cavities are drier, the peri-tuberculosis congestion less intense. The clinical symptoms follow those of the auscultation; as the patient expectorates less he is less feeble, coughs less, gains strength, and regains his spirits; but the tubercle remains untouched. The peri-tuberculous congestion only is diminished, as one may observe with the naked eye when Koch's lymph is employed in the amelioration of lupus. The peri-tuberculous inflammation disappears; the skin seems healthy, but the yellow tubercle remains as it was, and the patient is still uncured. Such are the limits I assign to *Bacillinum* in its action on consumption.

Far more potent is the part played by *Bacillinum* in non-tuberculous pulmonary affections, for the simple reason that the struggle is with a less redoubtable opponent. Ebersole, Young, Zoppritz, Burnett, James, Holmes, Jousset, Steinhauf have published cases of the cure of acute bronchitis, influenza diarrhœa, syphilitic eruptions, cystitis, ringworm of the scalp, nephritis, idiocy, retarded dentition, cretinism, gout, rheumatism, etc., with *Tuberculin* or *Bacillinum*.

If we wish to prescribe *Bacillinum* successfully in non-tuberculous affections, we must observe, on auscultation, symptoms analogous to those which are perceptible in tuberculosis. The peculiar characteristics which indicate *Bacillinum* for non-tuberculous maladies of the respiratory organs are, in my opinion, the two following: The first is *oppression*; the second, *muco purulent* expectoration. These two phenomena show themselves always in the last stage of tuberculosis; that is to say, together with the products contained in the preparation of *Bacillinum*. *Dyspnœa resulting from bronchial and pulmonary obstruction caused by a super-abundant secretion from the mucous membrane is marvellously relieved by Bacillinum.* I put forward this fact, not on the evidence of a single isolated observation, but on that of several cases conscientiously studied. Such expectoration leads to the auscultation of sub-crepitant râles, sounding liquid and gurgling, having some analogy to the moist sounds of tuberculosis.

This power of *Bacillinum* to relieve oppression in pulmonary catarrh is in no way surprising from the point of view of the law of similars; for in the acute and infectious stage of tuberculosis the dyspnœa is a characteristic symptom, and is far more distressing than the cough. I have read with pleasure in the work of Dr. Mersch, of Brussels, on *Tuberculin*, of a fact which corroborates my statement as to the influence of *Bacillinum* over catarrhal dyspnœa. After the sixth dose the patient, who was suffering from bronchial asthma, was seized with violent intercostal pains, with augmented cough; but the oppression entirely disappeared after the first day, and did not return even three months after the treatment had ceased.

In *L' Art Médical* of January, 1894, and in the *Hahnemannian Monthly* of July, 1894, I published the case of an old man of eighty years of age, suffering from broncho-pneumonia, who, in the last stage of asphyxia, had been saved by *Bacillinum*. Two years ago I was called upon to treat another octogenarian who, as the result of a cold, developed an obstruction in the bronchial tubes, and at the basis of the lungs. He passed sleepless nights in a sitting posture, striving to draw deep inspirations. *Phosphorus, Arsenic*, and *Stibium* produced no relief. I gave him *Bacillinum* 30th, and he slept the whole night through. Doses of this remedy, administered *at longish intervals*, always produced a remarkable amelioration. Last year I was called to the house of an upholsterer. He preferred not going to bed at all to passing the night in bed without closing his eyes. He had humid asthma with incessant cough, which ended by causing him to eject thick yellow and puriform mucus. For eight days he took *Arsenic* and *Blatta*, and for a whole week he passed the nights without sleeping. From the day he took *Bacillinum* he was able to sleep. I saw him again this year in good health. Once or twice he was attacked with the same bronchorrhea, and had my prescription made up at the chemists, with the same success. This year, too, I have given *Bacillinum* to several patients at the Hôpital St. Jacques for the same symptoms, and it has never yet failed me.

When I am called upon to treat a patient suffering from an obstruction of the bronchial tubes occasioned by mucus, which is frequently thick and opaque and puriform—an obstruction extending to the delicate bronchial ramification, and causing oppression more frequently than cough, I turn my thoughts at once to *Bacillinum*. *Bacillinum* is a drug for old people, or, at any rate, for those whose lungs are old; for those chronically catarrhal, or whose pulmonary circulation is enfeebled without regard to the age of the subject; for those who have dyspnœa, and who cough with difficulty from inaction of the respiratory ducts; for the humid asthmatic, the bronchorrheal, who feel suffocated at night; and, finally, for those who, after taking cold, are straightway attacked with pulmonary congestion. Here, I believe, is the exact sphere of action of *Bacillinum* as a homœopathic remedy.

Bacillinum has been stigmatized as an unstable product. I consider this reproach ill-founded. *Bacillinum* is no more unstable than *Psorinum*, which is an approved remedy in Homœopathy. Typical tuberculous lungs contain practically almost invariable elements. Do not the microbes produced by cultivation and the animal extracts show any variation in quality, and do they not change in the long run?

Like most homœopathists who have made use of *Bacillinum*, I think it is best given in the high dilutions and at long intervals. Dr. J. Compton Burnett and Van der Berghe recommended the higher potencies—the 1000th, 100,000, etc., whereas I content myself with the 30th, which satisfies every requirement. As regards the intervals which must elapse between the doses, certain writers recommend from one to two weeks. In acute cases I generally give six globules of *Bacillinum* 30th every two or three days; and in chronic cases of tuberculosis, etc., one dose about twice a week.

We are no longer permitted to include in the same description the tuberculosis of birds and that of mammals. Although the two bacilli, as far as form and color are concerned, are absolutely identical, the evolution of the two forms of tuberculosis presents characteristics so different that we are forced to study them separately. At this day the debate is a question of words, and experts discuss whether there are two distinct genera or merely two different species.

It is this characteristic of non-transmissibility from mammals to birds, and *vice versa*, which forms the chief difference between the two kinds of tuberculosis. Strauss failed in his endeavor to inoculate a fowl with tuberculosis by injecting fifty kilogrammes of tuberculous human sputa, whereas the fowl, absolutely impervious to human tuberculosis, became infected when treated with a very slight quantity of the avian tuberculosis. The guinea-pig, so sensitive to the human microbe, presented encysted abscesses when treated with the virus of birds; it dies of cachexia, but never, as far as the naked eye can discern, of generalized tuberculosis. Rabbits are more sensitive to the avian infection. Dogs are absolutely refractory. The monkey, so delicate in our climate, and which almost invariably perishes from tuberculosis, is uninjured by inoculation from avian virus. The parrot is a remarkable exception to the general rule; it is the only bird which resists avian tuberculosis, while, on the other hand, it is sensitive to that of man. Such facts as these irrefutably differentiate the two kinds of tuberculosis.

[H]	Tuberculosis of Birds.	Tuberculosis of Mammals.
Aspect of cultures.	Extreme softness on glycerine jelly or on serum.	Human tuberculous growths are adherent, hard and difficult to break up even with a strong platinum wire on glycerine jelly as well as on serum.

Medium of cultures.	Transferred from a solid to a liquid medium the bacillus grows rapidly, having the appearance of rounded grains.	Cultivation more difficult.
Temperature.	Develops at a temperature of 45° C.	Ceases to develop at temperatures under 41° C.
Odor.	Somewhat sour.	More subtle and fresh odor.
Duration.	Takes longer to develop, and may remain for a year or thereabouts.	Is with difficulty generated again at the end of six months. At the end of eight or ten months loses its vegetable character.
Seat of the tubercles.	In animals usually on the liver, the spleen, the intestines, and the peritoneum.	In the lung, generally in men, and in certain animals; in the spleen, the liver, and the glands in rabbits and guinea-pigs.
Transmissibility.	Only from one bird to another, except in the case of the parrot.	Mammals are unaffected by the tuberculosis of birds, and *vice versa*.

Ever since this variety of tuberculosis has been distinguished, attempts have been made to inoculate or cure human tuberculosis with that of birds. In our school the thing has been attempted at the Hôpital St. Jacques, where *Aviaire* has been administered in homœopathic dilutions, in potions or through punctures in cases of consumption. As a matter of fact, neither allopaths nor homœopaths have succeeded in obtaining a formula which will cure consumption with the virus of birds. Amelioration has been noted as with other remedies, but never a series of authenticated cures. Nevertheless, in every country experiments are continually being made; we must hope that they will end in a more decisive success than is at present the case.

Hoping to profit by the homœopathicity of an active virus, I was, I think, one of the first who employed *Aviaire* in non-tuberculous respiratory affections on the lines of *Bacillinum*, and I am bound to say that up to the present my faith in the law of similars has not been shaken by my experiments.

In *L'Art Médical* (August, 1895) I published a number of cases in which I successfully treated localized bronchitis, generally the result of influenza, and reproducing the symptoms of tuberculosis, with *Aviaire*. The most characteristic of all these observations is that of which I have spoken above. The patient was restored to health as if by magic with *Aviaire* within three weeks. Dr. P. Jousset, anticipating my observations, thus expressed himself in the number of *L'Art Médical* preceding the one which contained my remarks: "A young woman entered the Hôpital St. Jacques at the end of January, 1895, with feverish influenzal bronchitis. At first the patient was treated with small doses of *Sulphate of Quinine*, and a little later she took *Ipecac* and *Bryonia* alternately. The fever disappeared and the general condition improved considerably, and the sub-crepitant râles became confined to the top of the left lung. The patient continued to expectorate thick nummular and puriform sputa, as in the influenza. After some days the disease resumed its sway, the bodily forces diminished, the emaciation made great progress, and local and general signs indicated rapid consumption. Bacteriological analysis led to the detection of numerous Koch's bacilli. I gave over the case at this time, and some weeks afterwards I learnt with surprise that the patient was well and growing fat, and that the inoculation of the sputa had produced no effects. The cure has been maintained for three months, and the young woman has resumed her employment." I had prescribed *Aviaire* 100th, five drops a day, during the whole period of the disease, unaccompanied by any other remedy.

As I have said before, more than a year afterwards the young woman continued in good health.

Following this case, Dr. Jousset quoted two analogous instances in his practice, both of influential bronchitis, in which the sputa contained, for a certain period, Koch's bacillus. One was cured with *Aviaire* 6th and strong doses of *Sulphate of Quinine*, and the other with *Aviaire* 6th and twenty drops of *Tincture of Drosera*, a day.

"What conclusions must I draw from these facts?" says Dr. Jousset. "That the avian tuberculosis cured the consumption? I have failed too often in the treatment of ordinary consumption with this remedy to admit that." That is my opinion also.

Koch's bacillus has been found in the nasal secretions of healthy hospital nurses, and of students of medicine, as noted by Strauss. Would it not be possible to come across it accidentally in certain kinds of expectoration, just as the pneumococcus is found in saliva?

In one of the numbers of *La Médecine Moderne* of last year there appeared a short article on the "Influenzas known as pseudo-phymic." The writer remarked on the strong analogy which certain complications of pulmonary influenza presented to acute tuberculosis. He observed, among other forms: 1st, the influenzal bronchitis which affected one of the summits of the lung, the most difficult form to diagnose from tuberculosis; 2d, the broncho-pneumonic form; 3d, the pleuro-pneumonic form, bearing a close resemblance to tuberculous pleurisy. I might remark that this last form is still little known and ill-defined. The influenza microbe always imitates to a remarkable degree the microbe of tuberculosis in certain instances; and if we wish to effect a cure on the laws laid down by Hahnemann in certain forms of influenzal bronchitis, we must frequently seek for the simillimum in the virus of tuberculosis.

I have mentioned oppression as one of the characteristics of *Bacillinum*. Now influenzal bronchitis is markedly accompanied by an incessant cough and by grave general symptoms. There is more frequently acute than passive, obstructive and dyspnœic congestion. I am inclined to prefer *Aviaire* to *Bacillinum* in such cases, and I should like to briefly touch upon certain cases in my practice.

I have under my care a little girl of twelve years of age who has for two years developed an influenza which rapidly leads to pulmonary symptoms, always distinctly localized in the top of the left lung. The mother is tuberculous, and the child, who was born with forceps, has her left chest less developed than her right. The congestion which accompanies the influenza is sudden and severe; within twenty-four hours the lung is invaded, and fine râles are soon heard. Twice running, at intervals of a year, *Aviaire* 100th has stifled the symptoms in a few days. I have seen an analogous case, only with congestion of the base of the lung.

In my clinical report of the Hôpital St. Jacques (in August, 1895) I note ten cases of acute influenzal bronchitis with incessant cough, fever, and expectoration, rapidly cured with *Aviaire*. This year I have prescribed it with the same success as at the Hôpital St. Jacques in cases of influenzal bronchitis, with active congestion. I will mention two cases of the pulmonary complications of measles which were rapidly dissipated by this remedy; but I must also mention a third case of measles in which *Aviaire* failed and *Bryonia* proved successful. The child had an acute rubeolic laryngitis, and few pulmonary symptoms. *Bryonia* was in this case more decidedly indicated than *Aviaire*.

The dilution of *Aviaire* which I have always used is the 100th. I give usually five drops a day.

It seems that *Aviaire* does not act in diminishing the cough like an anodyne or a narcotic, but braces up the whole organism. The relief of debility and the return of appetite are the phenomena which I have observed in conjunction with the diminution of the cough.

I have given *Aviaire* 100th for weeks, and even for a month, regularly every day, without having observed excitement or aggravation. It would thus appear to be a remedy of long-lasting action, capable in certain cases of modifying the organism, and of bracing a constitution which has become enfeebled from the effects of influenza or of suspicious bronchitis.

In contrast with *Bacillinum* I have noted, in my observations on *Aviaire*, considerable cough and little dyspnœa—an acute inflammatory, extremely irritating cough, such as one meets with in acute diseases or sub-acute affections in young people; a cough which fatigues, and which leads to enfeeblement and loss of appetite—in a word, a suspicious cough. To conclude my remarks, the utility of *Aviaire* in *suspicious bronchitis*—an expression on which I again lay stress—I will recall certain indubitable examples of the cure (at the Hôpital St. Jacques) of bronchitis or of pulmonary congestion at the top of one of the lungs, or of bronchitis on one side only, or of congestion predominating on one side. These localizations on one side are sufficiently grave symptoms to warrant apprehension of the hatching of tuberculosis.

If I were myself attacked, as the result of influenza or measles, or of some weakening malady, with an incessant tickling and stubborn cough, with certain closely localized pulmonary symptoms; if I lost my strength and appetite; if, in a word, I were attacked by bronchitis whose upshot was highly doubtful, and which caused apprehension of tuberculosis, I should not hesitate a single moment, with the examples which I have had before me, to try *Aviaire* 100th upon myself.

Such is the conclusion of my clinical observations made at Hôpital St. Jacques in August, 1895.

What I said last year I can only repeat with renewed confidence in this; and I hope that the years which follow will not cause me to alter my opinion.

FOOTNOTES:

[C] *L' Union Homéopathique*, vol. v, No. 3.

[D] *Homœopathic World*, vol. xxvi, No. 304.

[E] "On Tuberculin," an extract from the *Journal Belge d' homéopathie*, 1895.

[F] *Pathogenese, sua importancia.*

[G] Dr. J. Compton Burnett, in his book, "New Cure for Consumption," p. 129, makes this remark: "The best way to get some really good *Bacillinum* is to take a portion of the lung of an individual who has died of genuine bacillary tuberculosis pulmonum, choosing a good-sized portion from the parietes of the cavity and its circumjacent tissue, as herein will be found everything pertaining to the tuberculous process—bacilla, *débris*, ptomaines and tubercles in all its stages (such was practically the origin of the matrix of my *Bacillinum*) and preparing by trituration in spirit. In this way nothing is lost."

[H] I have tabulated shortly their various characteristics.

BELLIS PERENNIS.

NAT. ORD., Compositæ.
COMMON NAMES, English Daisy. Garden Daisy. Hens and Chickens.
PREPARATION.—The fresh plant, in flower, is pounded to a pulp and submitted to pressure. The expressed juice is then mixed with an equal part by weight of alcohol.

(The following is from Thomas' *Additions to the Homœopathic Materia Medica*, 1858. To it we may add Dr. J. C. Burnett's statement that *Bellis* is a remedy for all ills that may be traced to a sudden wetting when overheated.)

Bellis perennis or daisy, formerly called *consolida*, on account of its vulnerary properties; the roots and leaves were used in wound drinks, and were considered efficacious in removing extravasated blood from bruises, etc. It is said to be refused by cattle on account of its peculiar taste. Lightfoot, in his *Flora Scotica*, says: "In a scarcity of garden-stuff, they (daisies) have, in some countries, been substituted as pot herbs." My first trial with this plant as a curative agent was in the autumn of 1856. While on a visit in the neighborhood of Bangor, a countryman, understanding that I was a "doctor," wished me to prescribe for his foot, which he had sprained very badly. Not having either *Arnica* or *Rhus* with me, I determined to try the effects of the daisy; so directed him to procure a handful of the leaves and flowers of the plant, chop them up small, boil them for a quarter of an hour in half a pint of water, and apply them in linen as a poultice round the ankle at night. The application was not made until the next morning, but in half an hour's time the ankle admitted of very fair motion. A piece of calico wetted and wrung out of the daisy water was then wrapped round the ankle, and the man put his shoe on and limped about all day, walking not less than five miles. He repeated the poultice at night, and found his ankle so much restored in the morning that he was able to walk four miles to his work without experiencing any difficulty. The success, in this instance, so far exceeded the previous use of *Arnica* and *Rhus*, especially in the time gained, that I had a tincture from the whole plant made for such uses, and have used it in sprained ankle from a fall—the ankle was well the second day. A sprain of the wrist, which had been a week ailing, yielded to the daisy in three days. I have also successfully used it in several severe whitlows; in every case the pure tincture was used externally. The only provings I have made with this remedy have been with the pure tincture in ten or twenty drop doses at a time. After taking the medicine for fourteen days without any symptoms, I suspended the use of it—in two weeks after leaving it off, for the first time in my life I had a large boil on the back of my neck (right side), commencing with a dull aching pain; some difficulty and a bruised pain in keeping the head erect; slight nausea, want of appetite, and a little giddiness in the head at times. Pain in middle finger of the left hand, as of a gathering, for a short time only; and at the same time pain in inner side of left forearm, as of a boil developing; two nights before similar pains in corresponding parts of the right arm—query, are these effects of *Bellis* (this was written December 11, 1856). The boil on the neck came December 7, 1856; began as a slight pimple with burning pain in the skin, increasing until in six days' time it was very large, of a dark fiery purple color, and very sore burning and aching pain in it, accompanied with headache, extending from occiput to sinciput, of a cold aching character; brain as though contracted in frontal region, dizziness, etc. (as before stated). I now set to work to cure myself, which by use of hot fomentations and lint dipped in θ tincture of *Belladonna* externally, taking at the same time 3d dil. *Belladonna* internally, was soon accomplished. Three days after this was cured, another made its appearance, which speedily succumbed to the same remedies. As I had never previously had a boil, and had not made any change in my diet, I suspected *Bellis* tincture to be the cause of the trouble. On the 12th of January, 1857, feeling my left foot somewhat strained after running, I applied *Bellis* θ to the strain, which for several days aggravated the feeling; and in five hours after the application I had another small boil (three weeks after disappearance of the last), which yielded to same treatment as the others, by January 19, 1857. On March 7, 1857, I chewed some daisy flowers. On the 11th, a small boil appeared at the angle of the inferior maxilla, right side; *Belladonna* θ, externally, cured it. The last trial I made with the third centesimal dilution of *Bellis*, taking three drops on Tuesday, 2d March, 1858, on the following Friday a small pimple appeared a little behind the angle of *left* inferior maxilla; it increased very much in size and pain by Saturday, when I treated it with *Belladonna* θ externally, to which it soon yielded. As at no other time in my life have I suffered from boils, I am inclined to think these are due to the use of the daisy.

BERBERIS AQUIFOLIUM.

NAT. ORD., Berberidaceæ
COMMON NAMES, Oregon grape. Mountain grape.
PREPARATION.—The fresh root and stem is pounded to a pulp and macerated in two parts by weight of alcohol.

(This unintentional proving was published in August, 1896, under the signature J. d. W. C. The paper referred to by J. d. W. C. was a clipping from the *Eclectic Medical Journal.*)

In the *Homœopathic Recorder* for March, 1896, p. 133, there appears an interesting article on the virtues of the plant named above—it starts out with: "From the fact that it will make a 'new' man of an old one in a short time it is an excellent remedy."

As I am now over sixty years old, it seemed high time to cast about for something possessing the virtue specified, viz., making "a 'new' man out of an old one"—and to my knowledge, as I have never had five days' illness confining me to bed, or even to my room, during the said sixty years, I considered myself an easy subject for the contemplated rejuvenation; besides all this, I am what some would call a homœopathic "crank;" and believed, and yet believe, if there be anything that can effect such a transformation it is to be found only within the lines of Homœopathy, I immediately ordered quantum suf. of the article in question from the celebrated firm of Boericke & Tafel, and started out on the trip to the "Fountain of Youth" in full confidence that *something* would come of it.

The first day I took two doses mother tincture 10-15 drops each; no special effect noticed—no youthfulness either! Second day, ditto; third day, one dose in morning; after bank hours went to friend's sanctum and engaged in a game of chess, and while so engaged felt a growing sense of nausea and thick-headedness—so much so, that I was obliged to excuse myself and hurry to my own quarters. *Berberis*, however, did not once occur to me—I had scarce reached my room when the sense of nausea (seven minutes' lively walk, since it became really oppressive) had *full sway*, and having eaten nothing whatever since the previous evening (as I do not eat unless I am hungry) the straining was rather severe, but exactly similar to some previous attacks of "biliousness"—in feeling, and color and taste of discharges—and still *Berberis* did not occur to me; as soon as the strain was over I was seized with a remarkable and peculiar headache; a thing of which I have no recollection whatever to have previously experienced in any shape—the sensation was that of a strong, well-defined, compressive band of iron (or some unyielding substance), about two inches wide, passing *entirely round the head, just above the ears*—it kept on growing tighter and tighter; I jumped from the reclined position on a couch, wet a folded towel in cold water, and passed it round my head so as to cover the "band;" but it gave little relief; about 10 o'clock I began to think over what I might have eaten to disagree with me so, and at last *Berberis* came plump into sight; I at once prepared a cup of strong, strong coffee (Hahnemann's antidote, and for which I had to send to a neighbor), believing it would antidote the *Berberis* (or rather hoping it might), and about 12 o'clock there was a slight diminution of pressure; then more coffee, black and strong, two or three mouthfuls, and again laid down; by morning the serious phase of the headache had disappeared, but I was exceedingly tremulous in nerves and unsteady in gait up to noon, when I ventured on some oatmeal and syrup— habitually, I do not eat meat, or drink tea or coffee, nor spirituous liquors, nor use tobacco, and have not for over thirty years.

Finally, I "made a good recovery," and now whenever I have a sensation of biliousness I touch my tongue to my finger after touching the cork of the mother tincture bottle of *Berberis aqui.*; with laid finger—and have no trouble compared to what I have usually had—I believe I may say, I am subject to bilousness by heredity, but it has removed much thereof, and this remedy, I think, is good enough for the remainder.

BLATTA ORIENTALIS.

SYNONYM, Indian cockroach.
CLASS, Insecta.
ORDER, Orthoptera.
COMMON NAME (Indian), Talápoka.
PREPARATION.—Triturate in the usual way.

(These two papers are by Dr. D. N. Ray, of Calcutta, India, and were originally published in the *Homœopathic Recorder* in the years 1890 and 1891. A number of papers from American physicians could be added confirming what Dr. Ray says of the drug.)

The *Blatta orientalis* is a common insect in India, where it is found abundantly in the dwelling houses. It has rather a flat body, from an inch to a couple of inches in length; deep brown color. It can fly a short distance. The wings reach beyond the body and cover it completely; the feet have several segments and are provided with prickles.

Preparation.—The live animal is crushed and triturated as under class IX of American Homœopathic Pharmacopœia, a tincture can be prepared as under class IV of the same Pharmacopœia.

This new unknown remedy has a curious anecdote connected with it. I call it new because it has not been mentioned in any of our medical works, although the use of *Blatta Americana* (American cockroach) as a remedy for dropsy has been mentioned in journals. The Indian cockroach is used not in cases of dropsy but in cases of *Asthma*, a most obstinate disease to deal with. In asthma it acts almost specifically. Before I further proceed to give an account of this new, invaluable drug I shall narrate here a short story how it came into use.

Some years ago an elderly gentleman had long been suffering from asthma; for over twenty years. He took all measures and tried different methods of both recognized and unrecognized medical treatments, but unfortunately all proved in vain. At last he gave up all treatment and was getting fits daily. He was brought to such a deplorable condition that he was left to suffer. He was in the habit of taking tea. One afternoon as usual he drank his cup of tea—afterwards he noticed that his oppression in the chest was much less and that he was feeling unusually better, so much so that he felt himself a different being. This led him and his friends to inquire into the cause of it. He immediately inferred that the relief was due to the drinking of the *tea*, although he habitually drank the same tea but never before had experienced any such changes. So this change he attributed to something in the tea. The servant who prepared the tea was sent for and questioned. His reply was that he made the tea as usual and there was nothing new in it. The residue of the teacup was carefully examined, nothing was found there, but on examining the tea-pot a dead cockroach was discovered. So it was concluded that this *infusion* of cockroach did the gentleman a world of good. The very day he drank that *cup of tea* he had hardly any fit of asthma at night, and in a few days he got entirely well to his and his friends' surprise.

The accounts of his Providential recovery were communicated to some of his friends—one of them, not a medical man, but quite an enterprising gentleman, took this into his head and resolved to try whether cockroach does any good to other asthmatic patients. For this purpose he got a lot of cockroaches, put them alive into a quantity of boiling water and mixed it after filtering the water when cool with almost the same quantity of the rectified spirit of wine, so that it might last for some time without getting soured. This new mixture (or tincture) he began to try in each and every case of asthma that he came across. The dose was a drop each time, 3 or 4 doses daily, and more frequently during the fits of asthma. Within a short time he made some such wonderful cures that people began to flock from different parts of the country to his door. Soon the number of attendants was so great that he had to manufacture the medicine by pounds and all this medicine he distributed to patients without any charge. He has records of some of the cases.

Some two years ago a patient of mine asked me whether we make any use of *Talápoka* (cockroach) in our Pharmacopœia. My reply was that we use many loathsome insects as our remedial agents. I told him also that *Blatta Americana* (American cockroach), I had heard, had been used in cases of dropsy, but I had no practical experience with it. He then said the Indian cockroach is used in cases of asthma and he knew several cases had been cured with it. This struck me and I determined to try this in cases of asthma whenever next opportunity occurred. For this purpose I got a lot of live cockroaches, killed them and pounded to a fine pulp and triturated according to class IX of American Homœopathic Pharmacopœia, that is, two parts by weight of the substance and nine parts by weight of sugar of milk, giving 1x trituration. Thus I prepare up to 3x trituration and I also make an alcoholic solution—a few live cockroaches were crushed and five parts by weight of alcohol poured over them—it was allowed to remain eight days in a dark, cool place, being shaken twice daily. After the expiration of that period the alcoholic solution was poured off, strained and filtered, when it was ready for use.

I began to try both the preparations—drop doses of the tincture and grain doses of 1x, 2x and sometimes 3x, 3 or 4 times daily when there was no fit and almost every fifteen minutes or half hourly during the severity of a fit. Both preparations began to answer well and I was getting daily more and more encouraged about the efficacy of this new drug. I had the opportunity of trying quite a number of cases of asthma within this short time, the reports of which I wish to publish in the future, but for the present I am glad to say in many cases it acted almost specifically, that is, the whole trouble cleared away within a fortnight or so without recurrence. In some cases the severity of the paroxysm was lessened and the recurrence of the fits took place at a longer interval; in others again only temporary benefit was observed. This failure to benefit all cases alike I attribute to many circumstances. Some people did not, rather could not, take the medicine regularly according to my directions owing to their untoward circumstances; some persons were suffering from other complications along with asthma; some again got temporary relief and in the meantime discontinued the medicine and came back again when there was a recurrence of the fits, that is, they did not continue the drug for sufficient length of time. Some cases again, not having derived immediate benefit, got impatient and discontinued the medicine without proper trial.

Besides all these, I think individual idiosyncrasy has a great deal to do. The season of the year has some influence. It is usually observed in this country that those who are subject to periodical attacks of asthmatic fits are more prone to an attack either during the full or the new moon, or at both the times. I believe if it is properly watched this fact will be evident all over the world. Same is true of some other diseases, as chronic cough, chronic fevers, rheumatism, either acute or chronic, gout, elephantiasis, other glandular enlargements, etc., get aggravated or are prone to aggravation during such changes of the moon. Then some people get more severe and frequent fits during the winter than the summer and the others more during the summer than the winter. Let me here tell you that the Indian summer is very different from either the English or the American. Some part of the Indian summer season is quite rainy and the atmosphere is saturated with moisture and other irritating ingredients, consequently a class of asthmatic people suffer more during this season. I noticed to this class of cases *Blatta orientalis* will prove most efficacious. I have used it in bronchial and nervous asthma with better success than the stomachæ.

SECOND PAPER.

I have of late tried *Blatta orientalis* indiscriminately in almost all cases of asthma that have come under my treatment, and I am glad to say I have received good results in most cases, as the reports of some of the clinical cases will show. I have not come to any definite use of this drug yet, but I shall only mention a few facts that I have observed during its use. It acts better in low potency and repeated doses during an attack of asthma; when the spasm subsides, the terminal asthmatic cough with wheezing and slight dyspnœa, etc., is better relieved with higher potencies; the low potency, if continued after the spasmodic period is over, will make the cough more troublesome and harassing to the patient and the expectoration tenacious, thick and very difficult to raise, but this will not be the case if the potency is changed. I had this difficulty in a few cases when I was less acquainted with the action of the drug, but now I manage my cases better. In four patients who continued the drug for some time in the low potency, during the paroxysm and after it was over, the cough became dry and hacking with little or no expectoration, the streaks of blood appeared in the sputa, which the patients had never observed in the course of their long illness. This appearance of blood in their sputa was the cause of a great anxiety to them and made them hurry over to my office. On inquiry I learned from two of them—one a lady and the other a young man—that while taking this remedy they felt a sensation all over the body, for four or five days previous to the appearance of the blood, as if heat were radiating from the ears, eyes, nose, top of the head, palms of the hands and soles of the feet. They attributed this sensation of heat all over the body and the appearance of the blood in the expectoration to the drug. I directed them to stop the medicine at once; this they did, and with the discontinuance of it the blood disappeared from the sputa as well as the sensation of heat, but to me it was an open question whether this appearance of blood in the expectoration was due to overdrugging, although I must say that the presence of the streaks of blood in the sputa of asthmatic patients is not an uncommon phenomenon. I resolved to give the same potency to the same patients after the lapse of some days. I did so, and to my surprise the blood-streaked sputa again appeared after they had taken the remedy ix, one grain four times daily. From this the patients understood it was the same medicine that had been given to them on the last occasion and begged me not to give it again, as the appearance of blood in the sputum frightened them, in spite of all my assurance. No more strong doses of the drug were given to them and they did not notice any more blood in the sputum. I have heard other patients complain of this peculiar sensation of heat whenever strong doses were given to them for some time. It acts better on stout and corpulent than on thin and emaciated persons. The asthmatic patients subject to repeated attacks of malaria derive less permanent benefit from the use of the drug. So, it seems to me, that in hæmic asthma, which is due to the abnormal condition of the blood, it is efficacious. I have also used this drug in troublesome cough with dyspnœa of phthisical patients with good result.

CLINICAL CASES.

CASE I. Baln R. M., aged fifty-five, thin, emaciated and irritable temperament, has been suffering from hereditary asthma for the last twenty-five years. For the last six or seven years he suffered from asthmatic fits almost nightly and a troublesome cough with a good deal of frothy expectoration. He said he had not known what sleep was for the last six or seven years, in fact, he could not lie down in bed, as that would immediately bring on a violent fit of coughing which would not cease until he sat up, so the recumbent posture for him was almost impracticable, and he used to sit up during the night and doze on a pile of pillows. He passed his days comparatively better, but the approach of the night was a horror to him, his struggle, commencing at 9 or 10 P.M., would last till the morning. He was the father of many children and was well taken care of, but his suffering was so great that he had no ambition to live any longer. He tried almost all systems of medicine without much good. For the last ten years he took opium, which afforded him slight relief at the beginning, using as high as forty-eight grains of opium in twenty-four hours. Owing to the constant sitting posture he became stooped, and the back of his neck stiff and painful. In April, 1889, he was suddenly taken ill with fever. The fever became protracted. After an illness of over a month his condition became so bad that all hope of his recovery was given up. During this illness he was treated by an old school physician of some repute, but his condition daily grew worse, the asthmatic attacks became very violent and almost incessant, and the difficulty of breathing very great. He became so feeble that he had not strength enough to enable him to bring up the expectoration; his chest was full of it; fever was less; there was general anasarca. He was sitting with head bent forward, almost touching the bed, as that was the only position possible to him day and night. He had become almost speechless, when I was sent for, at about 3 P.M. on the 23d of May, 1889. When I was entering the patient's room a medical man came out and hinted that there was no use of my going in as the patient was just expiring. I found the patient breathing hard; unconscious; jaws were locked and saliva dribbling from the corners of his mouth; body cold; cold, clammy perspiration on forehead; eyes partially opened; in fact, to all appearance, he looked as if he were dead, except for the respiratory movements. I felt his pulse and found it was not so bad as the patient was looking. I examined the back of his chest, as that was the only portion easily accessible, and noticed that the bronchial spasms were going on with loud mucous râle. From the character of his pulse I thought that the present state of the patient was *probably* due to the continued violent struggle and not deep coma, and that he had become so exhausted that he was motionless, speechless and completely unconscious. His bed was surrounded by many friends and relations, who had come to bid him a last farewell; and it was with surprise that they all looked at me when I proposed to administer medicine to a patient whose death was expected every minute and for whose cremation preparations were being made.

I got a big phial full of water and put in it *Blatta orientalis* 1x trit. a few grains and tried two or three times to give him a spoonful of it, but in vain; the jaws were locked and I could not make him swallow any of that medicine; then I put some powder dry in the hollow of his lips and asked the attendants to try to give him the medicine I left in the bottle. I was asked whether there was any hope of his recovery, of course my answer was "*no*," and I also said he could only live a few hours. I left the patient's house with the idea of not visiting it again, but at 9 P.M. a messenger came with the report that the patient was slightly better, he could swallow medicine and two doses of it had been given. I was asked to see the patient again. I could hardly believe what he said, however, I went to see the patient again. I noticed there was a slight change for the better, the pulse was steady, the jaws were unlocked, there was mobility of the limbs, he could swallow liquid with ease and was expectorating freely, the breathing though still difficult was slightly improved. There was the winking of the eyelids. On the whole he was looking less lifeless, but still I entertained no hope of his recovery. I left instructions to repeat the same medicine once or twice during the night, if required, at the same time to give milk repeatedly, one or two spoonfuls at a time, and to inform me next morning if he had survived the night. Next morning I really grew anxious to know what had become of my patient who had shown symptoms slightly better with this new remedy. A messenger came with the report that the patient passed a good night. I was requested to see him again. When I arrived at his place at 8 A.M. I was surprised to see him so much better, he had not only regained his consciousness, but was sitting quietly in his bed, could speak slowly, the difficulty of breathing was completely gone, but the cough occasionally troubled him and a good deal of expectoration of frothy white or sometimes of big yellowish lumps of mucus came up. He was given three doses of the same medicine 2x trit. during the day. He passed a fair day, but at night his difficulty of breathing again appeared in somewhat milder form. He had to take two doses of the medicine. Thus the medicine was continued for a week and his trouble daily became less and less until after the expiration of a week he was able to sleep at night for the first time in the last six or seven years. I treated him over a month, and his health improved so rapidly that he not only got rid of the asthmatic trouble, but was soon able to go out and even attend his business. The stooped condition of his neck with slight pain and slight chronic bronchitis did not leave him altogether. Besides *Blatta orientalis*, I also prescribed for him *Arsenicum alb. 6* and *12*, *Naja tri. 6*, *Ipecac 3*, and *Antim. tart. 3*, as they were indicated. He continued well for over a year, but in August, 1890, he had slight reappearance of the asthmatic trouble. He again took *Blatta orientalis* and got well.

CASE II. Mrs. Nundy, a thin lady, aged twenty-three, mother of three children, came from a village for the treatment of asthma, from which she had been suffering for the last eight years. For the first two or three years she used to get two or three attacks in the year, but gradually they were repeated more frequently, though the character of the attack remained the same throughout. It would last two days and two nights, whether any medicine was given to her or not. Nothing would alleviate her suffering during an attack—too much interference would increase her sufferings and prolong the duration of the attack, so, practically speaking, almost nothing was given to her during an attack. The great oppression of breathing, restlessness, profuse perspiration, inability to move or lie down and loud wheezing would be the most prominent symptoms in each attack. These would remain almost with equal violence for nearly forty hours, when the spasms would cease with slight cough and expectoration, and she would be perfectly at ease as ever, and there would be no trace of disease left, except slight wheezing sound on auscultation. But latterly these attacks were very frequent, almost every week or ten days. In August, 1890, she was brought here for treatment. It is worth while to mention that she took both allopathic and native drugs during the interval of attacks to prevent their recurrence, but without any effect. I saw her first on the morning of the 5th of August, during an attack. I prescribed *Blatta Orientalis* IX trit., one grain every two hours. It was to their surprise that this attack subsided unlike all others by the evening; that is, it disappeared within twenty hours. This encouraged the lady and her husband so much that she wanted to have regular course of treatment under me. I put her under tincture of *Blatta Orientalis* IX, one drop per dose, twice daily. She continued this medicine till the time of the next attack was over; that is, for ten days. After the expiration of this period she began to complain of a sensation of heat all over her body, so I changed it to 3x, one drop morning and evening. She kept well, and after a month she went home thinking she got well. A month after her going home she had an attack of asthma at night and took *Blatta Orientalis* IX as before, and by the next morning she was well. This was in October, and after two months of the last attack. She had another attack in winter and none since.

CASE III. A young man, aged thirty-four, had been suffering from asthma for some years. He was invariably worse during the rains and the winter, and a chronic bronchitis was almost a constant accompaniment. He tried allopathic and lots of patent drugs, with only temporary amelioration of the trouble. At last, in November, 1888, he came to my office. On examination of his chest I found there was a chronic bronchitis. He said that slight difficulty of breathing with hacking cough used to trouble him every night, besides a cold would be followed by a severe attack of asthma, so its periodicity of recurrence was irregular. I treated him with *Ipecac*, *Arsenicum alb.*, etc. The first-named medicine did him the most good, but he never got entirely well. So in July, 1889, I put him under tincture *Blatta orientalis* 3X, drop doses, three or four times daily. Under its use he began to improve steadily, and had only two or three attacks of asthmatic fits since he used this drug, which were promptly relieved by the same drug in 1x potency. *Euphrasia off.* was prescribed for his cold whenever he had it. He is free from all trouble for the last year and a half. His general condition is so much changed that there is no apprehension of the recurrence of his former illness.

CASE IV. Baln Bose, an old, corpulent gentleman, aged sixty-two, has been suffering from asthmatic attacks for some years. He never took any allopathic medicine, but had always been under treatment of native kabiraj (medical men), under whose treatment he was sometimes better and worse at others. Latterly he became very bad and passed several sleepless nights. He used to pass his days comparatively better, and it was at night and in the morning he used to be worse. On the 24th of July, 1890, at 9 A.M. I saw him first—there was a slight touch of asthma even then. I made him try to lie down in bed; this he could not do, owing to the coughing fit it excited while in that posture. On examination the chest revealed chronic bronchial catarrh, and there was also a harassing cough, with very little expectoration after repeated exertion. I prescribed *Blatta orientalis* IX trit., one grain every two hours. He passed the night without an attack, and the next morning when I saw him he complained that only the cough was troublesome last night and no fit of asthma. The cough was somewhat troublesome even when I saw him in the morning. I gave him tincture *Blatta ori.* 3x, one drop dose every two hours. He passed the day and night well. He continued the treatment for a fortnight and then went home, where he has been keeping good health, with the exception of an occasional bronchial catarrh.

CASE V. A shoemaker, aged forty-two, robust constitution, has been suffering with asthma for three or four years. He came to my office on the 6th of November, 1890. He had been getting asthmatic fits almost every night since October last. During the day troublesome cough, with slight expectoration and hurried breathing made him unable to attend his business. Tincture *Blatta orientalis* IX, one drop doses, six times daily, was given. The very first day he perceived the good effect of the medicine and continued the same for a month, when he got well and discontinued the medicine. He has been keeping well ever since.

CASE VI. Mr. G., aged forty, healthy constitution, had an asthmatic fit on the 4th of August, 1890, preceded by a violent attack of cold, from which he frequently used to suffer. He had this severe cold in the morning, and in the afternoon he began to experience a great difficulty of breathing and slight oppression and lightness of the chest—this, by 9 P.M., developed into a regular fit of asthma. I was sent for. On my arrival, at 10 P.M., I found he was sitting before a pile of pillows with elbows supported on them, and struggling for breath. There was also a great tightness in the chest, occasional cough, and inability to speak. I at once put him under *Blatta orientalis* IX trit., one grain every fifteen minutes, and less frequently afterwards if he felt better. On my visit next morning I found him much better, but he said his trouble at night continued, more or less, till 2 A.M., after which he got some rest. Now, there was a troublesome cough, slight oppression of the chest and great apprehension of a second attack in the night. The same medicine, 3x trit., was given to him during the day, and a few powders of 1x were left with him in case he was to get an attack at night. There was a slight aggravation of those symptoms at night, and he had occasion to take only two powders of 1x. The next morning he was every way better, except the cough, for which four powders of 3x were given daily. In four or five days he got entirely well and had no relapse.

CASE VII. Mrs. D., aged twenty, a healthy, stout lady, mother of one child, had been always enjoying good health, was suddenly attacked with a violent fit of asthma on the 8th of August, 1890. This was the first occasion she had a fit of asthma, the result of a severe cold. At about 2 A.M. she was suddenly seized with difficulty of breathing and a great oppression in the chest. She could not lie down any longer in bed and had to sit up, being supported on a pile of pillows. In the morning at 8 A.M. I saw her first. I noticed she was in great agony and almost speechless. On examination I could not detect much loud wheezing—the characteristic of an asthmatic attack—though the rapid movements of the walls of the chest were even quite visible to the bystanders. The patient was feeling almost choked up, and could not express what was going on. She only pointed out a point, a little over the pit of the stomach most painful. There was no cough— perspiration was pouring over her body. I could not at once make out whether it was a case of pure asthma, especially as she never had it before. However, I made up my mind to give her *Blatta orientalis* IX trit., a grain dose every fifteen minutes, and watch the effect myself. Three doses of it were given without much change for the better. I left a few more doses to be repeated half hourly and promised to see her again within a couple of hours. On my return I found her in a much better condition, and she had taken only one of those powders I had left, and they were not repeated, as she felt better. Now I thought it must have been an attack of asthma, and I continued the medicine unhesitatingly. There was no aggravation at night, but on the next morning she was better, and the usual asthmatic cough began with slight expectoration. There was pain in the chest and head with each coughing fit. *Blatta orientalis* 3x trit., four to six doses, was continued for a few days, when she got well. Again in November she had a slight tendency to an asthmatic fit, took two or three doses of the same medicine and got well. Since then she had not been troubled again.

CASE VIII. A gentleman, the keeper of a common shop, aged forty-four, belonging to a village, had been suffering from asthma for the last eight years and had always been under treatment of native kabiraj (medical men). In June, he came to the city, and I was called to see him on the 14th of June, to treat him for his asthma. The day previous he had an attack, for which he took no medicine. Each of his attacks usually lasted four or five days. I gave him *Blatta orientalis* IX trit., one grain every two hours, and left him six such powders to be taken during the day. He took them and felt better the next day. He stayed here two or three days more, and when well he wanted to proceed home, which was some couple of hundred miles. He took with him two two-drachm phials of *Blatta orientalis*, one of IX and the other of 3x trit. He continued the 3x, one grain doses, two or three times daily, for a month, and discontinued afterward. He had no more asthmatic fits. In January last, 1891, I had a letter from him, thanking me for his recovery and asking for some of the same medicine for a friend of his, who had been suffering from asthma. The friend of his who used the same drug, *Blatta orientalis*, was equally benefited.

CASE IX. Mrs. Dalta, a thin lady, aged thirty-eight, mother of several children, had been exposed to cold, which brought on an attack of bronchitis with fever. This, in the course of a fortnight, developed into a regular fit of asthma. She was all this time treated by an old-school physician, but when the husband of the lady saw that she was daily getting worse, and a new disease crept in, he made up his mind to change the treatment. I was called to see her in the morning of the 8th of June, 1890. She became very much emaciated, could not take any food, had fever with acute bronchitis, hurried respiration, difficulty of breathing; this she was complaining of bitterly, owing to which she could not lie down in bed, but had to sit up day and night. There was a prolonged fit of spasmodic cough at short intervals, with slight expectoration, but these coughing fits would make her almost breathless. This was the first time I prescribed *Blatta orientalis* IX in a case of asthma with fever and acute bronchitis. It answered my purpose well. She had only ten powders during the day and passed a comparatively better night. Next morning when I saw her she was better, except the coughing fits, which were continuing as before. The same medicine was repeated. On the 10th of June she had no asthmatic trouble at night, but there was not much improvement in her cough—*Anti. tart.* and *Bryonia* were needed to complete the cure.

BOLETUS LARICIS.

NAT. ORD., Fungi.

COMMON NAMES, Larch Agaric, Larch Boletus, Purging Agaric, White Agaric.

PREPARATION.—The dried fungus is macerated in five parts by weight of alcohol.

(Here are two typical cases out of thirteen by Dr. W. H. Burt, which we find in the *North American Journal of Homœopathy*, 1866, quoted from th *Medical Investigator* from a volume not attainable.)

CASE 1. Intermittent fever: Type Quotidiana Duplex. In a large lymphatic woman; weight about 180 lbs.; aged thirty-nine. November 4th. For the last five weeks has had the ague. At first it was a simple quotidian. Took Quinine, which broke it for four days, when it returned; took Quinine in massive doses, which checked it for one week. It returned two weeks since, in the form of a double quotidian. The chill comes on every day at 10 A.M. and 5 P.M.

The chill lasts from one to two hours each time; hands and feet get icy cold, chills run up and down the spine, with severe pains in the head, back and limbs; followed by high fever for three hours, and then profuse sweat. Tongue furred whitish-yellow, with large fissures in the tongue; flat, bitter taste; has had no appetite for five weeks; craves cold water all the time; bowels rather costive; has nausea during every chill, but no vomiting; very weak, can only sit up about one hour in the morning; great depression of spirits, cries during the whole examination; face very much jaundiced. Treatment: *Ars.* 2, every two hours, for three days. It produced constant nausea and lessened the chills, but aggravated the fever. I then determined to try the *Boletus* 1st, two grs. every two hours. Took two doses when the chills came on, she then ceased to take the medicine until 5 P.M. Took three doses, and then fell asleep. 8th. Says she is feeling a little better, continued treatment; 10 A.M., commenced to have a severe diarrhœa, an effect of the medicine; discontinued the powders until 5 P.M. The fever did not come on until 3 P.M.; had no chill; fever lasted three hours; perspired profusely all night; slept well for the first time in a number of weeks. 9th. Feeling much better. Fever came on at 4 P.M., had no chill; fever lasted four hours; nausea all the evening; sweat all night. 10th. Feeling quite well. Had no more fever, but had night sweats for a week after. Convalescence was very slow; notwithstanding she had no more fever it was three weeks before she felt perfectly well.

This case demonstrates the fact to us that the *Boletus* is superior to our *greatest remedial* agents in the case of intermittents. I believe if I had not been acquainted with the therapeutic properties of the *Boletus* I would have been compelled to treat this lady every few weeks for two or three months with our usual remedies.

CASE 2. Intermittent fever: Type quotidian. November 1st, Mrs. B., aged fifty-six. Temperament, nervous. Three weeks since had an abscess in left ear, which made her quite sick for a week. Since then has had a fever every afternoon and night; feels chilly whenever she moves; walking produces nausea; does not perspire any; tongue coated white; loss of appetite; bowels loose; very restless at night, cannot sleep any; getting very weak, keeps her bed most of the time. Gave *Boletus laricis*. Had the fever but one day after.

CALCAREA RENALIS PRÆPARATA.

PREPARATION.—There are two kinds of renal calculi, the phosphatic and the uric, which should be triturated as separate preparations.

(The *Homœopathric Examiner*, 1846, contained the following paper, by Dr. Bredenoll. We may add that the remedy is reported to be peculiarly beneficial in Rigg's disease of the teeth.)

My professional engagements do not permit me to spend much time in writing; the following case, however, I deem worthy of note.

Born of healthy parents, I remained quite healthy until my twenty-third year. I had no trouble in getting over the diseases to which children are generally liable. Some of them, scarlet fever and measles, attacked me when I was already engaged in my professional career. I am now fifty-seven years old.

In the year 1808, while vaccinating children, I caught the itch from one of them. Although I washed myself with soap water immediately, yet a pustule made its appearance in about eight days, between the little finger and ring finger of the left hand; afterwards a few more came on at the same place and some others between the ring and middle finger. I hastened to repel this eruption as fast as possible, which I unfortunately succeeded in doing within the period of eight days.

This suppression of the eruption was followed by a host of diseases: Liability to catching cold; frequent catarrh; rheumatic complaints; toothache; attacks of hemicrania, with vomiting; continual heartburn; hæmorrhoidal complaints, at times tumors, at times fluent; excessive emaciation; afterwards a pustulous eruption over the whole body; painful swelling of the joints, arthritic nodosities in different places; a copper-colored eruption in the face, especially on and about the nose, which made me look like a confirmed drunkard, etc., etc.

These affections tormented me more or less, until in the year 1833 I visited Hahnemann at Coethen, for the purpose of studying homœopathia with him. Hahnemann treated me for three weeks, and I continued the treatment at my native place. My health improved steadily, and at the end of a year I considered myself cured. This lasted until October, 1836, when I was attacked with violent colic in one night. The pain was felt in the region of the left kidney, lancinating, pinching, sore; retching ensued, resulting in vomiting of mucus, and lastly bile. I took a few pellets of *Nux v.* x; after this the pain disappeared gradually, and the vomiting ceased. Next day I was well again. Two days afterwards I discovered gravel in the urine, and my sufferings had vanished.

One year elapsed in this way; however, I occasionally experienced an uncomfortable sensation in the region of the left kidney, especially when riding on horseback, driving in a carriage, or walking fast; I took at times *Lycopod.*, at times *Nux v.*, in proportion as one or the other of these two remedies appeared indicated.

In November, 1837, I was suddenly attacked with vomiting, accompanied with violent lancinating, sore or pinching pains in the region of the left kidney. The horrible anguish and pain which I experienced extorted from me involuntary screams; I was writhing like a worm in the dust. A calculus had descended into the ureter and had become incarcerated in it. Repeated doses of *Nux* relieved the incarceration, and I distinctly felt that the calculus was descending towards the bladder. After twenty-four hours of horrible suffering the vomiting ceased, the pain became duller and was felt in the region where the ureter dips into and becomes interwoven with the tissue of the bladder: it continued for three days and then disappeared all of a sudden (the stone had not got into the bladder). Thirty-six hours afterwards the calculus entered the bulb of the urethra. I felt a frequent desire to urinate; the urine was turbid and bloody, until at last a calculus of four grains made its appearance in the urine. After this I frequently passed gravel and calculi, at times with slight, at times violent pains, sometimes accompanied with vomiting; I kept the larger calculi, with a view of using them hereafter as a curative agent.

Professor Nasse, of Bonn, where my son studied medicine at the time, has analyzed the calculi, and has found them to be urate of lime. He advised me to take *Merc. dulcis* and the *Sulphate of Soda* for some time; it is scarcely necessary for me to say that I did not follow his advice.

On the fifteenth of February, 1839, I felt the precursory symptoms of a new attack, which really did break out in all its fury on the 16th, and continued on the 17th and 18th. I now caused 5 grains of my calculi to be triturated in my presence with 95 grains of sugar of milk, according to the fashion of Hahnemann, and took 1/2 grain in the evening of the 17th, another 1/2 grain in the morning of the 18th. On this day I passed very turbid urine with a considerable quantity of gravel; however, in the region where the ureter dips into the bladder, I experienced an uncomfortable sensation, but was well otherwise. On the 19th I was obliged to visit a patient at the distance of two miles; on my journey I felt that the calculus was descending into the bladder; the urine which I emitted shortly afterwards was very turbid and bloody. That same evening, after returning home, I felt the stone in the bulb of the urethra, and on the morning of the 20th it came off during stool, but unfortunately got lost among the excrement. To judge from my feeling it must have been larger than any of the preceding calculi, and also rougher, for its passage through the urethra was very painful and followed by an oozing out of blood.

The uncomfortable feeling in the region of the left kidney never disappeared completely; it became especially painful when pressing upon that place, when riding on horseback or in a carriage, when taking exercise or turning the body. It seems to me that the whole pelvis of the kidneys must have been full of gravel and calculi. I now took 1/2 grain at intervals of eight days; the result was that I passed gravel and small calculi at every micturition. On the 30th of November my condition got worse, and I continued to take 1/2 grain of *Calc. ren. præp.*, at longer or shorter intervals, until October 18th, 1840. After this period I ceased to pass any gravel, and I felt entirely well. On the 3d of February I passed some more gravel. Another dose of 1/2 grain of *Lapis renalis*; another dose on June 3d. On June 17th precursors of another attack; on the 18th vomiting accompanied by all the frightful circumstances which I have detailed above; the vomiting of mucus, bile, ingesta, continued at short intervals until the 26th; my tongue was coated with yellow mucus, and my appetite had completely disappeared. *Bryon., Nux v.* and *Pulsat.* relieved the gastric symptom; on the 26th, in the afternoon, I passed a calculus of the size of a pea. I now resume the use of *Calc. ren. præp.* in 1/2 grain doses, at irregular intervals. On the 23d of October I passed a calculus of the size of a pea, without vomiting; there were no other precursory symptoms except the uncomfortable feeling in the region of the kidney a few days previous. I have felt well ever since and free from all complaint, although I continue the occasional use of 1/2 a grain of *Calc. ren. præp.*, lest I should have a relapse.

Every time I took a dose of *Calc. ren. pr.* I found that the so-called tartar on the teeth became detached a few days afterwards. A short while ago a nodosity, hard as a stone, which had appeared on the extensor tendon of the right middle finger, about nine months ago, and which threatened to increase more and more, disappeared. I consider the tartar on the teeth, calculi renales and arthritic nodosities very similar morbid products.

In conclusion I beg leave to offer the following remarks:

1. Hahnemann's theory of psora is no chimera, as many theoreticians would have us believe. I was perfectly healthy previous to my being infected with itch. What a host of sufferings have I been obliged to endure after the suppression of the itch!

2. Isopathy deserves especial notice.

It is true, the most suitable homœopathic remedies afforded me relief; the incarceration of calculi in the ureter especially was relieved by *Nux*; but they were unable to put a stop to the formation of calculi; this result was only attained by the preparation of *Calc. ren.*

CEANOTHUS AMERICANUS.

NAT. ORD., Rhamnaceæ.
COMMON NAMES, New Jersey Tea. Red Root. Wild Snowball.
PREPARATION.—The fresh leaves are pounded to a pulp and macerated in two parts by weight of alcohol.

(The following by Dr. Majumdar in *Indian Homœpathic Review*, 1897, illustrates the chief use of this "organ remedy.")

Recently I had a wonderful case of supposed heart disease cured by *Ceanothus*. I am indebted to my friend, Dr. Burnett, for the suggestion of using *Ceanothus*.

A thin and haggard looking young man presented himself to my office on the 26th of July, 1896. He told me he had some disease of the heart and had been under the treatment of several eminent allopathic physicians of this city; some declared it to be a case of hypertrophy of the heart and some of valvular disease.

Without asking him further, I examined his heart thoroughly, but with no particular results. The rhythm and sounds were all normal only there was a degree of weakness in these sounds. Dulness on percussion was not extended beyond its usual limit. So I could not make out any heart disease in this man.

On further inquiry, I learned that the man remained in a most malarious place for five years, during which he had been suffering off and on from intermittent fever. I percussed the abdomen and found an enormously enlarged and indurated spleen, reaching beyond the navel and pushing up the thoracic viscera.

The patient complained of palpitation of heart, dyspnœa, especially on ascending steps and walking fast. I thought from these symptoms his former medical advisers concluded heart disease. In my mind they seemed to be resulted from enlarged spleen.

On that very day I gave him six powders of *Ceonothus Amer.* 3x, one dose morning and evening. I asked him to see me when his medicine finished. He did not make his appearance, however, on the appointed day. I thought the result of my prescription was not promising. After a week he came and reported unusually good results.

His dyspnœa was gone, palpitation troubled him now and then, but much less than before. He wanted me to give him the same powders. I gave him *Sac. lac.*, six doses, in the usual way.

Reported further improvement; the same powders of *Sac. lac.* twice. To my astonishment I found the spleen much reduced in size and softened than before; I knew nothing about this patient for some time. Only recently I saw him, a perfect picture of sound health. He informed me that the same powders were sufficient to set him right. He gained health; no sign of enlarged spleen left.

CEPHALANTHUS OCCIDENTALIS.

NAT. ORD., Rubiaceæ.
COMMON NAMES, Button Bush, Crane Willow.
PREPARATION.—The fresh bark of branches and roots is pounded to a pulp and macerated in two parts by weight of alcohol.

(The item given below was contributed to the *American Observer*, 1875, by Dr. E. D. Wright.)

Proving—one-half ounce in a day.

First day—raw, sore throat; nervous, excited; felt light and easy, happy; bowels constipated.

Second day—the same dose. Hard dreams about fighting, quarreling; restless and tossing over; joints of the fingers lame; griping pains in the lungs(?); in body and limbs, especially in the joints; toothache; bowels loose, stool offensive; almost affected by the piles.

CURES.—Intermittent fever, quotidian and tertian fever; sore throat, quinsy—had very good effect.

Rheumatic fevers, with soreness of the flesh.

A teamster fell in the river. Cold, and inflammatory fever was cured quickly.

CEREUS BONPLANDII.

NAT. ORD., Cactacæ.
COMMON NAME, A variety of the night blooming cereus group.
PREPARATION.—The fresh green stems are pounded to a pulp and macerated in two parts by weight of alcohol.

(This paper, which we take from the *Homœopathic Physician*, 1892, was prepared by Dr. J. H. Flitch, of New Scotland, N. Y., the original prover. The proving is also found in the *Encyclopædia*, Allen's.)

Mind and Disposition.—An agreeable and tranquil state and frame of mind and body (first day, evening).

Mind perfectly composed.

Feel better when engaged at something or occupied.

Desire to be at useful work, desire to be busy (second day).

Desire to be employed.

Praying or disposition to be at prayer.

Ill at ease.

Rest (third day).

Doesn't know what to do with one's self.

Feels a strong desire to give away something very necessary for him to keep or have.

Feeling irritable (on rising).

Cannot keep himself employed at anything.

Very much disturbed in mind.

Passes the time in useless occupation (fourth day).

Very irritable; acts impulsively.

Spends the whole forenoon uselessly.

Difficulty in becoming devotional (at church).

Finds it easy to become devotional.

Feels well late in the evening (seventh day).

Thinks he is under a powerful influence.

Sensorium.—Vertigo followed by nausea.

Swimming of the head (sixth day).

Head.—Decidedly painful drawing sensation in the occiput, soon subsiding (first day).

Painful stunning feeling in the right frontal bone.

Pressive pain from without inward in the occiput high up on walking.

Slight painful pressure in the right occiput from behind forward (second day).

Disagreeable feeling in occiput, running down over the neck, followed by a slight qualmishness.

Slight heavy feeling in the top of the forehead.

Headache occipital, continued for a quarter of an hour.

Sensation, as if something hard like a board were bound against the back of the head, felt more especially on left side.

Head feels drawn to the left backward.

Pain in occiput running through lobes of the cerebrum.

Pain running from left ear through the head to right ear and right parietal bone.

Pain commencing in the medulla oblongata and running upward and expanding to the surface of the brain, worse on stooping or bending forward.

Pain along right external angular process of frontal bone.

Pain through or across the brain from left to right.

Feeling as of being pressed at left occiput and immediately thereafter a counter pain in left frontal bone, the latter continuing a minute or two.

Pain from left occiput verging around left parietal bone.

Pain through occiput.

Pain in right forehead (third day).

Pain in anterior portion of brain and extending in a backward direction.

Tenderness at the point of exit of the left supra-orbital nerve.

Pain in occiput (high up).

Occipital pain (fifth day).

Bad feeling, head (third day).

Eyes.—Pain over right eye, passing down over globe (first day).

Nauseated feeling commencing in throat, passing to stomach simultaneous with a congested feeling in both eyes.

Pain in orbits, running from before backward.

Pain in left eyelids when stooping low (second day).

On closing the eyes perception of a cluster of round-shaped, symmetrical, orange-colored spots.

Swimming eyes.

Capillary congestion of the conjunctiva.

Severe photophobia, producing a sticking pain through eyes.

Sore feeling through eyes as if exposed to strong sunlight.

Pain through globe of right eye.

Pain in the globe of left eye.

Nose.—Greenish (pale) mucus discharged from nostril.

Accumulation of mucus in nose as in nasal catarrh.

Stinging in nose, more especially right side.

Stinging in right nostril.

Sneezing.

Hardened mucus in left nostril.

Face.—Pain along right malar bone running to temple.

Looks haggard.

Yellowish face or countenance.

Mouth, etc.—Saliva in mouth when swallowed of no unpleasant taste (first day).

Feeling of coldness in the mouth (second day).

Feeling as of having eaten something tasting alkaline.

Water in the mouth.

Metallic taste in the mouth.

Watery saliva in the mouth (not disagreeable).

Slight metallic taste, feels as if having eaten something of a metallic taste.

Taste of green vegetables.

Watery taste.

Sensation as of a thread of mucus on the tongue.

Insipid, watery taste (third day).

Fetid breath (noticed by myself) (fourth day).

Fetid breath (noticed by others) (fifth day).

Tongue looks frothy (sixth day).

Tongue of a purplish red hue.

Tongue feels rough.

Throat.—Mucus adherent to the hard palate easily removed (first day).

Mucus in pharynx easily detached (second day).

Mucus in larynx easily detached.

Scraping of mucus, which seems to adhere to left side of pharynx.

Persistent accumulation of mucus in the pharynx, continually and recurring in considerable quantities and of a pale-green color.

Mucus easily expectorated or cleared from the throat.

Clearing of the hard palate of mucus.

Stomach, Appetite, etc.—Dry eructations (second day).

Thirstlessness.

Appetite diminished; ate very light breakfast (third day).

Relish of sweet things.

Abdomen, Stool, etc.—Slight rumbling in bowels, left side (first day).

Nearly or quite inefficient effort to evacuate bowels.

Fetid flatus passed from bowels.

Slight pain in epigastrium, coming and going at intervals of a few minutes.

Slightly painful sensation in epigastrium (second day).

Passed stool not easy, not sufficient at 6 A.M. (third day).

Natural stool at 6 A.M. (sixth day).

Urine and Urinary Organs.—Inclination to pass urine (first day).

Urine of a slightly brownish tinge (second day).

Urine smells strongly after a few minutes.

Yellowish urine.

Urine less than half usual quantity.

Urine normal.

Urine clear, small in quantity.

Urination frequent (at 4 P.M.) (second day).

Amelioration after urination.

Passed a small quantity saturated yellowish urine.

Sexual.—Slight increase of sexual desire.

Anæsthesia and dwindling of the sexual organs.

Kidneys.—Slight pain of a sticking character in right kidney (second day).

Pain in left kidney, long continued, as from the presence of a renal calculus.

Pain in left abdomen sharp and cutting, as from a calculus impacted in the ureter.

Slight pain in right kidney repeated after an interval (third day).

Sticking pain in right ureter.

More severe sticking pain in right kidney.

Soreness on external pressure over right kidney.

Pain on stooping, bending over in right kidney.

Pain in left kidney (fifth day).

Chest, Heart, etc.—Deep inspiration as if tired, although experiencing no fatigue whatever (second day).

Feels as if pained or oppressed at chest.

Slightly painful sensation at left chest, region of the heart.

Deep inspiration.

At intervals deep inspiration, as if the chest were laboring under an oppression hardly definable.

Slight feeling of oppression, or a weakness in the chest with the deep inspiration.

Tendency to expand the chest automatically and rhythmically, recurring very frequently.

The chest expands itself to its utmost capacity, seemingly, and in an instant collapses, the same process to be repeated.

Respiration measured, no interval between inspiration and expiration.

Sensation of uneasiness extending to lumbar region on deep inspiration (described above).

Slight pricking sensation of pain in the heart.

Sighing respiration (very frequent) (fourth day).

Tenderness of the anterior lower left intercostal muscles below the heart (third day).

Pain in chest and through heart, with pain running toward spleen, the latter momentarily, the former (heart pain) continuing.

Pain in left great pectoral muscle, worse toward the tendon.

Sighing respiration, noticed many times (fifth day).

Coughing on throwing off outer garments.

Somewhat persistent pains in the cartilages of the left lower ribs.

Long, deep, uneasy respiration, felt more acutely (sixth day).

The chest acts automatically, not according to will or whim.

Chest feels empty.

Pain at heart.

Pulse dicrotic, and several intermissions noticed within a minute (after rising 6 A.M.).

Deep inspiration and expiration, chest is emptied quickly.

Sensation as of a great stone laid upon the heart.

Sensation (soon after) as if the thoracic wall anterior to heart were broken out or torn away.

Pulse sharp.

Desire to remove clothing from chest.

Pain in chest and both arms.

Neck, Back, etc.—Painful sensation in the sides of the neck, left, at mastoid or below it, continuing longer than on right side.

Pain in left neck behind mastoid process, running backward and upward.

Pain through right shoulder blade (scapula).

Dorsal vertebræ feel painful (third day).

Tenderness along spines of cervical and upper dorsal vertebræ (fourth day).

Pain in muscles of thorax midway between scapula and sacrum (sixth day).

Pain on pressure of muscle of left side of the neck.

Back lame on stooping.

Pain in right scapula.

Pain in neck.

Pain in left side above and along clavicle.

Fatigue in lumbar region on riding.

Upper extremities.—Tired feeling in both arms (second day).

Drawing pain in index finger of both hands.

Pain in both upper arms.

Pain running across inner side of left arm, felt longest at bend of the elbow.

Pain in left shoulder like that produced by carrying a heavy load.

Pain running along the back down to the arms.

Dull pain in left elbow and forearm.

Pain with numbness in left forearm, ulnar side (third day).

Pain along inner side of right upper arm.

Pain with numbness of right arm while writing.

Pain in metacarpal bone of right thumb.

Pain (very noticeable) in metacarpal phalangeal joint of right hand.

Lameness in right forearm above wrist.

Drawing from end of right thumb upward, pain quite constant.

Considerable soreness on contact of anterior muscles of right arm.

Pain on ulnar side of left carpo-metacarpal joint (fourth day).

Pain in external border of left elbow joint.

Pain at and back of left shoulder joint.

Lameness of left little finger.

Pain over ulna posteriorly.

Pain above wrist.

Tenderness of the flexor muscles of both upper arms.

Pain in right ring finger at 3 P.M. and repeated (fifth day).

Pain at junction of second and third phalanx (last joint) of left index finger.

Pain in dorsum of right hand.

Pain in left forearm.

Pain in both arms and chest.

Pain in third phalanx of left index finger.

Pain in right little finger running through bone.

Pain in right ring finger.

Pain in right wrist.

Pain in first and second metacarpal bones (sixth day) of right hand.

Pain in the dorsum of left hand.

Pain in left little finger.

Pain on back of left wrist, running to forearm.

Pain in the anterior muscles of upper arm.

Lower Extremities.—Pain in right knee (second day).

Pain through right hip (fifth day).

Pain in right great trochanter.

Pain on the inner side of left knee (repeated).

Pain on left knee, inner and lower border.

Pain in both knees.

Pain in both knees on rising.

Pain in hamstring tendons of left thigh.

Pain in right hip (sixth day).

Pain in head of the right thigh bone.

Pain in right patella, very sore, difficult to touch without very considerable pain.

Pain above right external malleolus.

Pressing or pressive feeling, beginning at the sacrum and running down through both thighs down to feet.

Pain in different joints of the lower extremities.

Skin.—Itching of the nose (second day).

Itching on various parts of the body (general itching) (third day).

Itching pustule of face near ala of nose.

Itching of the right popliteal space, with roughness of the skin (fifth day).

Profuse shedding of the hair on combing the head.

Itching with roughness of the skin of a spot a few inches square above the left knee.

Itching of a spot a few inches below left scapula, with a condition of the skin like eczema periodically.

Sleep. Not sleeping late at night.

Not sleeping at 11 P.M., mind disturbed (fourth day).

Dreamed of dogs (fifth day).

Dream of a fracas which caused great excitement in the dreamer.

Drowsiness at 11 P.M. (sixth day).

Drowsiness (third day).

Slept pretty well (fifth day).

Awakes at 5 A.M. (sixth day).

Awakes at 9 A.M. (seventh day, Sunday).

Recurrence of old dreams of years ago.

Yawning (second day).

Generalities.—Feeling miserably on retiring.

Throws himself on bed without undressing.

Great yawning fit (third day).

Feels not pleasant.

Feels half sick.

Very dull in the morning, all morning.

Feels very badly, has an ill-defined bad feeling in the evening and at night.

Easily chilled in a room; better on disrobing for bed.

Alternations of symptoms of mind and bodily pains. When pains of the body are noticed, symptoms affecting the mind are suspended. The mind loses its characteristics, is clear, and one feels better.

REMARKS.—In looking over the above proving we find a number of illustrations of the alternate action of the drug. But perhaps what strikes the reader most forcibly is the way the symptoms follow Reuter's series. The most prominent symptoms early developed, catarrhal and gastric, have come and gone within three or four days, while those affecting the chest, heart, sensorium, eyes, brain, and nerves are more slowly developed, and are the ones that persist. Another thing to be noticed is the long duration of its action. The high-water mark in regard to its action was not reached (I mean its action on the nervous system) until nearly ten days after discontinuing to take it. It is an *antipsoric* of remarkable power. Some skin symptoms developed by it persisted off and on for years, two or three of which I will mention. "Itching of the right popliteal space," this after continuing for eight or nine years disappeared. I think some *Sepia* π I took had something to do with its disappearance. Another: "Itching with roughness of the skin, like eczema, above the left knee anteriorly." This still persists. I still have "Itching, with an eruption resembling at times herpes zoster below the left scapula." This is still present, although annoying. I have done nothing to cause its disappearance.

In regard to *verifications* I could report a goodly number. One of the first I ever had was a case of eczema of both hands, extending as far as the elbows. Cured in six weeks. The provings point in the direction of kidney troubles, and I have seen it speedily cause the disappearance of deposits in the urine that were giving much inconvenience. In a case of dropsy of cardiac and renal origin (albuminuria) in which there was great œdema, cured in two or three weeks. Sleeplessness, peculiar in its nature, corresponding to the proving, is relieved by it. Intercostal neuralgia, especially on left side. Anterior crural neuralgia, an aggravated case, promptly relieved. I need not say that the symptoms strongly point to rheumatism. I could say much on that part of the subject, and there is the sphere in which it has seemed to have been useful by the professional friend to whom I have furnished the medicine for trial. In a monograph by Dr. R. E. Kunge, of New York, and the writer, I ventured the prediction that *Cereus bonplandii* would prove of value in the treatment of insanity. I send you the report of two cases. I have one other still under treatment. A patient for fourteen years in the Middletown Insane Hospital, improving, called to see Ida Reamer, a young woman of eighteen, living in New Scotland, on what is called the Heldeberg Mountain or hill, on the evening of April 19th, 1884. For some time previously she had been living with a relative in Albany, attending school and assisting in household labor. Had studied hard and probably overtaxed her strength. Her friends noticing that she was not her former self, and that though usually amiable and cheerful, she had become gloomy and taciturn, brought her home. Rest did her no good, and I was called after she had been home for some time. On my visit I noticed she would not answer questions; was wandering aimlessly about the house; could not sit still, if seated, more than a few minutes. During my visit I think she changed her position a dozen or fifteen times. She would go to the water pail and get a drink, then in a minute or two would get up and go to the door. After standing a minute or two she would come in and sit down, only to rise up and repeat her restless wanderings. I could elicit nothing from the mother of anything wrong in regard to the menstrual function. Prescribed *Cereus bonplandii*, fourth decimal. Did not call again, but was informed by her friend that she soon regained her health. Was requested to call again to see Ida R. on November 29th of the same year. This time there was considerable mental disturbance; she had attended some entertainment which she had considered of a questionable nature, and had been worrying over it. Although living out at service, it did not appear that she had overworked. I found her sitting still; she would sit for hours. If any one disturbed her, she would curse, swear, throw boots and shoes or anything that came in her way, resisted attempts made by her friends to remove her to her home. Prescribed *Cer. bon.* 4. Saw her December 3d, 7th, 10th, at the end of which time she was entirely free from any mental manifestations, and although under observation has never experienced a return of them to the present date.

In the summer of 1879 was consulted in the case of Mrs. D. V., afflicted with melancholia for a year or two. The disease had appeared just subsequent to her confinement with her last child. Prescribed wholesome advice in regard to mode of life, etc., and very little medicine. In a few months she was apparently as well as ever. June 5th, 1884, was called to see Mrs. D. V. She had quite recently given birth to a child and was developing delusions, most of which were those of a spiritual nature. She thought she had committed the unpardonable sin, or that she had offended some of her friends, and was constantly worrying. Appetite very poor. Prescribed *Cer. bon.* 4, gave her nourishing diet with Maltine and Pepsin to aid digestion. On July 11th she was about the house attending to her household duties.

CHEIRANTHUS CHEIRI.

NAT. ORD., Cruciferæ.
COMMON NAME, Wall flower.
PREPARATION.—The fresh plant is pounded to a pulp and macerated in two parts by weight of alcohol.

(Dr. Robert T. Cooper, of London, contributed the following to the *Hahnemannian Monthly*, 1897):

A tincture is used made from a single dark-flowered plant. No proving of this remedy has come under my notice, yet I consider the following case worth reporting: T. T., age twenty, a clerk; admission date, 30th April, 1892; never heard well on the left side, but particularly deaf the last month, and deafness increases; watch, hearing contact only. History of much earache in childhood; left ear discharges, but the discharge does not run out. Wisdom teeth; left upper and right, lower and upper, breaking through. Gave *Cheiranthus cheiri*.

28th May, hears very much better; left, 3-1/2 inches. No medicine.

11th June, continues improving gradually; left, 15 inches.

25th June, continues to hear voices very fairly on the left side, but no improvement since last time; left, 15 inches. Gave *Cheiranthus cheiri*.

25th July, restoration of improving condition; left, 20 inches. No medicine.

CHIONANTHUS VIRGINICA.

NAT. ORD., Oleaceæ.
COMMON NAME, Fringe Tree. Snow-flower.
PREPARATION.—The fresh bark is pounded to a pulp and macerated in two parts by weight of alcohol.

(The following is the only proving, we believe, ever made of this drug; it was the thesis of Dr. John W. Lawshé, Atlanta, Ga., on his graduation, and was published in *North American Journal of Homœopathy*, May, 1883).

This being the first and only proving of this drug, Prof. Lilienthal requested a copy of it for publication, which I cheerfully agreed to give him.

Monday, July 10, 1882, 9:30 A.M., I took one drop of the tincture, after having taken the 12x and 6x potencies, one day each, without any effect. I continued taking the tincture each hour during the day, increasing each dose one drop till five were reached, then increased each dose five drops till twenty-five were reached, but without any effect whatever.

Tuesday, July 11th, I began with thirty drops at 9 o'clock A.M., and increased the dose five drops each hour till I reached one drachm, and took three doses of one drachm each. I retired at 10 o'clock feeling perfectly well.

I awoke at 4:10 A.M., Wednesday, July 12th, with a severe headache—chiefly in the forehead and just over the eyes—especially the left eye. Eyeballs exceedingly painful, feel sore and bruised.

Cutting twisting pains all through my abdomen.

I turned over and lay with my face downward, which seemed to relieve the abdominal pains some, and after awhile I went to sleep. I awoke again at 8:20 feeling very sick and badly all over. Head feels very sore all over and through it; heavy dull feeling in forehead and a drawing or pressing at the root of my nose. I felt so weak I had to sit down awhile before I could finish dressing; *never* before felt so sick at my stomach. Bitter eructations, great nausea and retching, with a desire for stool.

I finished dressing and looked at my tongue, which was heavily coated and of a dirty, greenish yellow color. I started down stairs and had a violent attack of nausea and a great deal of retching before I could vomit. It seemed as though there were a "*double suction*" in my abdomen, one trying to force something up and the other sucking it back, till finally, by quite an effort, I vomited a teacup full, or more, of *very dark green* bile, rather ropy, *I think*, and exceedingly bitter. The bile came up with a single gush and I was through. Immediately a cold perspiration broke out and stood in beads on my forehead, and I felt very weak. Desire for stool gone after vomiting.

I have a sore, weak, bruised feeling all over the small of my back; feels very weak when standing or moving about; better sitting or lying down.

No appetite for breakfast, but my stomach felt so weak and empty that I drank a cup of coffee and ate half a biscuit, which relieved to some extent.

9 A.M., am so nervous I cannot keep still and can hardly write down my symptoms.

9:30 o'clock, my back in lumbar and sacral region is so sore and weak I could hardly walk from the car to the office, every step seemed to jar my whole body and made my headache worse.

10 o'clock, have been quiet for half an hour and feel some better; have a pressing or squeezing sensation in the bridge of my nose; sore constricted feeling in the temples, with throbbing temporal arteries.

10:30 o'clock, just came from stool; the first passed was watery, but the last was more solid in appearance; stool terribly offensive, like *carrion*. Heavy, all-gone sort of feeling low down in hypogastrium; color of stool was dark brown with pieces of undigested food in it.

11:30, just got home and feel very bad and weak. My head and back ache considerably, and I feel "played out" generally.

12 o'clock, forehead and cheeks *very* hot and dry, radial pulse 114, chilly sensation darting through body from front to back, causing a sort of shivering or involuntary jerking, forehead feels like a hot coal of fire to my hand; headache in forehead and over eyes relieved by pressing with my hand, but I cannot bear it long for my head seems to get hotter from it; am exceedingly nervous, cannot lie still, involuntary jerkings in different parts of the body. Roof of mouth and tongue feel very dry, although there seems to be the usual amount of saliva present. No thirst at all.

I went to sleep about 12:20 P.M., and was awakened at 2 o'clock for dinner. Couldn't eat anything; I tried but it nauseated me; could only drink a cup of coffee; headache worse after waking; pulse 88; head not quite so hot, body feels chilly, and I had a shawl thrown over me; went to sleep again about 3:30.

I was told that at 4:15 my face and head were covered with a profuse perspiration, and my carotid arteries pulsated very hard and rapidly; I got up at 5 o'clock and bathed my face in cold water and felt somewhat better, though my head and back still ache considerably and feel quite sore; eyeballs feel bruised.

6:30. Weak, empty feeling about stomach, which was relieved for awhile by eating some crackers and drinking a cup of coffee. Pulse still 88.

At 8:15 had an action from my bowels; during stool griping and cutting pains in abdomen, about and below umbilicus; stool thin, watery, blackish-brown color and very offensive. I retired at 9:30 and had to have an extra covering thrown upon me, I was so chilly, while my room-mate lay without any covering at all. My head feels sore and bruised all over, and the small of my back is exceedingly weak and feels, when I touch it with my hand, as though the skin were all off.

Thursday, July 13th. I was very nervous and restless last night after going to bed; didn't go to sleep till after 12 o'clock, and woke up several times before daylight with pains in my head, abdomen and back. Got up at 8 o'clock. My head feels sore and bruised; the bruised feeling seems to go into my brain now; every time I move, cough or laugh it seems as if my head would split open and fly in every direction; my *back* is not so painful this morning; I couldn't eat much breakfast; stool this morning was quite copious, watery, *dark* brown and not so offensive as yesterday.

9:30. Headache better; several times this morning I have had attacks of cutting or griping pains in my intestines, in and about the umbilical region; my tongue is very heavily coated in the centre with a thick yellowish fur; the tip is slightly red, and on each side of the tip there are several little places that look as though blood was about to ooze forth from them; my tongue feels drawn and shriveled up the centre.

4:30. The only symptom at 11 o'clock was a dull, sore, aching feeling in the umbilical and iliac regions, occasionally changing for just a minute or so to a severe griping, which was relieved some by emission of flatus. My face has a yellowish appearance; from the outer to the inner canthus there is a reddish-yellow streak, about one-quarter of an inch wide, in the whites of both eyes; the blood vessels of the sclerotic coat are very much enlarged and distinctly visible.

Friday, July 14th. I suffered considerably after 5 o'clock yesterday afternoon and last night with pains in my abdomen, and they are more severe this morning than yesterday; it feels just like a string tied in a "slip knot" around my intestines in the umbilical region, and every once in awhile it was *suddenly* drawn tight for a minute or so, and then *gradually* loosened; stool this morning was very thin, watery and rather flaky; the flaky portion was dark yellow, the fluid portion *dark* green, with a *light* green foam or froth on top, streaked with a white, mucus-looking substance;

flatus and fæces passed together; some pain in my bowels during stool, and a hot, scalded sensation in anus, which lasted fifteen or twenty minutes after stool; during stool a cold perspiration broke out on my forehead and back of my hands; took quite a while to pass stool, and then only a small quantity passed; eyeballs feel bruised and the whites have a yellowish cast all over, though the "bands" are still very distinct; my skin is quite yellow to-day and I feel very much fatigued generally.

Saturday, July 15th. Stool about natural this morning; some feeling in my abdomen, though not so severe; no new symptoms.

Sunday, July 16th. The only thing unusual which I noticed to-day was the passage of considerable offensive flatus; a greater quantity after retiring than during the day.

I noticed no more symptoms after Sunday night.

(The following is from a letter of Dr. E. M. Hale):

Some time ago I received a letter from Dr. F. S. Smith, of Lock Haven, Pa., in which, referring to *Chionanthus*, he says:

"For the first time to-day I read your article on *Chionanthus* in the last edition of your Materia Medica of 'New Remedies.' I have been using this drug for over two years, as a specific for so-called sick headache. It has done wonders for me in that disease. I had been a victim from early childhood, and have suffered terribly. I have not had an attack for two years. If I am threatened, a few drops, timely taken, dissipates it at once.

"Dr. B., a dentist, aged 35, dark complexion, a victim to sick headache, had an attack on an average once in three weeks. Since taking *Chionanthus*, has not had more than two or three attacks in over two years, and then owing to a neglect to take the medicine. I have failed in but one case, and that was a menstrual sick headache.

"I prescribe it as follows: In cases of habitual sick headache, 5 gtts. of the 2x dil. three times a day for a week, then twice a day for a week, then once a day for a week, after which the patient only takes it when symptoms of the attack show themselves. I regard it almost a specific."

(*Chionanthus* is also, by some physicians, regarded as a specific in jaundice, either acute or chronic, and the proving seems to justify the belief.)

CORNUS ALTERNIFOLIA.

NAT. ORD., Cornaceæ.

COMMON NAME, Alternate-leaved Cornel or Dogwood. Swamp-walnut.

PREPARATION.—The fresh bark and young twigs are pounded to a pulp and macerated in two parts by weight of alcohol.

(The following proving of this remedy was made under the supervision of Dr. F. H. Lutze, Brooklyn. The *Cornus alternifolia*, or "swamp walnut," has a reputation among the people in certain localities as being a "sure" remedy for "salt rheum.")

FIRST PROVING BY R. E. ALBERTSON.

Commence at bedtime Tuesday, May 12, 1896.

Wednesday, May 13, 1896.—Awoke this morning after a very refreshing night's sleep, feeling as well as usual; and did not notice anything out of the ordinary during the entire day. Had stool, but somewhat scanty. Appetite fair.

Thursday, May 14, 1896.—Did not rest very well during night. Had dream I was spending summer in country. Did not get into anything like a sound sleep until near morning; and then was very reluctant about getting up; would have preferred to have had a couple hours more of such sleep. I have noticed nothing in the course of the day worthy of mention excepting a pain across the small of the back, which lasted only a short time and then disappeared. Stool to-day little better than yesterday.

Friday, May 15, 1896.—Another restless night; would get into a light sleep off and on until near morning. Dreamed again; this time of an exciting fire drill. Up to to-day had been taking *Cornus alternifolia* thrice daily; 3 drops 30th, commencing with this morning every three hours. Stool to-day at first hard and difficult, then loose. Nothing further noticed to-day.

Saturday, May 16, 1896.—Passed a very restless and sleepless night; guess I was awake at the striking of every hour. Tongue has been coated a yellowish white for a couple of days. Stool to-day, but scanty. Feel as well as usual, but don't seem to have the ambition to do anything for any length of time.

Sunday, May 17, 1896.—Experienced another very restless and sleepless night. Felt an aching in left shoulder and dull pain across forehead, more particularly on right side. Stool to-day and appetite fair.

Monday, May 18, 1896.—While I passed another restless night, it was not as bad as nights previous. Seem to hear every little noise and sound. When once awake, mind becomes active and then it is difficult to get into a sleep again. Have dreamed something mostly every night; some of which I do not remember.

Tuesday, May 19, 1896.—Rested somewhat better last night; though was awake off and on. Last dose taken at bedtime.

Wednesday, May 20, 1896.—Experienced another restless night; was awake most of the night until about 3 A.M., when I dropped off into a sleep.

Friday, May 22, 1896.—Noticed a little sore inside of mouth (left side), which by Saturday, Sunday, Monday and Tuesday had become very annoying. When eating anything that came in contact with it, or even when moving the mouth in a certain direction would cause a sticking, pricking pain. I also want to mention a few eruptions, small pustules on face and neck, which appeared during this proving.

SECOND PROVING OF "CORNUS ALTERNIFOLIA."

BY F. H. LUTZE, M. D.

February 1, 1896.—Took 5 drops of θ three times daily.

February 6, 1896.—Took 5 drops of θ every two hours. On second day had two loose evacuations in quick succession in the afternoon.

February 9, 1896.—A cold feeling in chest as if it were filled with cold air or ice; this continued for two days and was very disagreeable, but seemed to have no influence on action of heart or respiration.

A second proving, commenced on April 1st, reproduced the same symptoms in same manner. Have made no proving of 30th yet.

THIRD PROVING OF "CORNUS ALTERNIFOLIA" 30TH DILUTION.

Commenced at bedtime Sunday, June 7, 1896.

Monday, June 8, 1896.—Awoke after being awake the greater part of the night feeling as usual. Felt dull pain in right side region of liver about 11 A.M.

Tuesday, June 9, 1896.—Slept very little; tossed and turned mostly all night; could not get into any comfortable position. Tongue this morning coated a yellowish white. No stool to-day and appetite fair.

Wednesday, June 10, 1896.—While I rested somewhat better than nights previous, yet was awake considerable part of the night. Had two dreams;

one of dead rats mashed to a pulp; the other of coition, causing an emission. When I awoke this morning, felt a raw feeling in throat, which continued throughout the day; though not quite as bad as when I arose. Sneezed some, too, to-day; head partially stopped up toward night. About an hour or two after dinner, which I ate with a relish, a sick sensation came over me, a dull heavy feeling in forehead accompanied with a nauseous and dizzy feeling; could hardly pull one foot after the other on my way home from work; but after being a little while in the open air and walking, feeling subsided some, and when I reached home felt much better; and after supper had entirely left me; though when I retired that night I felt as though I had been doing a very hard day's work and was glad when my body touched the bed. Stool very scanty to-day; appears difficult to do anything; seems to be quite some gas.

Thursday, June 11, 1896.—Awoke very tired; sleep disturbed considerably; could not rest in any position. Raw feeling in throat still this morning, with a frequent desire to clear; a feeling as though something lodged there and should come out. Stool to-day, but scant. A dull ache in region of heart felt in afternoon. Feel tired and drowsy. All ambition seems to have left me. Appetite very good to-day.

Friday, June 12, 1896.—Feel very well this morning and slept fairly well during the night, though was awake a few times. To-day marks the first appearance of eruptions; one on the right wrist, the other on right side of chin; small pustules; in one case blind, all others forming pus.

Saturday, June 13, 1896.—Experienced another restless night. Another pustule has appeared on chin and also ringworm on forehead (right side); feel very well to-day.

Sunday, June 14, 1896.—Slept fairly well during night. Experienced nothing particular excepting toward night an awful uneasy feeling came over me; a feeling that something terrible was going to happen.

Monday, June 16, 1896.—Awoke very tired this morning; have a cough, with a feeling as though something heavy was lying upon my chest and throat.

Wednesday, June 17, 1896.—Slept pretty well during night; feel very languid and tired; a feeling as though my legs were unable to bear me up.

Sunday, June 28, 1896.—Toward evening felt very tired and drowsy with heavy sensation in head; about 9:30 lay down upon the lounge and dropped off into a doze; awoke a half hour afterwards with a feeling as though I wanted to vomit, and chills, which continued for an hour when I vomited, which seemed to relieve me some, after which fever took the place of the chill which abated some toward morning.

Monday, June 29, 1896.—Managed to get to my business, but was unable to do anything all day on account of the weak feeling and a violent pressing headache in forehead, which continued all day; worse on motion and on stooping felt as though everything would come out. About 5 P.M. diarrhœa set in which continued all night, every half hour to an hour, the same the day following and continued right up to Sunday night, July 5th. Lost in that time six pounds.

CRATÆGUS OXYACANTHA.

NAT. ORD., Pomaceæ.
COMMON NAME, White or May Thorn. English Hawthorn.
PREPARATION.—The fresh berries are pounded to a pulp and macerated in two times their weight of alcohol.

(The *The New York Medical Journal*, October 10, 1896, published a communication from Dr. M. C. Jennings, under the heading "Cratægus Oxyacantha in the treatment of Heart Disease," of which the following is the substance):

Dr. Green, of Ennis, Ireland, for many years had a reputation for the cure of heart disease that caused patients to flock to him from all parts of the United Kingdom. He cured the most of them and amassed considerable wealth by means of his secret, for, contrary to the code, he, though a physician in good standing, refused to reveal the remedy to his professional brethren. After his death, about two years ago, his daughter, a Mrs. Graham, revealed the name of the remedy her father had used so successfully. It is *Cratægus oxyacantha*. So much for the history of the remedy. Dr. Jennings procured for himself some of the remedy, and his experience with it explains Dr. Green's national reputation. He writes:

"Case I was that of a Mr. B., aged seventy-three years. I found him gasping for breath when I entered the room, with a pulse-rate of 158 and very feeble; great œdema of lower limbs and abdomen. A more desperate case could hardly be found. I gave him fifteen drops of *Cratægus* in half a wineglass of water. In fifteen minutes the pulse beat was 126 and stronger, and breathing was not so labored. In twenty-five minutes pulse beat 110 and the force was still increasing, breathing much easier. He now got ten drops in same quantity of water, and in one hour from the time I entered the house he was, for the first time in ten days, able to lie horizontally on the bed. I made an examination of the heart and found mitral regurgitation from valvular deficiency, with great enlargement. For the œdema I prescribed *Hydrargyrum cum creta*, *Squill* and *Digitalis*. He received ten drops four times a day of the *Cratægus* and was permitted to use some light beer, to which he had become accustomed at meal time. He made a rapid and apparently full recovery until, in three months, he felt as well as any man of his age in Chicago. He occasionally, particularly in the change of weather, takes some of the *Cratægus* which, he says, quickly stops shortness of breath or pain in the heart. His father and a brother died of heart disease."

Another case was that of a young woman, who, when Dr. Jennings appeared in response to the summons, was said to be dead. "I went in and found that she was not quite dead, though apparently so. I put five or six drops of *Nitrite of amyl* to her nose, and alternately pressing and relaxing the chest, so as to imitate natural breathing, I soon had her able to open her eyes and speak. I gave her hypodermically ten drops, and in less than half an hour she was able to talk and describe her feelings. An examination revealed a painfully anæmic condition of the patient, but without any discoverable lesions of the heart, except functional." Under *Cratægus* she made a good recovery. "Her heart trouble, though very dangerous, was only functional, and resulted from want of proper assimilation of the food, due chiefly to the dyspeptic state and dysentery."

Another case was that of a woman who "was suffering from compensatory enlargement of the heart from mitral insufficiency," was taken with dyspnœa when Dr. Jennings was called and was nearly dead. Under *Cratægus* and some other indicated remedies she made an excellent recovery. "In a letter from her, three months afterward, she said she was feeling well, but that she would not feel fully secure without some of the *Cratægus*."

"The forty other cases ran courses somewhat similar to the three cited— all having been apparently cured. Yet I am not satisfied beyond a doubt, that any of those patients were completely cured except those whose trouble of the heart were functional, like the second case cited. And it is possible and even probable that in weather of a heavy atmosphere or when it is surcharged with electricity, or if the patient be subjected to great excitement or sudden or violent commotion or exercise he may suffer again therewith. That the medicine has a remarkable influence on the diseased heart must, I think, be admitted. From experiments on dogs and cats made by myself, it appears to influence the vagi and cardio inhibitory centres, and diminishes the pulse rate, increases the intraventricular pressure, and thus filling the heart with blood causes retardation of the beat and an equilibrium between the general blood pressure and force of the beat. Cardiac impulse, after a few days' use of the *Cratægus*, is greatly strengthened and yields that low, soft tone so characteristic of the first sound, as shown by the cardiograph. The entire central nervous system seems to be influenced favorably by its use; the appetite increases and assimilation and nutrition improve, showing an influence over the sympathetic and the solar plexus. Also a sense of quietude and well-being rests on the patient, and he who before its use was cross, melancholic and irritable, after a few days of its use shows marked signs of improvement in his mental state. I doubt if it is indicated in fatty enlargement. The dose which I have found to be the most available is from ten to fifteen drops after meals or food. If taken before food it may, in very susceptible patients, cause nausea. I find also that after its use for a month it may be well to discontinue for a week or two, when it should be renewed for another month or so. Usually three months seem to be the proper time for actual treatment, and after that only at such times as a warning pain of the heart or dyspnœa may point out.

(The *Kansas City Medical Journal*, 1898, contained a paper on the remedy, by Dr. Joseph Clements, from which the following pertinent extracts are taken):

About twelve years ago I was suddenly seized with terrible pain in the left breast; it extended over the entire region of the heart and down the brachial plexus of the left arm as far as the wrist. I pressed my hands over my heart and seemed unable to move. My lips blenched, my eyes rolled in a paroxysm of agony; the most fearful sense of impending calamity oppressed me and I seemed to expect death, or something worse, to fall upon and overwhelm me. The attack lasted a short time and then began to subside, and soon I was myself again, but feeling weak and excited. I consulted no one; took no medicine. I did not know what to make of it, but gradually it faded from my mind and I thought no more of it until two years afterwards, when I had another attack, and again nearly a year later. Each of these was very severe, like the first, and lasted about as long and left me in about the same condition. I remember no other seizure of importance until about three years ago, and again a year later. These were not so terrible in the suffering involved, but the fear, the apprehension, the awful sense of coming calamity, I think, grew upon me. From this time on, two years ago, the attacks came frequently, the time varying from two or three months to two or three weeks between.

I took some nitro-glycerine tablets and some pills of *Cactus Mexicana*, but with no benefit that I could perceive. This brings me down to about fifteen months ago. I was feeling very badly, having had several attacks within a few weeks. My pulse was at times very rapid and weak, and irregular and intermittent.

(About this time he got hold of *Cratægus* with the following result):

After getting my supply I began with six drops, increasing to ten before meals and at bedtime. The results were marvellous. In twenty-four hours my pulse showed marked improvement; in two or three weeks it became regular and smooth and forceful. Palpitation and dyspnœa soon entirely left me; I began to walk up and down hills without difficulty, and a more general and buoyant sense of security and well-being has come to stay. During the three months that I was taking the medicine, which I did with a week's intermission several times, I had several slight attacks, one rather hard seizure, but was relieved at once on taking ten drops of the medicine.

(He adds that hypodermic of *Morphia* does not give relief from these heart pains as quickly and as surely as does fifteen drops of *Cratægus*. He also says, "of course I consider it the most useful discovery of the Nineteenth century." He also names a number of "the most reputable and careful men in the profession," who are having good results with this remedy.)

(Dr. T. C. Duncan contributes the following illustrative cases):

Mrs. A., a printer, came to me complaining of some pain in the side as if it would take her life. She did not have it all the time, only at times, usually the last of the week, when tired. I prescribed *Bryonia*, then *Belladonna*, without prompt relief. One Saturday she came with a severe attack, locating the pain with her right hand above and to the left of the stomach. The pulse was strong and forcible. On careful examination I found the heart beat below the normal, indicating hypertrophy. I examined the spine, and to the left of the vertebra about two inches I found a very tender spot (spinal hyperæmia). She told me that when a girl she had several attacks, and that her own family physician (Dr. Patchen) gave her a remedy that relieved her at once. She had tried several physicians, among them an allopath, who gave hypodermic injections of morphia, without relief. Hot applications sometimes relieved.

I now recognized that I had a case of angina pectoris, and that her early attacks were due, I thought, to carrying her heavy brother. Now the attacks come when she becomes tired holding her composing stick; at the same time she became very much flurried, so much so that she had to stop work because she was so confused.

I now gave her a prescription for *Cactus*, but told her I would like to try first a new remedy, giving her *Cratægus*, saturating some disks with the tincture (B. & T.). I directed her to take two disks every hour until relieved, and then less often. If not relieved to take the *Cactus*.

She returned in a week reporting that she was relieved after the first dose of *Cratægus*. More, that hurried, flurried feeling had not troubled her this week. Her face has a parchment skin, and the expression of anxiety so significant of heart disease was certainly relieved. I have not seen her since.

In my proving of this drug it produced a flurried feeling due, I thought, to the rapid action of the stimulated heart. One prover, a nervous lady medical student, gives to-day in her report "a feeling of quiet and calmness, mentally." This is a secondary effect, for it was preceded by "an unusual rush of blood to the head with a *confused* feeling."

"One swallow does not make a summer," neither does one case establish a remedy; but I think that as *Cactus* has a clearly defined therapeutic range, so it seems that *Cratægus* may prove a valuable addition to our meagre array of heart remedies.

CUPHEA VISCOSISSIMA.

NAT. ORD., Lythraceæ.
COMMON NAMES, Clammy cuphea. Tar-weed.
PREPARATION.—The fresh plant is pounded to a pulp and macerated in two parts by weight of alcohol.

(In 1888 Dr. A. A. Roth contributed the following concerning *Cuphea vis.* to the *Homœopathic Recorder*):

Two years ago, whilst battling manfully for the life of a child ill to death from cholera infantum, I was persuaded by a lady friend to use red pennyroyal tea, and to my delight I had the pleasure of seeing a marvellous change in less than twenty-four hours. The vomiting ceased promptly and the bowels gradually became normal. Impressed by this fact, and also the fact that it was used very extensively in home treatment by country people, I procured the fresh plant, and prepared a tincture as directed in the *American Homœopathic Pharmacopœia* under article "Hedeoma." This made a beautiful dark-green tincture, having an aromatic odor and slightly astringent taste. Of this I gave from five to ten drops, according to age, every hour until relieved, and then as often as needed, and found it act promptly and effectively. Feeling loath to add another remedy to our already over-burdened Materia Medica, I deferred any mention of the fact; but now after a fair trial for two seasons I feel justified in believing that the *Cuphea viscosissima* will prove a treasure in the treatment of cholera infantum. Out of a large number of cases treated I had but three square failures, and they were complicated with marasmus to an alarming extent before I began the *Cuphea*; one died and two finally recovered. *Cuphea* does not act with equal promptness in all forms of cholera infantum. Two classes of cases stand out prominently; and first, those arising from acidity of milk or food; vomiting of undigested food or curdled milk, with frequent green, watery, acid stools, varying in number from five to thirty per day; child fretful and feverish; can retain nothing on the stomach; food seems to pass right through the child. I have frequently had the mother say after twenty-four hours' use of *Cuphea*: "Doctor, the baby is all right," and a very pleasant greeting it is, as we all know. A second class is composed of cases in which the stools are decidedly dysenteric, small, frequent, bloody, with tenesmus and great pain; high fever, restlessness and sleeplessness. In these two classes *Cuphea* acts promptly and generally permanently. It contains a large percentage of tannic acid, and seems to possess decidedly tonic properties, as children rally rapidly under its use. It utterly failed me in ordinary forms of diarrhœa, especially in diarrhœas from colds, etc.; but in the classes mentioned I have frequently had it produce obstinate constipation after several days' use.

ECHINACEA ANGUSTIFOLIA.

NAT. ORD., Compositæ.
COMMON NAME, Pale Purple Cone-flower.
PREPARATION.—The whole plant including the root is pounded to a pulp and macerated in two parts by weight of alcohol.

(This rather famous drug first came to notice as "Meyers' Blood Purifier;" the proprietor did not know the name of the drug used and sent a whole plant to Professors King and Lloyd, of Cincinnati, who identified it as *Echinacea angustifolia*, commonly known as "cone flower," "black Sampson," "nigger head," etc. If we may believe all that has been printed about it the remedy is a veritable cure-all. The following, however, is a safe guide; it is taken from the paper by Dr. J. Willis Candee in Transactions, 1898, of the Homœopathic Medical Society of the State of New York, and credited by Dr. Candee to Dr. J. C. Fahnstock):

He (Dr. Fahnstock) refers to the clinical application of *Echinacea*, from personal experience, substantially as follows: Cases of shifting pains in rheumatism, for which *Puls.* had been unsuccessfully prescribed, rapidly disappeared under *Echin.* Several cases of acne resembling that caused by *Bromide of Potassium*, cured. "A great remedy." When boils progress to the stage where they appear about to "point" then stop and do not suppurate, *Echinacea* is the remedy. "In carbuncles with similar symptoms, a bluish-red color and intense pain, it will in a few hours make your patient grateful to you." It is of great value in very fetid ozæna. Beneficial in some cases of leucorrhœa with discharge bright yellow, as from a suppurating surface. Very serviceable in gangrene, where it may be classed with *Rhus* and *Arsenicum*, perhaps ranking between them. Has attributed to it unusually good results in a case of tuberculous disease of hip and in an old, well-dosed case of destructive syphilis of throat. "In suppurative processes *Echin.* is to be thought of."

In typhoid fever, diphtheria and appendicitis he has failed to substantiate the claims of other admirers of this remedy.

These clinical hints have been given place as naturally following report of the proving and also because of their coming from a closely observant homœopathist. It is unnecessary at this time to review in detail the alleged field of usefulness of *Echinacea*. All are familiar with the published testimonials and indications, some of which would lead one to think that little else is to be desired with which to combat degenerative processes in mankind.

On the other hand are those, who, having tried the drug without satisfactory results, are willing to cast it aside as worthless. To such it may be well to make these suggestions: 1, to ascertain whether they have used a reliable preparation, and 2, to refrain from hasty judgment until guides for prescribing, more accurate than perchance the label on a bottle, shall have been found and consulted.

My own limited experience would throw no particular light on the subject. It has, however, served to impress me with confidence in the remedy and its future. The gist of trustworthy clinical findings may be stated in two words, antiseptic and alterative.

(From an article by Dr. H. W. Feller, in the *Eclectic Medical Journal*, we quote the following generalities concerning this remedy):

If any single statement were to be made concerning the virtues of *Echinacea* it would read something like this: "A corrector of the deprivation of the body fluids;" and even this does not sufficiently cover the ground. Its extraordinary powers—combining essentially that formerly included under the terms antiseptic, antifermentative, and antizymotic—are well shown in its power over changes produced in the fluids of the body, whether from internal causes or from external introductions. The changes may be manifested in a disturbed balance of the fluids resulting in such tissue alterations as are exhibited in boils, carbuncles, abscesses, or cellular glandular inflammations. They may be from the introduction of serpent or insect venom, or they may be due to such fearful poisons as give rise to malignant diphtheria, cerebro-spinal meningitis, or puerperal and other forms of septicæmia. Such changes, whether they be septic or of devitalized morbid accumulations, or alterations in the fluids themselves, appear to have met their Richmond in *Echinacea*. "Bad blood" so called, asthenia and adynamia, and particularly a tendency to malignancy in acute and sub-acute disorders, seem to be special indicators for the use of *Echinacea*.

(The *North American Journal of Homœopathy*, December, 1896, contains a paper on the drug by Dr. Charles F. Otis, from which we quote the following):

I doubt if there are many physicians here assembled, who are general practitioners, who have not, at some period of their professional lives, come in contact with one or both of these diseases either in an epidemic form or isolated cases, and in instances, have met more than their match; have seen their patients with tongue so swollen that it protruded from the mouth; with membrane gradually extending from the throat into the posterior nares, possibly protruding from the nostrils, with the awful odor so characteristic; with a respiratory sound that told you too plainly that membrane was extending into the air passages and that the misery of your patient would soon cease, not because of your ability to afford relief, but because death would close the scene.

I need not complete the picture by mentioning the enormously high temperature, the thread-like pulse, the cessation of the action of the kidneys, the awful agonizing expression of the face, and, perhaps, in your efforts, intubation had been practiced without good results. It is in just this class of cases that *Echinacea* is king. So reliable has been its action in my hands that I am inclined to give a favorable prognosis, and if I am so fortunate as to be called early the application of the drug in question does not permit of the symptoms just enumerated. The whole case will usually be changed to one of a mild form followed by a quick recovery.

(This from a paper by Dr. W. H. Ramey in *Medical Gleaner*):

It is a specific, I think, for the condition of the system which sets up the boil habit. I never have found a case so bad, and I've had some very severe ones, that an ounce and a half of *Echinacea*, taken in ten-drop doses four times a day, would not cure. Try it in your cases of stomatitis with depraved conditions of the system, both internally and locally. It has done me valuable service in cases of old ulcers and unhealthy sores, both as local and internal treatment. Then in your typhoid cases, with the characteristic indication, it is simply a wonderful remedy. I have seen it step in and restore normal conditions when it seemed impossible for remedies to act quick enough to prevent a fatal termination.

(Dr. S. J. Hogan in *Chicago Medical Times*):

One other thing I would like to tell about it: I had a case I was treating. Among other things, the patient had on the scalp and at the margin of the hair on the back of the head a number of wen-like tumors; since taking *Echinacea* they have been entirely absorbed.

(Dr. Joseph Adolphus in *Medical Gleaner*):

I have seen its very beneficial action in two epidemics of smallpox. The remedy did certainly modify the severity of the disease, restrain suppuration, check the severity of the symptoms, and promote convalescence. I knew of several very desperate cases, which I think would have terminated fatally but for the timely use of *Echinacea*. I frequently saw cases of severe confluent type, wherein the symptoms were of a very serious kind, high fever, delirium; some with coma, abominably offensive odor of body and breath, urine nearly suppressed, eruption confluent, exceedingly abundant pus, steadily improve under *Echinacea* tea taken internally and used locally over the entire body. One of the very striking effects of the *Echinacea* was to abate the dreadfully offensive odor of the body and breath and modify the acute severity of the eruption.

(The following proving of *Echinacea*, conducted by Dr. J. C. Fahnestock, of Piqua, Ohio, was read before the American Institute of Homœopathy, at Atlantic City, 1899):

It becomes my pleasant duty to place before the American Institute of Homœopathy a collection of provings of *Echinacea angustifolia*.

Four species of this genus are recognized. Two of them, *E. Dicksoni* and *E. dubia*, are native in Mexico.

There are two native in this country, *E. purpurea*, *Mœnch*. Leaves rough, often serrate; the lowest ovate, five nerved, veiny, long petioled; the other ovate-lanceolate; involucre imbricated in three to five rows; stem smooth, or in one form rough, bristly, as well as the leaves. Prairies and banks, from western Pennsylvania and Virginia to Iowa, and southward; occasionally advancing eastward. July—Rays fifteen to twenty, dull purple (rarely whitish), one to two feet long or more. Root thick, black, very pungent to the taste, used in popular medicine under the name of Black Sampson. Very variable, and probably connects with *E. angustifolia*, described as follows: Leaves, as well as the slender, simple stem, bristly, hairy, lanceolate and linear lanceolate, attenuate at base, three nerved, entire; involucre less imbricated and heads often smaller; rays twelve to fifteen inches, (2) long, rose color or red. Plains from Illinois and Wisconsin southward—June to August. This is a brief description of the botany of the plant under consideration.

Your chairman, T. L. Hazard, in his usual characteristic manner, went vigorously to work and secured all the provers possible. I was also fortunate enough to secure a number of provers, besides proving and reproving it myself. The results of all these provings were handed over to me to present to you in such form as seemed best.

I must tarry just long enough to preface this collection and tell you that explicit printed directions were sent to all the superintendents of these provings. This being of too great length, I will give you the most important points in these directions, viz.: Let each prover be furnished with a small blank book, in which shall be written date, name, sex, residence, height, weight, temperament, color of eyes, color of hair, complexion; describe former ailments and present physical condition. In concluding give pulse in different positions, respiration, temperature, function of digestion, analysis of excretions, especially the urine; analysis of the blood, family history, habits, idiosyncrasy, etc.

The different colleges and universities were called upon to assist on these provings. The following institutions responded to the call: Cleveland, St. Louis, Minneapolis, the Chicago, Iowa City, and Ann Arbor. None of the eastern institutions responded; don't know whether dead or just hibernating.

I wish to publicly express my thanks to all who have taken part in these provings. I think it but just to state that the University of Michigan furnished the best provings. Thanks also are extended to Boericke & Tafel for remedy furnished in the θ, 3x, 30x, which were also used in the provings. One lady, who commenced the proving and had begun to develop valuable provings, contracted a severe cold and stopped, for which I am very sorry. All the rest of the provers were males; medical students or physicians. Only a very few symptoms were produced by the use of the 30x attenuation, a greater number of provers not recording any at all.

The symptoms here compiled were produced by the 3x attenuation and the tincture, using from one drop to thirty drops at a dose. In proving and then compiling the symptoms produced by this drug, I am fully aware of the many difficulties to be met on every side.

The one great trouble that I find is that those who are unaccustomed to proving do not observe what really is going on while attempting to make a proving, and are not capable of expressing the conditions so produced. I find that there are few who can take drugs and accurately define their effects. In selecting and discriminating the effects of drugs there must exist a mental superiority, and no man had this genius so highly developed as Hahnemann.

After making three different provings upon myself, I have undertaken to select those symptoms which to the best of my ability were found in all of these different provings.

I have taken special care not to omit any symptoms, even though it may have been noticed by but one prover; but in the majority of cases you will notice the symptoms occurred two or more times in different individuals, thus confirming the genuineness of the symptoms.

Not giving you the day-book records of these provers, a few remarks, showing its general action, may not be out of place. As stated before, only two recorded symptoms after the use of the 30x attenuation.

After taking the tincture, there is soon produced a biting, tingling sensation of the tongue, lips and fauces, not very much unlike the sensation produced by *Aconite*. In these provers there soon followed a sense of fear, with pain about the heart, and accelerated pulse. In a short time there was noticed a dull pain in both temples, a pressing pain; then shooting pains, which followed the fifth pair of nerves.

The next symptom produced was an accumulation of sticky mucus in mouth and fauces. Then a general languor and weakness followed, always worse in the afternoon. All the limbs felt weak and indisposed to make any motion, and this was accompanied by sharp, shooting, shifting pains. In quite a number of cases the appetite was not affected.

Those using sufficient quantity of the tincture had loss of appetite, with belching of tasteless gas, weakness in the stomach, pain in the right hypochondriac region, accompanied with gas in the bowels; griping pains followed by passing offensive flatus, or a loose, yellowish stool, which always produced great exhaustion. After using the drug several days the face becomes pale, the pulse very much lessened in frequency, and a general exhaustion follows like after a severe and long spell of sickness.

The tongue will then indicate slow digestion, accompanied with belching of tasteless gas. In most of the provers, however, there was a passing of very offensive gas and offensive stools.

You will observe that the remedy exerts quite an effect on the kidneys and bladder, but I am very sorry to say that the urinary analysis made did not show anything but the variations generally observed in ordinary health.

I must say that the provers did not go into the details as much as was desirable. Likewise, I may say the same of the blood tests made, but what was given is very valuable.

I could give you an expression of its special action, but will merely give you the symptoms collected and then you can make your own deductions.

ECHINACEA ANGUSTIFOLIA.

A collection of symptoms from twenty-five different provers, anatomically arranged:

MIND.

- 3 Dullness in head, with cross, irritable feeling.
- 2 So nervous could not study.
- 3 Confused feeling of the brain.
- 2 Felt depressed and much out of sorts.
- 3 Felt a mental depression in afternoons.
- 1 Senses seem to be numbed.
- 5 Drowsy, could not read, drowsiness.
- 2 Vertigo when changing position of head.

- 3 Drowsy condition with yawning.

- 2 Becomes angry when corrected, does not wish to be contradicted.

SENSORIUM.

- 5 General depression, with weakness.

- 8 General dullness and drowsiness.

- 4 General dullness, unable to apply the mind.

- 5 Does not wish to think or study.

- 3 Restless, wakes often in the night.

- 2 Dull headache, felt as if brain was too large, with every beat of heart.

- 5 Sleep full of dreams.

INNER HEAD.

- 5 Dull pain in brain, full feeling.

- 5 Dull frontal headache, especially over left eye, which was relieved in open air.

- 2 Severe headache in vertex, better by rest in bed.

- 5 Dull headache above eyes.

- 4 Dull throbbing headache, worse through temples.

- 3 Head feels too large.

- 1 Dull headache, worse in evening.

- 2 Dull headache, worse in right temple, with sharp pain.

-

- 3 Dull pain in occiput.

- 3 Dull headache, with dizziness.

OUTER HEAD.

- 3 Constant dull pressing pain in both temples.

- 2 Shooting pains through temples.

- 2 Dull occipital headache.

- 3 Constant dull pain in temples, better at rest and pressure.

- 2 Head feels as big as a windmill, with mental depression.

EYES.

- 2 Eyes ache when reading.

- 1 Tires me dreadfully to hold a book and read.

- 1 Eyes pain on looking at an object and will fill with tears, closing them relieves.

- 1 Sleepy sensation in eyes, but cannot sleep.

- 1 Pains back of right eye.

- 1 Sense of heat in eyes when closing them.

- 2 Dull pain in both eyes.

- 1 Lachrymation from cold air.

- 2 Sharp pains in eyes and temples.

EAR.

- 2 Shooting pain in right ear.

NOSE.

- 2 Stuffiness of nostrils, with mucus in nares and pharynx.

- 4 Full feeling in nose as if it would close up.

- 2 Full feeling of nose, obliged to blow nose, but does not relieve.

- 2 Nostrils sore.

- 2 Mucus discharge from right nostril.

- 2 Rawness of right nostril, sensitive to cold, which cause a flow of mucus.

- 1 Bleeding from right nostril.

- 1 Right nostril sore, when picking causes hæmorrhage.

- 1 Headache over eyes, with sneezing.

-

FACE.

- 2 Paleness of face when head aches.

- 1 Fine eruptions on forehead and cheeks.

- 2 Vomiting with pale face.

TEETH.

- 2 Darting pains in the teeth, worse on right side.

- 3 Neuralgic pains in superior and inferior maxilla.

- 2 Dull aching of the teeth.

TONGUE.

- 2 White coating of tongue in the mornings, with white frothy mucus in mouth.

- 2 Slight burning of tongue.

- 2 Whitish coat of tongue, with red edges.

MOUTH.

- 2 Accumulation of sticky, white mucus.

- 3 Eructation of tasteless gas.

- 2 Burning of the tongue, with increased saliva.

- 1 Dry sensation in back part of mouth.

- 2 Burning peppery taste when taking remedy.

- 3 Bad taste in the mouth in the morning.

- 3 A metallic taste.

- 3 Belching of gas which tastes of the food eaten.

- 2 Dryness of the mouth.

- 3 Sour eructation.

- 1 Sour eructation, which caused burning of throat.

THROAT.

- 3 Accumulation of mucus in throat.

- 1 Mucus in throat, with raw sensation.

- 1 After vomiting of sour mucus, throat burns.

- 2 Soreness of throat, worse on left side.

DESIRE.

- 5 Loss of appetite.
- 2 Desire for cold water.
-

EATING.

- 3 Nausea, could not eat.
- 5 Loss of appetite.

NAUSEA AND VOMITING.

- 2 Nausea before going to bed, which was always better lying down.
- 2 After eating stomach and abdomen fill with gas.
- 3 After eating belching, which tastes of food eaten.
- 2 Nausea, with eructation of gas.

STOMACH.

- 1 Stomach distended with gas, not relieved by belching.
- 4 Belching of tasteless gas.
- 2 Sense of something large and hard in stomach.
- 2 Belching of gas and at same time passing flatus.
- 3 Sour stomach, "heart burn," with belching of gas.
- 1 Relaxed feeling of the stomach.
- 1 Pain in stomach, going down through bowels, followed by diarrhœa.
- 3 Dull pain in stomach.

HYPOCHONDRIA.

- 5 Pain in right hypochondria.

ABDOMEN.

- 5 Full feeling in abdomen, with borborygmus.
- 2 Pain about umbilicus, relieved by bending double.
- 2 Pain in abdomen, sharp cutting, coming and going suddenly.

- 1 Pain in left illiac fossa.

URINE.

- 6 Desire for frequent urination.

- 4 Urine increased.

- 1 Involuntary urination "in spite of myself."

- 2 Sense of heat while passing urine.

- 3 Urine pale and copious.

- 1 Urine scanty and dark in color.

-

- 2 Pain and burning on urination.

MALE SEX ORGAN.

- 1 Soreness in perineum.

- 2 Testicles drawn up and sore.

- 1 Pain in meatus while urinating.

- 2 Pain across perineum.

- 2 Perineum seems stretched.

- 1 Pain in right spermatic cord.

FEMALE SEX ORGAN.

- 1 Mucus from vagina in evening.

- 1 Pain in right illiac region, which seems deep, lasting but a short time.

LARYNX.

- 2 Irritation of larynx.

- 1 Voice husky.

COUGH.

- 2 Constant clearing of mucus from throat.

- 2 Mucus comes in throat while in bed, must cough to clear throat.

LUNGS.

- 2 Full feeling in upper part of lungs.
- 2 Pain in region of diaphragm.
- 1 Pain in right lung.

HEART AND PULSE.

- 2 Slight pain over heart.
- 1 Rapid beating of heart.
- 4 Heart's action increased.
- 2 Heart's action decreased.
- 2 Anxiety about the heart.

CHEST.

- 2 Pain in pectoral muscles.
- 1 Sore feeling in the chest.
- 1 Feels like lump in chest.
- 2 Feeling of a lump under sternum.
-

NECK AND BACK.

- 3 Pain in small of back over kidneys.
- 6 Dull pain in small of back.
- 3 Pain in back of neck.
- 4 Pain in lumbar region, worse from stooping.

UPPER LIMBS.

- 3 Pain in right thumb.
- 2 Sharp pain in left elbow.
- 2 Pain in right shoulder, going down to fingers.
- 2 Sharp pain in left arm, going down to fingers, with loss of muscular power.
- 2 Cold hands.
- 4 Pain in wrists and fingers.
- 2 Pain in left shoulder, better by rest and warmth.

LOWER LIMBS.

- 2 Cold feet.
- 2 Pain back of left knee.
- 2 Sharp shooting pain in legs.
- 1 Extremities cold.
- 3 Left hip and knee pains.
- 2 Pain in right thigh.
- 2 Pain in right leg.

LIMBS IN GENERAL.

- 7 General weakness of limbs.
- 1 Pain between shoulders, which extend to axilla and down the arms.

POSITION.

- Pains and sickness of stomach better by lying down.

NERVES.

- 7 Exhausted, tired feeling.
- 5 Muscular weakness.
- 2 Felt as if I had been sick for a long time.
- 6 General aching all over, with exhaustion.
-

SLEEP.

- 2 General languor, sleepy.
- 3 Sleep disturbed, wakes often.
- 5 Sleep full of dreams.
- 1 Dreams about exciting things all night.
- 2 Dreams of dead relations.

TIME.

- Worse after eating.
- Worse in evenings.

- Worse after physical or mental labor.

- Better at rest.

CHILLS.

- 1 Chills up the back.

- 1 Cold flashes all over the back.

- 2 General chilliness with nausea.

SKIN.

- 3 Intense itching and burning of skin on neck.

- 1 Little papules on skin, with redness, feeling like nettles; this occurred on the fifth day of the proving.

- 1 Skin dry.

- 2 Small red pimples on neck and face.

BLOOD.

- 2 After proving found a diminution of red corpuscles.

EPIGEA REPENS.

NAT. ORD., Ericaceæ.
COMMON NAMES, Trailing Arbutus. Ground Laurel. Gravel Root.
PREPARATION.—The fresh leaves are pounded to a pulp and macerated in two parts by weight of alcohol.

(In the subjoined paper by Dr. E. M. Hale, *North American Journal of Homœopathy*, 1869, the old doctrine of signatures seems to crop out again.)

The *Gravel Root* has long had some reputation in urinary difficulties, and even in calculous affections. The common appellation of "Gravel root" shows that the popular belief points in the direction of its use.

I have never tested its virtues but in one instance, and its effects seemed to be so decided and curative that I deem the case worthy of publication.

A young man, aged twenty-three, applied for treatment of a long array of symptoms, some of which seemed to indicate *enlargement of the prostate*, and others a *vesical catarrh*.

The *quantity* of urine was nearly normal.

The *quality* was decidedly abnormal. It contained a large amount of mucus, the phosphates, some blood, and a little pus. It was dark red, colored blue litmus paper red (showing its acid condition).

The pain was similar to a vesical tenesmus, a pain in the region of the neck of the bladder and prostate gland. Pressure in the perineum was painful.

He had been under the most atrocious allopathic treatment; had been drugged with copaiva, spts. nitric.-dulc., turpentine, tincture muriate of iron, and other diuretics in enormous doses.

I commenced the treatment with *Sulphur* 30th, three doses a day for a week.

By this time he had eliminated the drug-poisons from his system, and the real symptoms of the malady began to appear uncomplicated. The blood and pus disappeared from the urine, there was less mucus, and the urine was of a lighter color.

A red, sandy sediment, however, remained. This sediment was not "gritty" under the finger, at least no such sensation was perceptible.

Second prescription: *Lycopodium* 30th and 6th, the former in the morning, the latter in evening, for a week. No improvement except a slight diminution of the sediment.

No medicine was given for four days, at which time there appeared dysuria, pain in the region of the prostate, mucous sediment, and itching at the orifice of the urethra.

While undecided as to the next prescription, I happened to take up a vial of tincture *Epigea repens*, which I had prepared from the fresh plant, while on a visit to Mackinaw six months before. Knowing the high estimate placed on this plant, by the people, in the treatment of gravel I resolved to test its virtues. Ten drops of the mother tincture were prescribed, to be taken every four hours.

Two days afterwards my patient brought me several small brownish particles, having the appearance of fine sand. When crushed and pressed between the fingers they had a decidedly gritty feel. Under the microscope they had the appearance of rough coarse sand. The discharge of calculi kept up for nearly a week, under the use of the *Epigea*, and then ceased, and with it all the symptoms of irritation of the bladder.

It is just possible that the discharge of gravel may have been a coincidence. It is equally possible that the *Lycopodium* acted curatively; but I am inclined to believe their disintegration and expulsion was caused or aided by the use of the last medicine.

Further observations are needed to place the curative powers of this plant on a certain basis.

ERYNGIUM AQUATICUM.

NAT. ORD., Umbeliferæ.
COMMON NAMES, Button Snakeroot. Water Eryngo.
PREPARATION.—The fresh root is pounded to a pulp and macerated in two parts by weight of alcohol.

(Although a well-known remedy, the following concerning its early history may not be out of place here. It is from Thomas' *Additions*.)

"For spermatorrhœa properly so called, or emission of semen without erections, there is no remedy which has yet received the sanction of experience."—*Repertory*.

"We have one, however, to propose for trial—it is the *Eryngium aquaticum*, which has two remarkable cures, reported by Dr. Parks (Pharmacentist, Cin.), to recommend it.

"CASE I.—A married man injured his testicles by jumping upon a horse; this was followed by a discharge of what was considered semen for fifteen years, during which time he was treated allopathically and homœopathically. Dr. Parks exhibited a number of the usual remedies without permanent benefit. He then gave a half-grain dose, three times a day, of the third decimal trituration of the '*Eryngium aquaticum*.' In five days the emissions were entirely suppressed, and have not returned to this time (over two years ago). The emissions were without erections day or night, and followed by great lassitude.

"CASE II.—A married man, not conscious of having sustained any injury, was troubled for eight or ten years with emissions at night—with erections. The semen also passed by day with the urine. The loss of semen was followed by great lassitude and depression, continuing from twelve to forty-eight hours. There also partial impotence. Had been treated allopathically. Dr. Parks gave him Phos. acid for two weeks, without material benefit. He then exhibited the *Eryngium aquaticum*, as above, with the like excellent and prompt result."[1]

I used this remedy with a patient who was quite broken down from spermatorrhœa; the emissions left him, but he suffered from vertigo and dim-sightedness whenever he took a dose of the medicine. He is now well through the use of other medicines. Our English *Eryngo*—the *E. maritimum*, is noted as an aphrodisiac, and is very similar in appearance to the *Eryngium aquaticum*.

FOOTNOTES:

[1] Drs. Hill and Hunt, Homœopathic Surgery.

EUPHORBIA COROLLATA.

NAT. ORD., Euphorbiaceæ.
COMMON NAMES, Milk Weed. Wild Ipecac. Blooming or Flowering Spurge.
PREPARATION.—The fresh root is pounded to a pulp and macerated in two parts by weight of alcohol.

(In *North American Journal of Homœopathy*, Dr. E. M. Hale has, among other things, the following to say of this drug):

Its action on the system is intense and peculiar. It is called by the country people by the expressive name of *Go-quick*, referring to its quick and prompt action. I am indebted to Dr. A. R. Brown, of Litchfield, Mich., for many interesting facts relating to its action. It is considered, by those who use it, as the most powerful "revulsive agent" in their Materia Medica, in all cases of local congestion, especially of the lungs and head; also in inflammation of the pleura, lungs, and liver, and is used as a substitute for bleeding and Calomel. Its admirers allege that it will certainly *arrest* the progress of the above affections in a few hours, and break up all simple fevers. This is of course erroneous, but it reminds one of the Helleborine of the ancients, so graphically described by Hahnemann. In fact no drug with which I am acquainted so much resembles the *Veratrum album*.

FAGOPYRUM.

NAT. ORD., Polygonaceæ.
COMMON NAME, Buckwheat.
PREPARATION.—The fresh mature plant is pounded to a pulp and macerated in two parts by weight of alcohol.

(The following paper was published in the Transactions of the Homœopathic Society of Maine in 1895. It is by Dr. D. C. Perkins, of Rockland, Me.)

There is, perhaps, no well proven remedy in the Materia Medica, of equal value to that of which I present a brief study, that has been so wholly overlooked by the homœopathic profession. There certainly is none which possesses a more marked individuality, and which more fully fills a place by itself. It is safe to say that not one in ten of those who practice the healing art has ever used it or is familiar with its pathogenesis. Having not unfrequently cured cases with it, which had refused to yield to other remedies apparently well indicated, I have come to regard it as among the important drugs in our super-abundant Materia Medica. Its effects upon mental conditions are marked by depression of spirits, irritability, inability to study, or to remember what has been read, bringing to our minds *Aconite*, *Bryonia*, *Chamomilla*, *Coffea*, *Colocynth*, *Ignatia*, *Lachesis*, *Mercury*, *Nux vomica*, *Staphisagria*, *Stramonium*, and *Veratrum*. Its effects upon the head are deep-seated and persistent. There is vertigo, confusion, severe pain in many parts of head, with upward pressure described as of a bursting character. The pain may be in forehead, back of eyes, through temporal region on either side, but always of a pressive or bursting nature. For congestive headaches it is as valuable as *Belladonna*, *Glonoine*, *Nux vomica*, or *Sepia*.

In and about the eyes there is itching, smarting, swelling, heat and soreness; the itching being especially marked and usually regarded as characteristic. The last named symptom is no less prominent in affections of the ears, as has often been shown in the efficacy of buckwheat flour in frost-bites, or erysipelas of those useful organs, from time immemorial. Here the similarity to *Agaricus* will readily be recognized. The nose does not escape. It is swollen, red, inflamed and sore. There is at first fluent coryza with sneezing, followed by fulness, dryness and the formation of crusts. Nor is the burning absent which has been elsewhere noted. There is much soreness and somewhat persistent pain from even gentle pressure.

The face is pale or unevenly flushed, with dark semi-circles below the eyes. Later, the face becomes swollen, hot and dry, as though severely sunburnt, and the lips are cracked and sore. The mouth feels dry and hot, and yet saliva is not wanting. There is soreness and swelling of roof of mouth, and the tongue is red and fissured along its edges. The bad taste in the morning reminds us of *Pulsatilla.*

In the throat, there is soreness with pain just back of the isthmus of the fauces, a feeling of excoriation and soreness extending deep down in the pharynx. The uvula is elongated, the tonsils are swollen and red, there is a sensation of rawness in the throat strikingly reminding us of *Phytolacca.* Externally, there is scarlet redness of the neck below the mastoid process, throbbing of the carotids, the neck feels tired, the head heavy and the parotid glands are swollen and painful. It is unnecessary to name the remedy having similar symptoms.

While the symptoms produced on the digestive tract are not characterized by that intensity noted elsewhere, they are still valuable. There is persistent morning nausea which should lead us to study this remedy in the vomiting of pregnancy. Contrary to *Lycopodium* and *Nux moschata* the appetite is improved by eating. The empty or "all-gone" feeling at the stomach is like that of *Sepia.*

In the abdomen there is fulness and pain but no rumbling. Discharges of flatus are frequent and annoying. The region of the liver is painful, tender and there is aggravation from pressure, compelling the patient to lie on the left side. The stools are pappy, or watery, profuse, offensive and followed by tenesmus.

On the male genital organs there is profuse perspiration of an offensive odor. The urine is scalding, and pain extends from testicles to abdomen. In females the drug acts with force upon the right ovary, producing pain of a bruised or burning character, noted particularly when walking. There is pruritus with slight yellow leucorrhœa, the discharge being more noticed when at rest than when exercising. So far as known this latter symptom does not occur under the action of any other remedy.

In the chest we find a heavy, pulsating pain extending to all its parts. This is persistent, and is worse from a deep inspiration. Around the heart there are dull pains with oppression and occasional sharp pains passing through the heart. Pressure with the hand increases the oppression. The pulse is increased but is extremely variable. There is reason to believe that *Cactus grandiflora,* or *Spigelia* are often given in affections of the heart, where *Fagopyrum,* if given, would accomplish better results.

On the muscular system the action of the remedy stands out in bold relief. There is stiffness and soreness of all the muscles of the neck, with pain, and a feeling as if the neck would hardly support the head. Pains extend from occiput to back of neck and are relieved by bending the head backward. There are dull pains in small of back, with stitching pains in the region of the kidneys. Pains with occasional sharp stitches extend from the arms to muscles of both sides of chest. Rheumatic pains in the shoulders of a dull aching character. Stinging and burning pains extend the whole length of fingers, aggravated by motion. Streaking pains pass through arms and legs with sharp pains extending to feet. Pains extend from hips to small of back, and these also frequently run down to the feet. In the knees there is dull pain and weakness, while deep in the limbs there is burning and stinging. There is numbness in the limbs, with dragging in the joints, especially right knee, hip and elbow. Stooping to write causes constant severe pain through chest and in region of liver. This group of symptoms gives *Fagopyrum* a striking individuality and establishes it in an uncontested position among the long list of remedies prescribed for rheumatic complaints.

Scarcely less important are the symptoms of the skin. There is intense itching of the arms and legs, becoming worse toward evening. Blotches like flea-bites appear in many localities, sometimes all over the body, are sore to the touch and are multiplied by scratching. These eruptions are persistent and the itching is intense. Blind boils may be developed and attain a large size. The itching of the face is especially marked about the roots of the whiskers. Itching of the hands which is "deep in" is persistent and annoying, this condition being supposed to be the result of irritation of the coats of the arteries.

The sleepiness is unlike that of *Belladonna, Nux vomica, Sepia* or *Sulphur*, occurring early in the evening and characterized by stretching and yawning. It is not profound, and when the mind is diverted the patient gets wide awake, but soon relapses unless conversation is continued. In bed, sleep is disturbed by troublesome dreams and frequent waking. Aggravations occur after retiring, ascending stairs, from deep inspiration, walking in bright sunlight, lying on right side, riding in cars, and when stooping or writing. Ameliorations occur after taking coffee, from cold applications, from motion in cold air, and from sitting still in warm room.

FAGUS SYLVATICUS.

NAT. ORD., Cupuliferæ.

COMMON NAME, European Beech.

PREPARATION.—The Beech Nuts are pounded to a pulp and macerated in five parts by weight of alcohol.

(In volume XIII of the *American Observer*, Dr. E. W. Berridge, contributes the following concerning the action of *Fagus sylvaticus* or Beech nuts):

BEECH NUTS. (From *Medical Museum—London, 1781—vol. ii., pp. 97, 294.*) From a dissertation on hydrophobia, by Christian Frederick Seleg, M. D., of Enbenstoff, in Saxony, printed in Eslong, in 1762.

A boy aged 13 had eaten four days ago a large quantity of beech nuts. I found him in great pain, languid, and terrified with apprehensions of present death. Pulse very unequal, sometimes extremely quick, sometimes languid and intermittent; skin burning violently; mouth flowing with froth and saliva, intolerable thirst, entreating for drink, but as soon as any liquid was brought he seemed to shudder with equal horror, as if he had been eating unripe grapes. Soon after eating the nuts he had been seized with torpor, gloominess and dread of liquids. He had not been bitten by any rabid animal.

Next (5th) day, early in the morning, he was the same, but seemed to talk more in his wildness and perturbation of mind, and his mouth flowed with foam more abundantly; the urine he had voided by night was red and firey, depositing a copious turbid white sediment, resembling an emulsion of beech nuts, subsiding as deep as the breadth of the finger at the bottom of the vessel. A few hours before he died he vomited a porraceous bile, after which he died quietly.

The author in the *original* work gives a number of fatal cases of *spontaneous* hydrophobia. This work should be examined.

John Bauhin (*Hist. Plants*, vol. i, pp. 2, 121) says that the nuts will disorder the head like darnel; hogs grow stupid and drowsy by feeding on them.

Ray (*Hist. of Plants*, tom. ii, p. 1382) and Mangetus (*Biblioth. Pharm.*, vol. i, p. 910) says the same.

FRAXINUS EXCELSIOR.

NAT. ORD., Oleaceæ.
COMMON NAME, European Ash.
PREPARATION.—The fresh leaves are pounded to a pulp and macerated with two parts by weight of alcohol.

(In the *Union Médicale*, November, 1852, two French physicians detailed several cases of gout and rheumatism treated with *Fraxinus excelsior*, or ash leaves, one of Rademacher's favorite remedies. Of the two physicians, one of them, Dr. Peyraud, was himself relieved of the gout by this treatment.)

Ash-leaves were highly recommended by Rademacher, and have been quite extensively used in Germany on his suggestion. In the *Union Médicale* for Nov. 27, 1852, two French physicians, Drs. Pouget and Peyraud, detailed several cases of gout and rheumatism cured by an infusion of ash-leaves in boiling water. Dr. Peyraud himself was one of those relieved.

"In 1842, Dr. Peyraud had his first attack of gout, which was severe, and lasted for twenty-five days. During the three following years the attacks increased in frequency and severity. Having derived little benefit from the remedial means which he had resorted to, he listened to the suggestion of one of his patients, an inhabitant of the department of Dordogne, in France, who advised him to try an infusion of ash-leaves, informing him, at the same time, that his forefathers had been cured by this prescription, and that many of the country people got rid of 'their pains' by employing it. Dr. Peyraud took the infusion of ash-leaves and from 1845 to 1849 had no fit of gout. He then had an attack, which yielded in five days to the infusion of ash-leaves, used under the observation of Dr. Pouget. These circumstances recalled to the recollection of Dr. Pouget a fact which he might otherwise never again have considered. It was this: that when he was a physician at Soréze, in 1824, the peasants of that place had spoken to him of the great power which an infusion of ash-leaves had in driving away pains. He afterwards discovered that it had been used forty years ago as a gout-specific by the peasants of Auvergne.

"A commercial traveller, who had been gouty for twenty years, and had saturated himself with the syrup of Boubée and other vaunted specifics, consulted Dr. Pouget. At this time he was an almost constant prisoner in his room with successive attacks. After eleven days' use of the infusion, he was able to walk two kilomètres (one and a quarter English miles); in fifteen days he resumed his journeys, and was able to travel without suffering, by diligence, from Bordeaux to Quimper.

"Several other cases are detailed, some of them acute, and others chronic. Articular rheumatism, in numerous instances, was also benefited by the infusion of ash-leaves."

FUCUS VESICULOSIS.

NAT. ORD., Algæ.
COMMON NAMES, Sea-wrack. Bladder-wrack. Sea-kelp.
PREPARATION.—The fresh alga gathered in May or June are pounded to a pulp and macerated in two parts by weight of alcohol.

(The following letter, by Dr. J. Herbert Knapp to the *Homœopathic Recorder*, was published in 1896):

After treating many cases of exophthalmic goitre, I have come to the conclusion that I have found a specific for that disease in *Fucus vesiculosis* (sea-wrack). I might record one case. Mrs. Mary B., æt. 24 years, German, came into my clinic at the Brooklyn E. D. Homœopathic Dispensary to be treated for swelling of the neck of several years' duration. I gave her the tincture of *Fucus ves.*, thirty drops three times a day. The treatment began December 1, 1895, and patient was discharged cured, on October 2, 1896. Would be pleased to hear from any others who have had any experience with *Fucus vesiculosis*.

(The foregoing brought out this by Dr. R. N. Foster, of Chicago):

It gives me great pleasure to be able to say a word confirmatory of the remarks made in your December issue by J. Herbert Knapp, M. D., respecting the above named drug.

Twenty years ago, while turning over the pages of that very useful book, "The American Eclectic Dispensatory," by John King, M. D., I chanced to notice the following sentences: "*Fucus vesiculosis*, sea-wrack, or bladder-wrack,... has a peculiar odor, and a nauseous saline taste.... The charcoal of this plant has long had the reputation of a deobstruent, and been given in goitre and scrofulous swelling."

So far as I now remember, this is the only hint I ever received which led me to try the drug in goitre. At the same time, I do not feel sure of this. Perhaps I had met in some medical journal a statement respecting the relation of this drug to goitre, which fact led me to look it up in the "Eclectic Dispensatory." But if so, I cannot recall the authority. At all events, I was led to try the remedy in a pronounced case of goitre, with such good results that I have never since given any other remedy for that disease, either in the exophthalmic or in the uncomplicated form. And what is more, I have never known it to fail to cure when the patient was under thirty years of age. After that time of life, or about that period, it seems to be no longer efficacious.

I have now used it on more than twenty-four cases, with the same unvarying result, and never with any other result—that is, no unpleasant consequences have ever accompanied or followed its use.

I published this fact in the *Medical Investigator* after I had used it in a few cases, and again announced it in the Chicago Homœopathic Medical Society still later; and again have frequently repeated it with growing confidence and of greater numbers of cases in medical societies, in colleges, and in private conversation with physicians.

And yet the fact is so utterly unknown that your journal publishes Dr. Knapp's inquiry respecting it, which shows how easily a good thing may be forgotten, and how readily a genuine specific may be superseded by a host of abortive procedures right under the eyes of the profession. It is most probable that more real good things have been forgotten or cast aside in medicine than it now, or at any one time, possesses.

Respecting this *Fucus vesiculosis* and its use in goitre, I would like to add a few words. The drug is of variable quality. If one specimen fails to give satisfaction it ought to be discarded and another tried. The pharmacist must be importuned to make special efforts to give us an article that is not inert, but contains all the activity that belongs to the drug.

Time is required for effecting a cure. This varies according to the age and size of the goitre. Three months may suffice for a small goitre of one year's growth. Six months may be required for one twice as large and of longer standing. A year and a half is the longest period during which I have had to continue the medicine. But during all that time the goitre was manifestly diminishing.

The dose is a teaspoonful of the tincture twice or three times daily, in a well-developed case. Half a teaspoonful twice a day will answer in recent cases.

Smaller doses seem not to produce any effect.

The medicine is very unpleasant to the taste, but causes no disturbance after it has been taken. It ought to be taken, each dose in about two ounces of water, and preferably between meals.

GAULTHERIA.

NAT. ORD., Ericaceæ.
COMMON NAME, Wintergreen.
PREPARATION.—The distilled oil from the leaves of Gaultheria procumbens is used and dispensed in one or two drop tablets.

(These two papers were contributed to the *Homœopathic Recorder*, 1894, by Dr. Benj. F. Lang, York, Nebraska, on the action of *Gaultheria*.)

My attention was first called to its use about ten years ago in southern Ohio, where I received most pleasing results in the treatment of inflammatory rheumatism. Afterwards to a somewhat more disagreeable class of complaints in form of neuralgia. While I am not a champion of any specific, I want to say that this drug has given me the quickest and most satisfactory results of any remedy in the Materia Medica. If there is anything that a man wants relief from quick and "now," it is from these excruciating pains. Often was I called to treat some obstinate cases of ciliary neuralgia, or facial, or in fact nearly every form of neuralgia, and found my skill taxed to its utmost to bring out the balm. Did I find it in the homœopathic indicated remedy? I trust so, but not in any Materia Medica. I don't say but what I got some results from them, but I found it in this a "helper;" it came to my relief immediately and to the great comfort of the patient. In severest cases of neuralgias of the head and face it would do its work quick and well. Equally well has it served me in very severe cases of neuralgia of stomach and bowels, while for the past few years it has done faithful work in ovarian and uterine neuralgias following or preceding difficult menstruation. I have many a dear friend to-day whose relief from suffering was found in this remedy.

I am satisfied that it should be given a prominent place in our Materia Medica. Lest this article should become tedious, I will cite a few cases.

Mr. A., travelling man from Chicago, a few years ago called on me for temporary relief of a severe case of ciliary neuralgia; said he had suffered for many years with it, every spring especially, and that he had consulted great numbers of physicians of Chicago, Milwaukee and Cincinnati, and, as he said, "had taken bushels of drugs, both old and new school," with only temporary relief. So he expected nothing more, as he was told he must wear it out. I told him I thought I could give him relief. I furnished him one-half ounce of *Gaultheria*, with directions to take; did not see him again for two years, when he came into my office one day and greeted me by saying I was the only man that could ever give him any permanent relief from his sufferings; that he never had any return after first day taking medicine, and unlike most patrons wanted to make me a present of a $5 (five dollar bill), which of course no doctor refuses. I cite this first, as it was of long standing and had tested the ability of a number of prominent men.

Miss B., dressmaker, came to me suffering terribly with facial neuralgia and greeted me similar to No. 1; that she expected nothing but temporary relief, as she had been afflicted for a long time. Gave her two (2) drachms of oil W.; told her to take one dose immediately and another in two hours if the pain did not quiet down. She was careful to ask if it was an opiate, as she objected to that. I assured her it was not; saw her next day, said that pain disappeared and had not returned. I was acquainted with the lady for three and one-half years, and she only had one return of the disease, which the same remedy relieved immediately. Many cases more could I cite in which it never has failed me.

Mrs. G., No. 3. I was called to relieve a severe case of neuralgia of stomach and bowels this last summer, who had been under the care of two of my worthy competitors. They had exhausted their pill case, and for about three weeks the poor woman had suffered everything but death itself. After diagnosing the case I put her on this remedy, and in two hours she was relieved and after two days was able to be about, and was cured shortly by no other remedy than it. I want to say you will find a true friend in this remedy in all forms of neuralgia, and only give a few suggestions now; but if it should be necessary could give scores to prove its value.

I mentioned in the beginning that it had been of great value in inflammatory rheumatism. So it has, and will give later many cases of immediate and permanent relief if it would be of any value to the profession. A word as to the best way of giving the drug. I have found that the dose should never be less than five drops, and if pain is severe fifteen drops repeated in half hour; afterward two hours apart. For adult it may be necessary to give twenty drops at first. It always should be dropped on sugar and taken.

One suggestion: I would like to have it put in a tablet of about two to five drops pure oil, as I think it could be taken more satisfactorily. While the crude oil is very pleasant to take at first, yet, on account of its strong odor, will nauseate after awhile if not removed from room. I am confident that if you make this into a tablet and place it among your remedies you would have a weapon that you could place into the hands of doctors of untold value in these troubles.

(The latter part of the foregoing communication was addressed to Messrs. Boericke & Tafel, homœopathic pharmacists. This was followed by a second communication reading as follows):

Since the few lines written for the last issue of *Recorder* on *Gaultheria* in treatment of neuralgia, I have been asked to write my experience with it in inflammatory rheumatism.

It has never failed me in this terrible disease to give relief. My experience with it dates back to the fall of 1884, in Ross county, Ohio, where I was called to treat a very stubborn case, then under the treatment of one of my old school friends. The patient, a lady about fifty years old, had suffered with two previous attacks, lasting about three months each time. At the time I was called to treat her she had been confined to bed about four weeks. She was suffering intensely, the joints of upper and lower limbs being swollen and extremely tender; in fact, so sensitive that one could scarcely walk about the bed without causing great suffering; temperature, 103; pulse weak and intermittent. At my first visit, 2:30 P.M., I ordered all of the joints to be wrapped with cotton, to exclude all air. I then gave her *Bry.* On my return, next day, I did not find much improvement, excepting the nausea, which was due to heroic drugging she had been subjected to. Continued *Bry.* The next day the appetite some better, but joints still very tender; temperature and pulse about the same; some difficulty in respiration. I then resolved to try *Gaultheria*. I left one drachm vial of the remedy and ordered the same to be divided into two equal doses, one-half at one o'clock P.M., the balance at five o'clock P.M.

At about 7:30 of the same evening a messenger came into town in great haste, saying my patient was failing very fast, and requested me to come out as soon as possible. On my arrival at the home I found the patient sitting by the fire. The husband informed me that he thought she was losing her mind. I asked her why she was out of bed; she said she saw no reason for staying in bed after a patient was well, and further said that about one hour after taking the first dose she began to move easily, and after taking second dose all of the soreness and swelling left the joints. She also said she was all right; that we need not feel alarmed about her. I made only one visit after; continued the same remedy; there were no relapses.

No. 2. A prominent woman in Nebraska had been under treatment for ten days with free old-line medication, Dover's powders and *Morphia* as palliatives. Husband consulted me to know whether anything could be given to relieve her suffering. I called and found her with temperature 102, pulse 105, left (hand) fingers and elbow joints swollen, very sensitive to touch or movement. I at once assured her that I thought she would get relief without any more *Morphia*. Gave her one-half drachm *Gaultheria* and requested her to take twenty drops in two hours if pain and soreness was not relieved. This was about 4 P.M. I met her husband next morning on street on my way to visit her again and he said "that he hardly thought it necessary, as his wife was relieved in about one hour after taking first dose and felt no pain after second, and that she was up dressing her hair when he left home." She had a slight return on account of overwork, but remedy always gave relief and made firm patrons of one of our best families for me. I always advise patients to wrap the joints with cotton to exclude air and advise them to keep quiet.

No. 3. Young man, twenty-eight; had two attacks before, one lasting three months, the second ten weeks. This was the worst case that I have ever treated. As the heart was very weak, pulse intermittent, I put him on the remedy, *Gaultheria*, with almost immediate relief, but second day there was relapse, which again responded immediately to treatment by same remedy; with this, or in connection with this remedy, I used some *Bry*. 3 and *Rhus tox*. 3. I dismissed him in ten days, more than pleased, as we were always able to control the pain immediately without any other remedy than *Gaultheria*.

I cite these cases among the many that I have had, and have never failed to get good results in any; will say that I give any other remedy after soreness and swelling are removed that may be indicated, always taking the necessary precaution to exclude all air from parts affected and to keep them warm. About three hours apart is as often as I give remedy, and always careful to give it on sugar and remove it from room, with *spoon used*.

No. 4. Since my article on neuralgia I had a quite severe case of sciatica that had taxed the skill of one of my worthy competitors for nearly two months without any good results; he was about to go to Hot Springs for some relief. Meeting me on the street, wanted to know if I thought any of my "little pills or drops would give any relief." I assured him that I was quite positive that I could. He could hardly move about, and suffered very much if he did; he came and got a prescription and found relief to his great astonishment almost immediately; has had it refilled twice and has worked every day; he takes the remedy morning and night; there is no pain or soreness, nor has there been any after first day, only if he sneezes or gets the leg cramped there seems to be slight contraction of nerve, but the remedy has done most satisfactory work in this case and gained a valuable family.

I hope these few cases may be of some benefit to the readers of the *Recorder*. 1. Be careful to observe the rule that if remedy should nauseate cease giving for twelve or twenty-four hours. 2. Always give on sugar or in tablets. 3. Remove it immediately from room after administering. 4. Cover joints to exclude air and keep them warm. 5. Give any other indicated remedy.

HELODERMA HORRIDUS.

PREPARATION.—The virus, obtained by irritating the animal and allowing it to bite on glass, is triturated in the usual way.

(Dr. T. L. Bradford furnishes us with the following classification of this reptile):

The heloderma is classed as follows: Order: Saurii. Lacertilia. Lizards. Sub order: 5. Fissilinguia. Family: Lacratidæ. Heloderma horridum of Mexico; the crust lizard; the Mexican Caltetopen. Called heloderma from its skin being studded with nail or tubercle-like heads. The Gila monster is a native of Arizona, New Mexico and Texas. It is smaller than the Mexican variety, and is called, by Cope, Heloderma Suspectum. It is the only lizard whose character is not above reproach, hence the name. Zoology says: An esquamate-tongued lizard with clavicles not dilated proximally, a postorbital arch, no postfront-osquamosal arch, the pre and post frontals in contact, separating the frontal from the orbit, and furrowed teeth receiving the different ducts of highly developed salivary glands.

(There has been considerable difference of opinion as to whether the Heloderma is poisonous or not; but the following abstract from a paper on the subject read before the College of Physicians, Philadelphia, 1883, by S. Wier Mitchell, together with the provings made later, ought to very effectually settle all dispute on this point; the conclusions are the result of experiments on animals):

The poison of heloderma causes no local injury. It arrests the heart in diastole, the organ afterwards contracts slowly—possibly in rapid rigor mortis.

The cardiac muscle loses its irritability to stimuli at the time it ceases to beat. The other muscles and nerves respond to irritants.

The spinal cord has its power annihilated abruptly, and refuses to respond to the most powerful electrical currents.

This virulent heart poison contrasts strongly with serpent venom, since they give rise to local hæmorrhages, causing death chiefly through failure of respiration and not by the heart unless given in overwhelming doses. They lower muscle and nerve reactions, especially those of the respiratory apparatus, but do not cause extreme and abrupt loss of spinal power. They also produce secondary pathological appearances absent in heloderma poisoning.

The briefest examination of the lizard's anatomy makes it clear why it has been with reason suspected to be poisonous, and why it poisons with so much difficulty. Unless the teeth are entire, the poison abundant, and the teeth buried in the bitten flesh so as to force it down into contact with the ducts where they open at the crown of the teeth, it is hard to see how even a drop of poison could be forced into the wounds. Yet it is certain that small animals may die from the bite, and this may be due to the extraordinary activity of the poison, and to the lizard's habit of holding tenaciously to what it bites, so as to allow time for a certain amount of absorption.

(The provings and the clinical cases that follow were from the virus of the Gila monster obtained by Dr. Charles D. Belden, of Phœnix, Arizona, in 1890, who suggested it as a possible remedy for paralysis agitans and locomotor ataxia. He obtained the virus from a captive monster by irritating it and then letting it strike, or bite, a piece of heavy glass; by this means he obtained a few drops of a pasty yellowish fluid. In his letters Dr. Belden quotes Sir John Lubbock as follows):

This animal does not bite frequently, but when it does it is understood that the result is a benumbing paralysis like to paralysis agitans or to locomotor attaxia. There is no tetanic phase, being, as I apprehend, a condition almost reverse in objective symptoms to hydrocyanic acid or strychnia.

(Dr. Belden also writes):

It seems to me that it (the poison) differs in so many points from all present known venoms that it is worth our having. In the first place it is alkaline, and all other poisons of reptiles are acid. Second, its effect is not always sudden but is lasting—causing sickness for months and death even after a year. Again, although it does not produce paralysis it is not the tonic spasm, but rather the slow creeping death from extremities. It does not seem to excite but to depress.

(A supply of this poison was sent to Dr. Robert Boocock at his request for proving, and he made three different trials of it, the results of which were published in the *Homœopathic Recorder* for March and April, 1893; but as Dr. James E. Lilienthal has arranged the matter in schema form we will here only give fragmentary quotations from Dr. Boocock's papers, which are quite long, covering nearly thirty pages. The following is from Dr. Boocock's paper):

I am in my sixtieth year, sanguine, bilious temperament, fair complexion and weigh 160 pounds; height, 5 feet 6 inches. My normal pulse rate is 72, full, round and regular. I am in very good health. I do not drink alcoholic beverages of any kind, neither do I smoke nor drink strong coffee, or tea, or cocoa. My usual and favorite beverage is hot water with a little milk and sugar in it. If much sugar or salt is used my stomach gets very sour, and water-brash is the result. I therefore use very little of either, though I am very fond of sweetmeats.

When I received the first bottle of *Heloderma horridus*, I took a one drachm vial and filled it with the 6x trit., and dissolved it in four ounces of diluted alcohol, of which I took a few drops, dried my fingers on my tongue, and a severe feeling of internal coldness, so intense as to cause me to fear being frozen to death, ensued. I had some twitches about my heart, as if the blood was hard to get in or out. I was somewhat alarmed, but as I had no trembling I sat over the register and tried to get warm. The day was a very cold one, but my office was comfortably warm, and I had no consciousness of having taken cold.

I was not surprised at feeling this so soon after taking the few drops, for I know that I am very sensitive to any medicine and have a bad habit of tasting medicine, but never without being conscious of its effects, sometimes very unpleasantly so.

Now, to-day is warm and damp, thunderstorm this morning, although it is December 9th. The storm lasted three or more hours; lightning very vivid. I had already taken one drop of the 30th, with a very severe nervous headache, but I forgot that when I took the medicine. I have medicated 2 oz. No. 35 globules with 30th dilution, and having taken six globules as a dose before they were dry.

A feeling of heat in head and face, some headache over the right eyebrow. Cold feeling in my legs; after two hours a numb feeling around and down my left thigh; feeling very drowsy, so took a short nap in my chair. Was awakened suddenly with a jerking in my head. Central part of frontal bone so queer as to awaken me.

When my office bell rang it threw me into a startled and trembling condition, something new to me. At 5:30 took four globules more.

8 P.M. The pressure at my heart and in my head and scalp is very great. A feeling of great heat and some pressure. Not so much burning in my face, but a feeling on my left cheek as if being pricked with points of ice. A very severe and tired feeling, with coldness of legs and feet. A slight dryness of my lips, with a tingling feeling and great dryness in my throat. Gurgling in the region of the spleen.

9:30 P.M. The pressure and heat on the top of my head appears like an inflammation of the meninges. It does not affect my mind; that remains clear, and I can think and read as well and as long as ever. No more medicine. * * *

December 29, 1892. No medicine. Some trembling, but not so great or so extensive; it does not now extend along the whole limb. Parts of right arm and left thigh hemiplegial; no acute feeling. But some muscles will twitch and tremble for a few seconds. Just enough to arrest my attention and amuse me, and feel like saying, "Hello, *Heloderma hor*! have you not done with me yet?" For it is a great surprise to me how these feelings will come on and creep over me. And I am inclined to ask myself, can it be that all these strange and to me new feelings can be the effects following the taking of these few doses? And yet, if it were necessary, I could swear they were. I have my fears if I will ever be free from these nervous trembling spells, and the feeling in my head and heart.

(The foregoing gives the gist of the first trials. The third and last now follows. It was made with repeated doses of the 30th potency.)

12 meridian. Sensation as if a cold, freezing wind were blowing upon me from the bend of my knees. Head feeling as if the scalp were being drawn tight over my skull, and my facial muscles were being drawn very tight over the bones. A giddiness and a cold pressure from within the skull. A cold, running chill from superior maxillary down to the chin. Trembling of limbs. Coldness extending from the knee into the calf of the leg. Pain and pressure within the skull from crown to occiput, and from back forward over the left eye. A very drowsy feeling. I could sleep if I gave way to the feeling. * * * *

January 4, 1893, 7:45 A.M. Took another dose of six globules. Pulse, 72. Temperature, 97 3·5. A flush of heat in my face. A feeling as if I were walking on sponge or as if my feet were swollen. Dull headache. The arctic cold feeling is more in my right arm, elbow joint, and right thigh and left foot. A great trembling of my arm. It is hard work to steady my hand, which holds my book, enough to continue reading or writing.

The feeling of swelling in my feet of walking on sponges sensation continues; a springiness, with a sense of looseness in stepping out, which requires some caution, as if I were not sure of my steps. The trembling of my hands is on the increase; feeling of soreness in my heart, more under left nipple; pain in my back, lumbar region. Some little scalding of urine; flow not so free and full, intermitting slightly, as if I had some calculus in the bladder which interfered with continuous flow. Stool more free and full.

Earwax, which had been very dry, now flows from both ears, but is more free on the left side. Left nostril sore; ulcerated. Throat sore and tender to outside touch. * * *

9 P.M. Very weak feeling, with pain in my heart; same place, under left nipple. Head aches and arctic rays in various parts of my body. * * *

January 5, 12 noon. Took twelve more globules. Numb feeling in my head. A feeling as if I would fall on my right side. A good drive this morning in the snowstorm; and felt a desire to bear to the right side and could not walk straight because of this, and had repeatedly to stop or step to the left to get a straight course on the causeway. A good deal of the same feeling, but very weak and sleepy; was compelled to lie down, but did not sleep, although feeling very drowsy; laid very quiet, as if I was in a stupor; the old feeling in various parts of my body, only more acute; a feeling in various parts as if a needle were being thrust into my flesh.

4:45 P.M. Took thirteen globules. A very stiff neck the most prominent feeling. All the previously recorded feelings, only more intensely. I have a painful boring feeling in the middle third of left thigh. * * *

8:30. Flushed, hot feeling in my head and face, but no increase in color; but then I have just come out of the storm.

9:30. Took twelve globules more and retired to rest; very tired; slept very profoundly until 1 A.M., then could not sleep. My back, in the lumbar muscles, ached so and my left leg that I could not sleep for hours, and my brain felt as if scalded; an intense burning feeling in the meninges, for this did not affect my power to think. This hot feeling commenced and spread down my back. An intense pain over left eyebrow, through my left eye to base of brain and down my back. The pain in the back of my head caused me to bore my head deep into my pillow, and reminded me of cases I have seen of cerebro-spinal meningitis. An intense weakness, as if I had no power to move, and no wish to do so, and yet I was afraid I could not attend to my business. Yet, strange to say, I was not alarmed, but passively indifferent. I could not open my eyes without great effort; it was hard work to keep them open and the easiest thing for them to close, as if there were a great weight upon them, keeping them down. I begged to be allowed to remain in bed until some one wanted me professionally, and yet I could not thus give way to my feelings, and so got up.

7 A.M. Feeling very weak and giddy. Staggering about my bedroom trying to dress. It was all that I could do to lift a hod of coal to the stove. The pains in my head and lumbar muscles, back of my head near atlas and middle third of left thigh and right elbow are the most noticeable from the great pains; and arctic coldness in my feet and hands and arms; have had a

transient feeling of pain in the little finger and little toe of right side. Very feverish or parched in the night, and my breathing was hard and sounded as if I was drawing my breath through iron pipes. I feel that I must not take any more medicine at present. When I remember what a long time I was in getting to the end of the previous proving, I feel that I dare not go any further.

The dose I have been taking, a No. 35 globule, is as large as ten such as is ordinarily used for the 30th or for high dilutions, so that I have taken as good as sixty high dilution globules as a dose, and lately as high as one hundred and twenty-four and sometimes oftener daily.

I was surprised at these hot flushes and burnings in my head and along my spine. And these strongly reminded me of some feeling a proving of *Gelsemium* caused, only that has sweat, whilst this has no moisture, everything being dried up. Saliva, tears, nostrils, and earwax; the great weakness and pain in the body reminds me of cerebro-spinal meningitis.

My pulse rate is 68. 8:15. Temperature, 97 only.

1 P.M. What fearful aching in my body! Arctic feeling throughout my body, except my head and face, and oh! so tired. A feeling as if it were almost impossible to keep my eyes open. While out on my professional rounds a feeling came over me as if it would be far easier to lie down in the snowy streets than to keep trying to get along. The trembling is very persistent.

9 P.M. Oh! this bad feeling in my head, the aching, aching in my bones, in every part of my body, head to feet; no part entirely free from pain, my body so cold; a feeling as if I had holes in my garments, and cold, frosty winds were blowing through and freezing my flesh; cold penis and testicles, no feeling but coldness. A slight gluey discharge; a fluent discharge from nose, with great sneezing. * * *

January 9th, 8 A.M. Pulse rate 68; is not so full or jerky, but it is some. Temperature under the tip of the tongue, 96; deeper in, 97. This morning awoke at 3 A.M. and got up to urinate, but I could not stand without I had hold of something. Oh, such a weak, giddy feeling! I never fainted but once, from loss of blood, and these sensations are similar. Plenty of strength to hold me up, but unable to balance myself, and when I put forth an effort I staggered about like a man trying to walk with paralysis or locomotor ataxy. This idea was the most prominent in my mind, but I have a patient recovering from paralysis who has to swing his body as he walks, to get his feet forward, and is very weak and shaky about his knees, and these sensations very strongly reminded me of his efforts. His weakness is in his knees, but mine was from the base of my skull—cerebrum—where the pains have been so persistent near the atlas extending downward. When I arose, at 7 A.M., it was very hard work for me to balance myself enough to complete dressing myself, and very hard work to carry my head. If I bent forward, then it required great effort to keep from falling on my face or backward. This lack of balancing power was accompanied by a sensation of nausea, as if I were going to vomit. I persisted in my efforts to work, in hopes of shaking off these very alarming sensations, and by effort got through my morning work. Whilst shaving a severe jerk of my right arm caused me to gash my face; very strange, but I ought not to have tried to do this. I have now some numbness in my right hand and arm, and a good deal of trembling. Arctic feeling in my feet and in various parts of my body. This feeling of want of balancing power does not entirely leave me; a full, pressing feeling in all parts of my head. And when I walk I notice I lift my feet higher than usual, or than is necessary, and I put my heel down hard, as if I was not sure of holding on to the ground. I notice some twitching, as if my feet would spring up, making me walk as if I had the cock's gait, as it is described. * * *

7 A.M., January 10, 1893. Thank God I began this day with more comfort and more control of myself; my limbs are easier to manage; a little giddiness and staggering, and stiff, bruised sensation in my back and lower limbs. My cervical vertebra is less sore and have little pain; and altogether feel very much better. My pulse rate is 80 this A.M.; full and round; no jerks perceptible. Temperature 98 under the tongue, by the root. Mercury very slow in rising; had to keep the thermometer in a long time. I have a flushed, hot feeling in my face and head; no trembling, less staggering, and can manage my limbs fairly well. I feel as I dared not trifle with myself any further, for I am very weak. A very little exertion would make me feel very ill. I am feeling like a man who had just come from under a deadly risk; am very weak and prostrated, with every nerve on the jump. Oh, so very weak! A sinking feeling. A parched thirstiness in my throat and mouth. My tongue is clean; bowels regular; a good deal of flatus, very fetid; pale yellow, greenish urine (specific gravity 1008), smelling very fetid; same smell as the flatus; more like the smell of rotting sweet fruit or vegetables. * * *

January 14, 1893. Could not get out of bed at my usual time; very severe pain in head and back of neck, going down my back and right leg; twitches, with cold, stinging, ice-needle pricks. My right hand is feeling as if it were frozen. Pulse rate 64; full, round, but appears to have a pendulum motion or twitch. Temperature 96 3-5. Mind clear, but very weak in my body, and I can not get warm over a hot register or with hot fluids. This constant arctic cold is very hard to bear and makes me this morning feel as if I had a cake of ice on my back. My hands are blue with cold and my feet feel like lumps of ice. Headache and giddiness; could not keep from trembling while some patients were in my consulting room, and had a good deal of difficulty in steadying and controlling my voice; when excited could not get hold of the right words I wanted and dropped some when speaking, from a want of flexibility or a catch in my tongue. Pains in various parts of my body; the same locations and character. Quite a rush of business to-day and very ill-fitted to attend to it. My hands and feet blue and aching with cold, even while I was sitting over a hot register that scorched my boot leather, yet no feeling of warmth in hands or feet. A good deal of throbbing and aching in the upper part of my kidneys, the right one the sorest. Sharp pains in my bowels, near the cæcum; some trembling (when asleep it awoke me) in my right arm and left leg, with a sharp pain near the ankle joint. * * *

January 20. Awoke this morning in a shivering fit. Trembling, giddiness and headache, but not very severe. Cold arctic feeling. Pulse 68. Temperature 97 1-5. My feet, 8 A.M., cold. Severe pain in left testicle, extending through to the back to anus. Bleed very much from old piles. An aching at end of penis, and no sexual desire. A feeling as if the testicles were swollen and painful, as in orchitis; this is only a transient pain, and comes and goes at infrequent periods, or remittent in their character. I notice my urine is taking on the greenish-yellow again, and my right arm is chilly from the arctic rays. My feet are cold, and the coldness creeps up higher in my legs. A great deal of arctic feeling in and around my heart. My breath is cold. Headache, but mind clear. Cold chills run over me in various parts of my body. My hands tremble very much at times, so that I can not write. Pain in testicles and coldness, as if they were frozen. Pass a large quantity of urine. * *

January 21. 8 A.M. Did not get up before, owing to the pressure in my skull, as if it were too full; dropsy or some swelling of my brain; giddiness, and a numbness down my left leg, and a jerking upward in both of them. Some trembling and coldness around my heart, and in my lungs and down my arms. My feet were very hot in the night until 5 A.M., when they became cold, numb and jerky, upwards. My pulse rate is very slow this morning, only 56 beats. Temperature is slowly forced up to 98. I have a sensation as if my left cheek were swollen, but it is not so. Trembling very much in my hands.

2:30 P.M. Have not been warm yet to-day; very intense arctic sensation in my body and heart and lungs. Slight cough. Numbness in my right arm. Much trembling, and a sensation of inward trembling in all parts of my body. Generative organs frozen cold, and this coldness extends up my back. My feet so cold that I have burned my boots, and yet cannot get them warm. Coldness extends up to my knees. Stiffness and pain in left thigh. Cold arctic band round my head, with fulness in skull. Pulse 60. Temperature 97 4-5. Good appetite. Mentally clear, although very weak;

very tired and discouraged that these feelings last so long. They seem to be all beginning over again; worse now than they were a week ago. I feel more like giving up and going to bed sick, but I cannot afford to do so, so I brace up and resist this temptation to try and find an antidote for these recurring series of feelings. * * *

January 23. Slept well until 5 A.M.; then awoke with pains in head and burning in my feet, with some trembling and stiff feeling in my lungs and heart, as if they were tied or unable to move. As I lay awake I could hear my heart pounding away, but, oh! so slow. Felt very weak and wanted to stay in bed, but after some hard thinking I got up. 7 A.M. Very weak; staggered about while dressing. Pains in the base of the brain. Pulse 64 and irregular in its beats, some of them failing altogether to declare themselves only by their absence to respond. Temperature, after being held under my tongue ten minutes, 97 2-5. Very cold in my back and over my shoulders; hands and feet are blue with cold. Itching all over my body, and as if I was bitten with fleas or bugs were crawling over me. Skin of my hands very rough and cracks are in them. My ears have a feeling as if wax were running out of them. * * *

January 26, 10 P.M. It has required a mighty effort to keep up this day. My pulse 56, slow and irregular; temperature 98. Headache, yet mind clear; backache. Weakness in all my body; my limbs so weak in walking that it was difficult to keep going, and felt as if I could lay down or drop down anywhere. What heart failure symptoms are I do not know, but fear I came very near it and yet I have resisted this feeling, and kept awake and about. Have felt very ill all the day, and am so now on retiring, 11 P.M. * * *

January 29. 9 A.M. Just after breakfast, pulse 68, temperature 99; slept very heavy, but dreamed of treating many cases of black diphtheria. Awoke, slept, dreamed the same dream again, and again the same dream, three separate times. How very singular! During these provings, I have done this three separate times. Three dreams in one night—the same dream, the same disease, the same families in my dream. This singularity caused me to lay awake wondering what this can mean. I have not any patients suffering from this disease, and I do not know of any in the town, and nothing that I know of to bring this disease to my mind. Awoke feeling very stiff and sore. * * *

January 30. Head pains again, the same old character. Sensation of swelling in my face and pain in nerves of teeth, molars. Hot feeling. Pulse, 68. Temperature, 99. Very weak, but my mind clear. Much trembling and the oppression round my heart and chest producing a suffocating feeling that makes me afraid, and I must now seek some means to arrest this difficulty and give me some relief. I know it looks cowardly to give up, but my family compels me to do something to enable me to keep about. I cannot do any more; this heart oppression makes me think of heart failure. Pulse, 56, and temperature 96. Very weak. I hope it will wear away and this trembling improve. They have been caused by this drug, one of the most powerful. I gave up and went to bed very ill. I had to keep it from my family, but I was afraid my heart would stop beating and had a very restless night. I took acetic acid, as vinegar I had in some pickles I thought changed or relieved the first class or effort of provings and caused me to stop and begin again. I think it did help me. Next day very prostrated but did not take any note of my pulse or temperature, because I had began to try to find an antidote, and this vinegar and lemon juice has relieved many of them. I fear sometimes that the trembling in my hands may never fully leave me now.

February 12, 1893. Copying my notes has brought so vividly to my memory that I can almost feel the old arctic rays through my body, and the giddiness and staggering gait of the *Heloderma hor.* days. I hope that you may have many others more courageous than I have been, whose provings will compare or improve upon this poor effort of mine.

CLINICAL.

The case of paralysis that I spoke of, whose staggering gait was called to my mind by my feelings, is now taking *Heloderma.*

In the following case, Mrs. Ford, eighty-one years of age, has been my patient several times during the last four years. She suffered from erysipelas and dropsy in the legs. In September I was again called in for the same old trouble; the usual remedies were effectual. In October she caught cold, and had also a bad fall; her symptoms were those of pneumonia, fever, delirium and cough, pain in chest and hard work to breathe, blueness of lips, tongue and cheeks, cold extremities and was very low in appetite, and appeared to be sinking. Pulse, fifty; temperature, ninety, and to all human appearance was rapidly dying; all said so, and I fully believed so, but left *Heloderma horridus*, one powder in water, and ordered her tongue to be moistened with a feather dipped in this every half hour. I did not call the next day until evening. I was waiting to be notified of her death, but no such notice coming called to see, and, to my surprise, found everything changed. I then gave *Helo. hor.* 200, every four hours, with placebos. All the bad symptoms gradually disappeared, breathing became natural, heart gained strength, pulse increased to seventy, temperature to ninety-eight and appetite became better, asking frequently for food. This continued so long as she was taking this medicine. She was so well that I ceased to attend, she having no aches or pains, was eating and sleeping well, bowels moved regularly and night watching was given up. All who saw the recovery were pleasingly surprised, and so was I, and have frequently asked myself could anything else have done this. *Lachesis* has changed a slate colored tongue, and has aroused those who appeared to be dying for a short time, but to extend the life of one as good as dead for thirty days is a triumph for the *Helo. hor.*

(To the foregoing we may add that some have thought that the proving was too sensational, but other evidence that has not appeared in print leads to the conclusion that it is essentially true, and that the proving was made by one peculiarly susceptible to the remedy. We know of one gentleman who laughed at it and in bravado took a number of doses during an afternoon. He felt no immediate effects, but during the night awoke with some very peculiar feelings that he could attribute to nothing but the *Heloderma*, and they were of such a character that he refused to take any more. It would be well to use the remedy with caution until the practitioner has gauged its powers.)

(Dr. Charles E. Johnson wrote as follows to Dr. Boocock concerning the remedy):

"I have had under treatment a case that has been pronounced incurable by many physicians. She has had most of the symptoms developed in your proving, that awful coldness being most pronounced. She has had two doses of the 200th. I learn through a neighbor that she is delighted with the result of the last medicine. The coldness has nearly disappeared, leaving a comfortable glow upon the body. She tells her neighbors this without having been informed by me what results I expected from the medicine."

(Dr. Erastus E. Case contributed the following detailed clinical case to the *Medical Advance*, July, 1897):

An auburn haired woman, 55 years of age, had numbness in the feet two years ago. It has gradually extended upward until it now includes the lower part of the abdomen.

Tingling, creeping sensation on the legs as if from insects.

Worse when lying in bed at night.

Worse from exposure to cold air.

Worse from touch; she cannot endure to place her bare feet together.

Legs insensible to an electric battery.

Legs wasting away, skin very dry and inelastic.

Ankles turn easily when trying to walk.

Numbness of the arms from the hands to the elbows.

Forgetfulness.

Melancholy with weeping.

Worse in stormy weather.

Worse when thinking of her ailments, cheered by company.

Pain in the forehead in the morning, aggravated by turning the eyes.

Tongue dry and cracked in the morning.

Swallowing difficult.

Empty eructations, especially before breakfast.

Empty, gone sensation in the stomach.

Dislikes sweet things and worse from taking them.

Sensation of constriction about the whole abdomen.

Constipation from torpor of the rectum.

Hemorrhoids and itching of the anus.

Burning in the urethra during and after micturition.

Burning and dryness of the vagina.

Palpitation and dyspnœa from slight exertion.

Drawing sensation in all the extremities.

Yellow skin.

April 11, 1895. *Heloderma horridus* four powders, one every four hours.

April 23, 1895. Decidedly more cheerful and memory is better.

Bowels more active.

Legs more reliable, with the numbness and tingling.

No medicine.

April 26, 1895. Alarmed because the palms and soles are swollen and itching.

No medicine.

May 22, 1895. She gained rapidly in both flesh and strength, until a week ago.

Heloderma horridus one powder.

Soon after this an itching eruption came all over her, which subsided without any further medication. She was restored to a fair degree of health so that she has taken care of her house and family up to the present time.

(The following arrangement of Dr. Boocock's proving was made by Dr. Lilienthal):

Mind.—No inclination for exertion in any way.

Difficulty in remembering the spelling of simple words.

Depressed, feels blue.

Head.—Sensation of heat in head; heat on vertex.

Headache over right eyebrow.

Pressure in head and scalp; pressure in skull as if too full.

Soreness and stiffness in occiput, extending down neck; sore spot in various parts of head.

Intense pain over left eyebrow, through eye to base of brain and down back.

Aching at base of brain.

Sharp, digging pains.

Benumbed feeling all over head.

Burning feeling in brain.

Throbbing on top of head; head sore and bruised.

Sensation of band around head.

Cold band around head.

Sensation as if scalp was drawn tight over skull.

Bores head in pillow.

Vertigo and weakness when moving quickly.

Dizziness, with inclination to fall backward.

Eyes.—Itching of eyelids, lachrymation.

Weight of eyelids, difficult to keep them open.

Ears.—Pressure behind left ear; pressure in ear from within outward.

Copious flow of wax.

Ears dry and scurfy.

Nose.—Left nostril sore; ulcerated.

Dry, itching scurfs in nostrils.

Severe attack of sneezing. Fluent discharge.

Face.—Sensation of heat. Flushes of heat.

Cold, crawling feeling from temple down right cheek.

Sensation as if pricked with points of ice.

Sensation as if facial muscles were drawn tight over bones.

Stiffness of jaw.

Mouth.—Dryness of lips.

Soreness.

Very thirsty.

Tongue tender and dry.

Throat.—Dryness; parched sensation.

Tingling.

Soreness, tenderness to touch.

Stinging, sore feeling in right tonsil.

Stomach.—Acid burning in stomach.

Hypochondria.—Gurgling in region of spleen.

Abdomen.—Sharp shooting pain in bowels, more on left side.

Pain across pubic bones, extending down into left testicle.

Stitching pains in bowels.

Throbbing in bowels.

Rumbling in bowels.

Stool.—Loose, copious stool, lumpy, preceded by stitches in abdomen.

Stool loose, mushy with considerable flatus.

Stool soft, dark, difficult to expel.

Hæmorrhoids swollen, itch and bleed.

Urinary Organs.—Bladder irritable, frequent urging to pass urine.

Tenderness in urethra, with sensation of discharge.

Urine not as free as usual, muddy.

Intermittent flow.

Urine, specific gravity, 1010; greenish-yellow, fetid (decaying fruit).

Sexual Organs.—Erections.

Cold penis and testicle, with gluey discharge.

Pain and enlargement of left testicle.

Female.—

Respiratory Organs.—Slight, hacking cough, with pain in left scapulæ.

Fulness in chest, requiring an effort to inflate the lungs.

Oppressed for breath from least exertion.

Chest.—Sharp stitch through right nipple to inside of right arm.

Cold feeling in right lung.

Heart.—Pressure at heart.

Tingling around heart.

Trembling and coldness around heart.

Oppression around heart.

Sticking pains, shooting from left to right.

Stitches in heart.

Soreness in heart, more under left nipple.

Pulse, 56-72; full and jerky.

Back.—Stiff neck; aching in bones of neck.

Painfulness of upper neck.

Coldness across scapulæ.

Chill in back from base of brain downwards.

Pain in back; pain in lumbar muscles awakening him.

Aching in right kidney; stitch pain in right kidney.

Upper Extremities.—Numbness of right arm and hand with trembling.

Tingling in arms and hands.

Tingling in palm of left hand and along fingers.

Drawing in left hand, followed by tingling and prickling.

Pains in hands, if holding anything for some time.

Trembling of hands.

Hands blue, cracked and rough.

Lower Extremities.—Numb feeling around and down left thigh.

Pain in left thigh and calf as if bruised.

Numb feeling down right leg.

Coldness extending from knee to calf.

Coldness of legs and feet.

Boring sharp pain on tibia of right leg.

Sensation of tight hand around left ankle.

Trembling of limbs. Jerking of limbs.

Tingling and burning of feet as if recovering from being frozen.

Burning in feet, preventing sleep, had to put them out of bed.

Sensation as if walking on sponge and as if swollen.

Staggering gait.

Tendency to turn to right when walking.

When walking lift feet higher than usual and put down heel hard.

Skin.—Itching of skin as from insects.

Sleep.—Drowsiness, but inability to sleep.

Restless sleep; awakens at 3 A.M.

Awakened from sleep by jerking in head; trembling of limbs; pain in lumbar muscles.

Fever.—Internal coldness.

Severe chill ran down back.

Cold rings around body.

Cold waves ascend from feet, or downward from base of brain.

Nerves.—Startled easily. Trembling.

Tired feeling; very weak and nervous.

Intense aching in bones and all parts of body.

Trembling of left side; hands shaky.

Trembling can be controlled by effort of will.

Generalities.—Stretching relieves pains in muscles and limbs.

Stitch pains going from left to right.

Weak, giddy, making it difficult to stand.

Unable to balance myself.

Movement does not increase the pain.

Throbbing all over body.

Bone pains.

JACARANDA GUALANDAI.

NAT. ORD., Bignoniaceæ.
COMMON NAME, Carroba.
PREPARATION.—The dried leaves are crushed and macerated in five parts by weight of alcohol.

(Of this South American remedy the *Dispensatory* says it is used in Brazil and other South American countries for syphilis; sometimes under the name *Carroba*. Its value was also asserted in *British Medical Journal*, 1885. The following letter from Dr. J. F. Convers, of Bogota, to Messrs. Boericke & Tafel, throws some further light on its use; the letter is dated November 24, 1888):

Dear Gentlemen: Please to accept the leaves of a tree of the Bignoniacea family, called *Jacaranda gualandai*, that I send you with this, because it is very much used by our natives to cure illness of a syphilitic character. I have used the mother tincture (5 drops *pro dosi*), and the 3d dilution of it, in the treatment of blennorrhagia and chancroids with the greatest success. In my experience I have found that this medicine is a complementary and antidote to *Merc. v.*

Mr. José M. Reyes, who proved the θ and the 2x dilution during more than one month three times a day, found the following results:

HEAD.—Vertigo on rising after stooping, with momentary loss of sight, and sensation of heaviness in the forehead. Weakness of memory and inability to study.

EYES.—*Pains and inflammation of the eyes, with redness more marked in the left eye. Sensation of sand in both eyes.* Ophthalmia, which begins in the left eye, with lachrymation and night agglutination of the eyelids. Weakness of sight. Syphilitic-like ophthalmia.

STOOL.—Diarrhœa with dark mulberry-colored stools without pain or tenesmus, but with mucus.

URINARY AND SEXUAL ORGANS.—Increased secretion of the urine. Pain in the penis. *Blennorrhagia* with a discharge which stains the linen a dirty yellow color. *Chancroids.*

THROAT.—Pain and burning of the larynx, when laughing or reading aloud, and small vesicles in the pharynx.

BACK.—Weakness of the lumbar region.

These are not doubtful symptoms.

N. B.—This remedy acts on the head at first, afterwards on the intestines, and on the eyes last.

Please try it, and make it known to our colleagues. Should it prove to be there as good as here, I assure you it will be a valued remedy.

(Dr. J. S. Whittinghill contributed the following, *Eclectic Medical Journal*, concerning *Jacaranda*):

Let me give the results of my experience with *Jacaranda*. I believe it to be a true specific for certain kinds of rheumatism. Its first trial was given a patient suffering as follows: She had had rheumatism for about ten years— never became serious. Sometimes she was nearly relieved from it; again lost much rest and sleep from it. Her wrist would become painful and very weak from ordinary labor. She always suffered very much in the morning upon any motion, and complained of being stiff. Had to have assistance in dressing. Upon sudden motion, sensation in the muscles as of tearing and being bruised—even painful upon pressure.

I gave her different remedies as they seemed to be indicated, with no results towards removing the trouble. I thought there could be nothing lost by trying *Jacaranda*. It met with decided success. She was entirely relieved of muscular pains in a few days. Had the recurrence of some symptoms in about six weeks after; tried *Jacaranda* again with the same decided success. Some eight weeks have elapsed since, with no recurrence of muscular pains. I have tried it on three other patients with the same peculiar morning stiffness and soreness of muscles. All were relieved in a few days. They have no more muscular trouble. So I put morning soreness and stiffness of muscles as the guide in prescribing *Jacaranda*.

LAC CANINUM.

PREPARATION.—The fresh milk from a bitch is triturated in the usual way.

(The late Dr. Sam. Swan had a proving of this remedy, dog milk, in the Materia Medica he attempted to publish, but of which only one volume appeared. The work is now very rare. The following clinical cases were contributed by Dr. Philip Rice to the *Medical Century*, Vol. IX, No. 24):

Lac caninum is a remedy of undoubted value, though not very thoroughly understood and consequently not very extensively used in this dread disease. And since a proving has never been made, and since we have to depend entirely upon clinical reports I feel it my duty to report a few cases in which a clear demonstration of the value of this remedy was made.

CASE I.—Bruce McG., æt. 15, dark hair, gray eyes, spare habit, rigid fibre, nervous, quick, active, called at my office in the evening complaining of sore throat, worse on right side, and on swallowing. Headache dull and heavy, slight fever. Inspection revealed tonsils and fauces congested and angry looking. On right tonsil a patch of membrane the size of a split pea was seen.

Lycopodium 30x was given. The next morning the entire trouble seemed to have gone to the left side; with it had come, also, stiff neck and tongue; profuse flow of saliva; temperature 101 F. Membrane somewhat larger. *Mercurius ruber* 30x was given. In the evening the trouble was worse again on right side, the membrane now entirely covering both tonsils, temperature 102 F. Limbs ached, back ached, and patient was restless. Remembering the symptom, "membrane alternates between right and left sides," and this having been so characteristic, I gave *Lac caninum* in the 30th potency. Improvement began immediately and at the end of the third day the membrane was entirely gone and case discharged as far as medicine was concerned.

CASE II.—Louisa McG., æt. 13, in temperament exactly like her brother, the preceding case. Was irritable and listless for two days, but owing to the fact that the fair began in a few days, to which she was determined to go, she did not complain. The third day, however, her mother noticed that she was truly sick and, there being a number of cases of diphtheria in town, looked into her throat. She found both tonsils covered with a membrane. I was called and as no other symptoms could be elicited I gave *Sulphur* 30x and told them I would call again in the evening, which I did and found symptoms rapidly developing. Aching in all the limbs; headache; pain in the throat on swallowing; worse on the right side; neck and tongue stiff; membrane just the same. Temperature 101.5; same remedy continued.

Next morning the membrane was the same, pain now in left side, throat internally and externally œdematous, fauces and uvula glossy or varnished in appearance. Temperature 102, urine scanty, no thirst. *Apis* 30x was now given. In the evening pain back in right side again. Temperature 102.5. Membrane spreading; stiffness of neck and tongue more marked and saliva profuse. Not having seen the case till the membrane had quite generally formed, but the patient being in temperament like her brother and the pain shifting from side to side, as in his case, I decided to give her *Lac caninum*. Improvement began immediately and at the end of four days the membrane was entirely gone.

CASE III.—The servant girl in the family where cases one and two had been, Anna B., æt. 17. In temperament the very opposite to the other cases, being fat, fair and flabby. Complained of pain in right side of throat on swallowing, neck stiff, tonsil slightly congested. Felt as if she had a bad cold. Advised her to come to the office and get some medicine. She had, however, some "dope" on hand and said she guessed she would take that first. Next evening I was called and found her with throat much worse. Membrane covering left tonsil entirely, also a narrow strip of membrane on posterior wall of pharynx, pain in left tonsil on swallowing, neck and tongue stiff, saliva quite profuse. Temperature only slightly above normal. *Lac caninum* 30x was given. Patient never went to bed and at the end of the second day no trace of membrane could be seen.

Now, the symptoms common to all three cases and the only ones characteristic in each case were, first, both pain and membrane shifting from side to side; second, stiffness of neck and tongue; third, profuse saliva; fourth, aching in limbs marked; fifth, entire absence of prostration; sixth, character of pain was "as if throat was burned raw." Now, the question will arise in the bacteria man's mind, was this real diphtheria; were the German's bacteria present? I will answer candidly, I don't know; I never looked for them.

LAPIS ALBUS.

SYNONYM. Silico-Fluoride of Calcium.

PREPARATION.—The residue obtained by evaporation, from the waters of the mineral springs of Gastein, Germany, is triturated in the usual way.

(It was Von Grauvogl who first called attention to this drug, the product of certain mineral springs in Germany, that have reputation for curing ulcers, cancers, tumors, etc. In the Transactions of the American Institute of Homœopathy, 1896, will be found the following by Dr. W. A. Dewey):

My experience with this remedy, and I have been somewhat interested in it, dates from about 1876. At that time a member of my own family had an enlargement of one of the cervical glands. It was nearly as large as a hen's egg, and had a soft, doughy feel. Under *Lapis albus* 6, prescribed, I believe, by Dr. G. E. E. Sparhawk, now of Burlington, Vt., the swelling speedily and completely disappeared. A peculiar and unusual symptom noticed by this patient while taking the medicine was a marked increase in the appetite; it became ravenous.

Since that time I have used the remedy in many cases of scrofulous enlargement of the cervical glands, and find that it is almost specific where the glands have a certain amount of elasticity and pliability about them, rather than a stony hardness, such as might call for *Calcarea fluorica*, *Cistus* or *Carbo animalis*.

One case in particular which I recall was a young lady, about twenty years of age, a natural blonde, skin fair, bluish white, showing prominent veins, who had a glandular enlargement in the right supra-clavicular region, nearly the size of a goose egg, and one somewhat smaller a little farther back in the interval between the sterno-cleido mastoid and trapezius muscles. These had a certain amount of hardness, but they were movable. Others of the cervical chain were also enlarged, the right side being the only one affected. As the young lady was engaged to be married, these unsightly lumps were very distressing. *Lapis albus* 6, a powder four times a day, in a week caused a marked diminution of the size of the glands, and in three weeks they were not noticeable, and eventually entirely disappeared. This patient also had a ravenous appetite while taking the remedy, an unusual thing for her. Her anæmic color and complexion were also greatly improved.

The most remarkable effect of the use of the remedy I have had was in the case of goitre in a lady of about thirty-five, blonde, who had for over a year noticed a gradual increase in the size of the thyroid gland, until it was as large as a good-sized fist, when she came to me. Both halves of the gland seemed to be equally involved. It did not appear to be of the encapsulated variety. This patient had received previous homœopathic treatment, having had *Spongia, Iodine, Thuja,* as well as some other remedies. *Lapis albus* 6 was prescribed, a dose every three hours. The swelling began to disappear at once, and continued to diminish in size until it completely disappeared, and at the present time over five years have passed with no return of the trouble.

LATRODECTUS MACTANS.

PREPARATION.—The spiders are triturated in the usual way.

(The following paper by Dr. Samuel A. Jones appeared in the *Homœopathic Recorder*, July, 1889, under the title, "Latrodectus Mactans: a Suggested Remedy in Angina Pectoris"):

"The great result of the grim doctor's labor, so far as known to the public, was a certain preparation or extract of cobwebs, which, out of a great abundance of material, he was able to produce in any desirable quantity, and by the administration of which he professed to cure diseases of the inflammatory class, and to work very wonderful effects upon the human system."—*Dr. Grimshawe's Secret.*

I do not know that the doctor who is the direct occasion of this paper was *grim*, nor do I imagine he ever dreamed of such an application of his paper as I purpose to make. I never met him; though he wore the gray and I the blue during a struggle wherein fate might easily have thrown us together. It was not until the autumn of '76 that I became aware of his existence, and then by a contribution of his to a medical magazine—the special copy of which was found amongst the multifarious waifs of a bookstall. I could not "decline the article," although I was then entering upon a field of labor that would leave little time for such quiet research as the old doctor's paper so powerfully suggested, so I bought the odd number, and fourteen years later I am making such use of it as my sense of its significance enforces.

It is due Mr. A. J. Tafel to state that but for his most efficient services this paper of mine would never have been written. To his endeavors, stretching through some years, I owe the identification of the remedy, without which I should not have put pen to paper; and having secured this, from unimpeachable authority, too, he never rested from his labors until he had put in my possession dilutions of the poison itself. If, then, this *magis venenum* shall prove itself *magis remedium*, most assuredly the *pars magna* of its introduction is his.

From the days of Dioscorides and Pliny to the present a venomous quality has been ascribed to "the fluid emitted from the orifice in the fangs of the arancidæ." That this quality was even lethal has been both believed and questioned. *Insect Life*, Vol. I., No. 7, pp. 204-211, Washington, 1889, contains "A Contribution to the Literature of Fatal Spider Bites," in which the credulity of mere medical observers and the emphatic incredulity of professed "entomologists and arachnologists" are dwelt upon, and concerning which its author cautiously concludes as follows:

"It will possibly appear to the reader that after collecting this testimony we are as far from the solution of the question—'Do spider bites ever produce fatal results?'—as we were before; but it seems to us, after analyzing the evidence, that it must at least be admitted that certain spiders of the genus Latrodectus have the power to inflict poisonous bites which may (probably exceptionally and depending upon exceptional conditions) bring about the death of a human being. Admitting in its fullest force the argument that in reported cases the spider has seldom if ever been seen by a reliable observer to inflict the wound, we consider that the fact that species of the Latrodectus, occurring in such widely distant localities as South Europe, the Southern United States, and New Zealand, are uniformly set aside by the natives as poisonous species, when there is nothing especially dangerous in their appearance, is the strongest argument for believing that these statements have some verification in fact. It is no wonder that a popular fear should follow the ferocious-looking spiders of the family Theraphosoidæ; but considering the comparatively small size and modest coloring of the species of Latrodectus so wide-spread a prejudice, occurring in so many distinct localities, must be well founded." P. 211.

Is it indeed an *argument* that "in reported cases the spider has seldom if ever been seen by a reliable observer to inflict the wound?" How an Orfila, a Christison, and a Caspar would smile when asked if the evidence of a poisonous quality depended upon the administration of the poison being "seen by a reliable observer." Toxicology detects a poison by the physiological test as well as the chemical. Strychnia in quantity too small for the coarse chemical test is revealed by the tetanized muscles of a frog whether that "arch martyr to science" be in "South Europe, the Southern United States, or New Zealand," and that infinitesimal fractions of Strychnia will display its characteristics whether or not its administration is "seen" by a Christison, or a college janitor. Of course, a Christison would recognize Strychnia from and in the phenomena, while a college janitor (and here and there an over-scientific entomologist) might not.

It is neither the aim nor the purpose of this paper to establish the lethal property of spider poison; though I must acknowledge that, until I read the paper in *Insect Life*, I had no thought that its possession of such a property would be called in question. I shall content myself with calling attention to the pathogenetic quality of the poison of *Latrodectus mactans*, leaving my reader to discern the resemblance of its *tout ensemble* to an attack of angina pectoris, and therefore to infer its homœopathic applicability in that dread disorder. I shall not enter upon the pathology—various and much confused—of that cardiac seizure, because, as I get older, I find the "like" more and more of a "pillar of cloud by day and pillar of fire by night," whilst in my short life I have found "pathology" as changeable as a dying dolphin—and every one knows that a dead fish "stinks and shines, and shines and stinks."

BY G. WILLIAM SEMPLE, M. D., HAMPTON, VA.[1]

"Spider bites are of rare occurrence in this vicinity, but are generally productive of grave symptoms. [Isn't it bad taste for doctors to use the words grave symptoms?] I will report all that have occurred to me in a practice of forty years:

"CASE I. September 4, 1853. I was called to see Mr. D., at Old Point, who had been bitten by a small, black spider on the prepuce, whilst on the privy seat, at 12:30 o'clock. The bite at first caused only itching of the prepuce, with a little redness of the part, but in less than half an hour *nausea*, followed by *severe abdominal pains*, ensued. A messenger was dispatched in haste for me to Hampton, three miles off. Before I reached the patient, at 2:30 o'clock, *violent præcordial pains extending to the axilla, and down the* [left] *arm and forearm to the fingers*, with *numbness of the extremity*, had succeeded, attended by *apnœa*.

"In consequence of the violence of the symptoms, Dr. Stineca, surgeon of the post, had been sent for, who had given two doses of *Laudanum* of ʒj each, and two of rectified whiskey of ℥ij each, and, being in ill health and unable to remain, had ordered his steward to apply four dry cups over the præcordia. This had just been done when I arrived. I saw the *blood, thin and florid*, fill the cups like water oozing through the muslin. When the cups were removed, the *blood*, emptied into a basin, *did not coagulate*; and blood continued to ooze slightly from the surfaces to which the cups had been applied until the next morning, though a solution of *Tannin* was applied.

"I found the patient *suffering extremely from the most violent præcordial pains and from apnœa*, and also *violent pain in the left* arm, which was almost *paralyzed*. His *pulse* was 130 *and very feeble*, his *skin cold* as marble, and his *countenance expressive of the deep anxiety* he felt and expressed in words. The laudanum and whiskey seemed to have produced no effect—the nausea and abdominal pains having subsided before they were administered. There was no pain, inflammation, or swelling where the bite was received. Even the itching of the part had subsided. I gave the patient every half hour for several hours ʒj of aromatic spirits of ammonia, and as much whiskey and water as he could be induced to take, and afterwards gave them every hour; also pediluvia of hot mustard and water, frequently repeated, until the next night.

"September 5th, 8 A.M.—The symptoms continued unabated; indeed, the patient grew worse until 2:30 o'clock, twenty-six hours after he was bitten, for his *pulse* had then become *so frequent that it could not be counted, and so feeble that it could scarcely be felt*. He then *vomited black vomit* copiously—a quart or more. Soon afterwards reaction set in, his pulse gradually gained force, and became less frequent, the pain subsided and the respiration improved. At 8 P.M., the pulse had gained considerable force, and the patient slept until some minutes after 12; his pulse was pretty full at 1:10; his surface warm and perspirable, and he felt almost free of pain. After a short interval he again fell asleep, and slept quietly until morning, when he awoke—his respiration healthy, pulse 80, regular and with sufficient force, and entirely relieved of pain. He soon afterwards had *two pretty copious evacuations from the bowels*, similar to the black vomit he had vomited. After this he said he felt quite well, and took a light breakfast and dinner, and returned that evening to his residence in Portsmouth, and in a few days went to work at his trade.

"In thirty-six hours from the time he was bitten, he took three and a half quart bottles of the best rectified whiskey—about three quarts without showing the least symptom of intoxication."

I have cited this case at full length in order to present the *evolution of the symptoms*, on which alone depends the resemblance of the action of the poison to the chief symptoms of an attack of angina pectoris—a closer resemblance than half a lifetime of somewhat wide reading has enabled me to find in the effect of any other noxious agent. In fact, after much searching, I find this case to be unique. In other cases of spider bite I can find evidence that assures me of its genuineness, but, to my knowledge, its *order of symptom evolution* is as solitary as it is singular and significant. This feature of *uniqueness* will cause many to regard it with suspicion. I think they will do wrong; for some experience in proving work has taught me that one positive result from a drug out-weighs any number of negative.

In the case of *Latrodectus mactans* we shall find, from other poisonings, that, as a rule, it displays an affinity for the præcordial region as the *locus* of its chief attack; and having assurance of that fact, we shall not find it difficult to accept a clue from even a solitary instance.

Of the remaining cases in Dr. Semple's paper I shall cite only the symptoms, and be it observed that in all the cases as here given the italics are my own.

CASE 2. A man "was bitten in the groin, and complained of only a slight prickling and itching at the spot where he was bitten, but was complaining [when Dr. S. saw him] of *severe abdominal pain*, with *nausea*, and a *sinking sensation at the epigastrium*; and his *pulse*, in a few minutes after the bite, had already become *quick and thready*; and the *skin very cold*." The man soon recovered under ammonia and whiskey—two quarts of the latter produced no symptoms of intoxication.

CASE III. A lad of eighteen years of age. "There was no pain, but only itching and redness at the part bitten at first; but *violent pain soon commenced there* [on the back of the left hand] *and extended in a short time up the forearm and arm to the shoulder and thence to the præcordial region.*"

CASE IV. "A tawny woman [daughter of a quadroon mulatto woman] about twenty-two years old, the mother of two children." "Found her *apparently moribund;* her *skin as cold* as marble; *violent pain extending from the bite on the right wrist up the forearm and arm to the shoulder, and thence up the neck to the back of the head on the right side;* more *violent pain in the præcordia, extending thence to the shoulder and axilla on the left, and down the arm and forearm to the ends of the fingers,* and *this extremity partially paralysed;* added to this, *apnæa was extreme; the respiration only occasional—gasping;* the *pulse could not be felt in the left radial,* and I was not sure that I felt it in the right."

In about fifteen minutes after the intra-venous injection of 13 minims of undiluted *Aqua Ammoniæ,* the doctor "was astonished at the calm and painless expression of her *countenance,* so lately *expressive of anxiety and pain.*"

CASE V. A healthy young girl of 13. She felt a stinging sensation on the [right] wrist, accompanied by itching and redness at the spot [bitten]. For several minutes there was but little pain, but in half an hour a *painful sensation* began to be felt at the spot, which quickly *extended up the arm to the shoulder,* and, in the course of an hour, *along the neck to the back of the head.* * * * *Pain in the præcordial region, with apnæa* coming on, I was sent for. When I arrived she was screaming fearfully with *pain,* and frequently exclaiming she would *lose her breath and die.* The *pulse* had become *thready* and the *surface cold.*

From these *data* the poison of *Latrodectus mactans* is suggested for trial in *angina pectoris,* in that its physiological action presents the closest *similimum* yet found.

FOOTNOTES:

[1] *Virginia Medical Monthly*, Vol. II., No. 9, pp. 633-38, 1875. "He was commissioned surgeon in the Confederate army, July 1, 1861; served until August 1st in the field on the peninsula; then placed in charge of hospital in Williamsburg; afterwards ordered to Richmond and placed in charge of an hospital, and remained until close of war." Failing to find any further trace of him I am led to believe that he has been mustered out of service by the Grand Commander.

II.

It may be well to offer a critical examination of the foregoing cases. If they are genuine effects of the poison of *Latrodectus mactans*, they must afford a *recurrence of corresponding symptoms*. They may differ in *degree*, because the quality of the venom may vary; first, from the season in which the bite occurred (and judging from cases I, IV and V, the poison of *Latrodectus mactans* is most virulent in the month of September), and, secondly, from the more thorough elaboration of the venom. It is known that the poison of *Crotalus horridus* differs in intensity according to the frequency with which the snake has bitten in a given period of time; of four successive "strikes" in four different organisms, and at brief intervals, the intensity of the action will vary, so that while the first wound is lethal the last is not—on which fact depends the vaunted reputation of many an antidote to the bite of the rattlesnake. That this may be also true of the spider poison is the only explanation I can offer for the fact that many naturalists have allowed themselves to be bitten by spiders of reputed poisonous species, and with impunity.

RECURRENCE OF CORRESPONDING SYMPTOMS.

(Arabic numerals refer to the Cases.)

I.	Nausea	1	2		
II.	Abdominal pain	1	2		
III.	Countenance anxious	1		4	
IV.	Pain up arm to shoulder, thence to back of neck			4	5
V.	Præcordial pain extending to				

		1	2	3	4	5
	left axilla, and down arm to finger ends	1			4	
VI.	Left arm almost paralyzed	1			4	
VII.	Pain up arm to shoulder, thence to præcordia			3	4	5
VIII.	Apnæa	1			4	5
IX.	Præcordial pain	1		3	4	5
X.	Pulse feeble, thready	1	2		4	5
XI.	Skin cold	1	2		4	5
XII.	Sense of impending dissolution	1			4	5

While Dr. Semple's reports do not precisely state it, I think we may safely infer a *sense of impending dissolution* in cases I, IV and V. The girl exclaimed she "would lose her breath and die;" the man in case I "expressed in words" "the deep anxiety he felt;" the woman in case IV was found "apparently moribund" with "gasping respiration," and therefore incapable of speech, but who can doubt that she had *a sense of impending dissolution?*

ISOLATED SYMPTOMS.

- *Numbness of the arm*, 1.
- *Black vomit*, 1.
- *Alvine evacuations similar to the black vomit*, 1.
- *Sinking sensation at epigastrium*, 2.
- *Respiration only occasional—gasping*, 4.

It must be admitted that many of our accepted provings cannot as well bear a similar test.

III.

There is another feature that the believer in the law of similars should find no insuperable difficulty in accepting as a criterion of the validity of a proving, namely: *the similarity of the drug symptoms to certain disease symptoms.* I am not ready to believe that drug symptoms are only the result of a "fortuitous concourse of atoms," nor can I for one moment imagine that they are the product of blind and aimless chance. I plainly discern in them the result of law, and I am wholly unable to conceive of existing law without the absolutely necessary *pre*-existing law maker. The consequent must have its antecedent. Therefore, in a drug symptom I see a purpose, and by the light of the law of similars I find the purpose of a drug symptom in an analogous disease symptom—they answer to each other as face unto face in the refiner's silver—and behind and beyond them both is another purpose, of wisdom inscrutable, of love unfathomable. In a word, my reader, the problem of the visible universe forces upon me the alternative that weighed upon Marcus Aurelius—"either gods, or atoms." With atoms only I cannot account for law; with God and in God both atoms and law find a meaning and a purpose.

If I were submitting these convictions, or, if you will, this "working hypothesis," to a Sir Thomas Browne, or a William Harvey, or a Thomas Sydenham I should feel no momentary hesitation; as it is, I can only hope that the spirit that filled these worthies is not extinct in days when the "spiritual colic" that disordered an imaginary *Robert Elsmere* is thought to disturb the eternal Verities. I much doubt if they who mistake an eclipse for an annihilation will get any good from this poor pen of mine.

The resemblance between the symptoms of angina pectoris and the effects of the poison of *Latrodectus mactans* are so striking as to justify the presentation of a comparison; and it is hoped that physicians of wide reading will pardon what may seem to them a piece of supererogation for the sake of many a humbler practitioner whose opportunities have not been so happy. At the same time, the widest reader must admit that he has not found any one authority who has given a complete picture of angina pectoris. Nor is it essential that such an all-including "composite" shall now be presented; on the contrary, we shall offer only salient points substantiated by observers of the highest order.

It will be well to start from an authority whose scholarship has never been excelled—*Copland.* Of all our medical writers he may be called the *Great Definer*—his readers will know what that means.

"*Acute constricting pain at the lower part of the sternum, inclining to the left side, and extending to the arm, accompanied with great anxiety, difficulty of breathing, tendency to syncope, and feeling of approaching dissolution.*"

Copland presents a group of constants, and, for a terse definition, has well covered the principal phenomena. As variants he has omitted the pulse and the surface temperature. He errs on the side of dogmatism in defining the character of the pain as "constricting;" "aching, burning, or indescribable," and "generally attended with a sense of constriction" is more in accordance with the actual condition. Of Copland's seven constants, Case 4 presents an analogue for each in symptoms IX., V., III., VIII., XII., and the "tendency to syncope," which is not included in our table because Dr. Semple did not put the fact in express words. If to this group we add the *thready pulse* and *cold skin*, we shall have "covered" nine of the most prominent symptoms of angina pectoris; a pathological "composite" with a most striking pathogenetic *similimum*.

But all the elements of Copland's group are not of equal importance; two of them, at least, are pathognomonic. "The two constituent elements of the paroxysm," says Latham, are "the sense of dissolution and the pain." "Pain with one awful accompaniment may be everything." "This mixture of the sharpest pain with a feeling of instant death." According to Fothergill "the two prominent subjective phenomena are pain in the chest and a sense of impending death." Eulenburg and Guttmann include another element: "We regard the substernal pain, the feeling of anxiety, and the disturbance of the heart's action, as the essential symptoms of angina pectoris." Romberg notes the companionship of these two elements: "The patient attacked with angina pectoris is suddenly seized with a pain under the sternum in the neighborhood of the heart, accompanied by a sense of anxiety so intense as to induce a belief in the approach of death."

We have laid the emphasis of these various citations on the "essential symptoms" in order to assert, with equal emphasis, that their analogues occur in not only one case of *Latrodectus mactans* poisoning. The præcordial pain is noted in Cases 1, 3, 4 and 5, and the sense of impending dissolution in Cases 1, 4 and 5. And that disturbance of the heart's action which Eulenburg and Guttmann consider an essential element is found in Cases 1, 2, 4 and 5; so that the *tout ensemble* presented by Case 4 is corroborated.

Another important element, though it is one subject to variations, is the direction of the extension of the pain. It most generally extends to the left axilla, and down the arm to the fingers; as variations it sometimes affects the right axilla and the back of the head. In Cases 1 and 4 the spider poison followed the direction of the disease, and in Cases 4 and 5 it also affected the back of the head. In Case 1 it produced the numbness of the arm and hand that is sometimes observed in the diseases.

Copland includes "difficulty of breathing" amongst the elements of angina pectoris. Trousseau does not regard this difficulty as real. "Although patients think they are going to be suffocated during a paroxysm, the chest is normally resonant on percussion, and if it be auscultated as they draw in breath again vesicular breathing is heard everywhere." Watson says, "the patient is not necessarily out of breath. It is not dyspnœa that oppresses him; for he can, and generally does, breathe freely and easily." Stokes is decided: "Respiration is *secondarily* affected; there may be slight dyspnœa or orthopnœa, with lividity of the face, yet by an effort of the will (if the patient dares to encounter the pang this commonly produces) the chest may be pretty freely expanded, and the breathing relieved for a brief space; dyspnœa is not a primary symptom of angina." Eulenburg and Guttmann say, "Our own experience leads us to adopt Parry's conclusion, that the changes in the respiration are principally, perhaps even solely, due to the pain." Bristowe speaks of the sufferer as "fearing to breathe." We can readily see that the "apnæa" observed by Dr. Semple in Cases 1 and 5 had physical origin, but in Case 4 he says "apnæa was extreme; the respiration only occasional—gasping." This shows to what an extreme extent the action of the spider poison had gone—even to implicating the diaphragm; and it is noteworthy that Anstie records a case of angina pectoris (*Neuralgia and its Counterfeits*, p. 67, London, 1871), in which "there was so marked a catching of the breath as to make it almost certain that there was a diaphragmatic spasm."

Of the changes in respiration accompanying angina pectoris we have, then, both the general, and the rarest, form, produced pathogenetically by the poison of *Latrodectus mactans*.

IV.

In its physiological action the poison of *Latrodectus mactans* resembles angina pectoris vasomotoria—a purely functional derangement. The similitude of the physiological action to pure angina pectoris corroborates the accepted pathology of the latter condition, because the phenomena of *Latrodectus* poisoning were educed from previously healthy organisms, and in pure angina pectoris there is no pre-existent organic change occasioning the attack. According to the accepted pathology, we have in angina pectoris vasomotoria, sudden spasms of the arterioles; from this an increase of the arterial tension; to overcome this is more forcible and rapid action of the heart; as the arteriole spasm persists and doubtless deepens in intensity, distension of the left ventricle follows, and from overdistension the agonizing breast-pang, and even death from stoppage of the heart's diastole. But we must include another element—spasm of the coronary vessels. "When there is a sudden rise in the blood-pressure in the arteries, due to vasomotor spasm of the peripheral systemic arterioles, and the heart-walls are strong and well nourished, palpitation is evoked; when the coronary branches are involved in the vasomotor spasm then angina is produced, and the heart-walls, acutely distended with blood, can scarcely contract in the face of the opposition presented to their contraction by the high arterial tension. When this sudden systemic arteriole spasm extends to the coronary vessels in a heart whose walls are diseased, a fatal attack of angina with the heart full of blood may be induced. The danger increases with the extent of the structural degeneration of the heart-walls. Sudden rises of blood-pressure in the arteries will tax hearts in their textural integrity, and lead to painful distension; such sudden demands on decayed hearts lead to agonizing angina pectoris, and the sense of impending dissolution is frequently followed by sudden death."

Spasm of the arterioles and coronary vessels, rise of blood-pressure in the arteries, embarrassed action of the heart, and painful distension are just so many consecutive links in the phenomena produced by the poison of *Latrodectus mactans*, as Cases I and IV amply testify.

The spider poisons are akin to the serpent poisons in their property of producing a disorganization of the blood. In Case I, thin and florid non-coagulable blood continued to ooze from the cut surface despite the application of tannin. It may be a question whether this condition of the blood is directly toxicological, or a pathological result of stasis in the peripheral vessels. I incline to regard it as due to the latter condition, and I believe this explanation also holds good in the case of serpent poisoning.

The hæmorrhage recorded in Case I was of gastric origin; splenic congestion existed, and the vasa brevia—branches of the splenic artery—gave way under the pressure. I once met a similar hæmorrhage in a case of intermittent fever in a child, and I recorded the fact as a possible hint for the applicability of *Latrodectus mactans* in a similar condition.

In all the year that the stray copy of the old magazine was in my possession I felt it a duty to write up this remedy. I have done it lamely, but as well as I was able. Reader, where my duty ends yours begins. May you discharge it more worthily than I.

(There have been a number of cases reported in which *Latrodectus mac.* acted as Dr. Jones predicted; from them we select the following by Dr. E. H. Linnell, *North American Journal of Homœopathy*, December, 1890):

S. L. G., a man fifty years old, of bilious temperament, a dentist by profession, had slight attacks of angina after severe exposure and overexertion during "the blizzard" in March, 1888. He did not consider them of sufficient importance to consult a physician about them, but some months later he had a suppurative prostatitis, which was followed by considerable prostration, and the attacks of angina became very severe. I never could get a satisfactory description of the character of the pain, and I never saw him during a paroxysm. The pain was brought on by exertion of any kind, and was especially frequent soon after dinner. The pain was sometimes felt in the left arm, but was usually confined to the cardiac region. I once or twice detected a slight aortic obstruction sound, but aside from this failed to find any evidence of organic disease. The usual remedies gave no relief, but *Latrodectus* 3c was of great benefit. Under its use the

- 172 -

attacks gradually became less frequent and less severe. He has taken no medicine now for at least six months, and he tells me that although he occasionally has a little reminder of his former trouble, the attacks are so slight that he pays no attention to them. I have given the remedy in another similar case, with even more gratifying success. The attacks were very promptly arrested and have not returned, although nearly a year has elapsed. I think we have in this remedy, to which Dr. S. A. Jones directed attention in one of the issues of the *Homœopathic Recorder*, a very valuable remedy in this painful affection. It is probably, as Dr. Jones suggests, in angina pectoris vasomotoria that it will be found especially serviceable.

LEMNA MINOR.

NAT. ORD., Lemnaccæ.
COMMON NAME, Duckweed.
PREPARATION. The fresh plant is pounded to a pulp and macerated in two parts by weight of alcohol.

(The following is by Dr. Robert C. Cooper, of London, and appeared in the *Hahnemannian Monthly*, 1894):

"The lowest form of phœnogamous vegetation. It consists," says Lindley, "of lenticular floating fronds, composed of stem and leaf together and bearing the flowers in slits in the edge." It forms the green scum found on stagnant ponds and dykes. It is found in two varieties, the *Lemna minor* and the *Lemna gibba*.

Before going any further I may as well at once make a bald as well as a bold statement, and say that the special province of *Lemna minor* is to pitch with vigor upon the nostrils; from the very moment I began prescribing it this was beyond question evident. I can think of no possible source of error except that this beneficial action may be due to the germs adhering to the fronds of the *Lemna* rather than to the pure plant-force.

To guard against this I have carefully filtered my tincture, but this has not made the slightest change in its beneficial influence.

CASE I. Woman aged seventy-four; admission date, September 24, 1892. Nose never clear; breath very unpleasant; for twelve hours nose bled continuously last Christmas; unable to smell properly; hearing for the past seven or eight weeks bad; watch not heard on contact. Prescribed *Lemna minor* θA. October 1, 1892: Feeling of cold in nose is better; sense of obstruction nearly gone; can smell better; hears on contact on both sides; no medicine. October 22: Decided, though slight improvement in hearing; nose, throat and all parts around more comfortable. Last attendance.

In proceeding with the consideration of the action of this remedy, I must consider myself fortunate in having the following case to bring forward:

1. A boy of fourteen, whose nose was completely blocked up for the last two years, and whose nostrils were full of polypi, the nose itself being broadened, and in whom the nose had been cleared out by operation a year ago at St. Bartholomew's Hospital, was sent to me by my colleague, Dr. J. H. Clarke. The boy never remembers having smelt anything, and the polypi can easily be seen blocking up both nostrils.

From the 26th of November, 1892, to the 4th of March, 1893, four doses of *Lemna m.* θA were given at regular intervals without much change, then *Calcarea carbonica* 200 was given, and two weeks after, as he had faceache, *Mercurius* 3d dec., and on the 8th of April following the faceache was better but the nose in no way improved.

Then *Lemna* was given again, and this time with the most pronounced relief; the nose became much clearer, and he went on taking it, and it alone with scarcely an exception, in fortnightly doses, till the 14th of March last, when his nose was quite clear, with none but a very small polypi visible; he could breathe freely and his sense of smell had completely returned.

The delay in the manifestation of remedial change from November to March arose from complete blockage of the nose, and until the space created by the subsidence in the size of the polypi sufficed for a passage of air the patient had no reason to acknowledge relief.

In the treatment, both of swollen tonsils and in that of nasal polypi, the prescriber will be led away at the onset who accepts the testimony of the patient alone; he should make careful inspection of the parts, and be guided by what is often but a slight local change, as well as by concomitant, and it may be remote, symptoms.

2. The next case I have to bring forward is one of ozœna in a girl of sixteen, who had been three years under the treatment of a colleague who kindly sent her on to me for treatment at the London Homœopathic Hospital. The girl, whose occupation was a teacher, has had ozœna since three or four years old. The odor complained of was horrid, and the discharge excessive; a most unpleasant smell in the nose and nasty taste in the mouth; she takes cold easily if out in the night air or damp, and her nose, at times, gets stuffed up; bowels irregular; catamenia only twice— once three months ago and two months before that.

On December 30, 1893, I prescribed *Lemna minor*, and she returned to me from the country, where she was living, on the 31st of the following March, imploring me for another powder, as she had been almost well for two weeks after the last and then had relapsed to her old state; breathing is short and is low spirited.

21st of April, very much better; odor not nearly so bad, discharge much less; unmedicated pilules, three times a day.

19th of May, 1894, kept better for a month; took cold two weeks ago, and since then throat has felt thick and nose has discharged with a horrid odor. Catamenia regular. Breathing is better; crusts coming from both, worse on the left side. To have *Lemna minor*.

This patient came from a distance which prevented frequent attendance, but the above is quite sufficient evidence of the power possessed by *Lemna m.* in acting upon the nasal mucous membrane.

In both these cases relief was immediate after the administration of the dose, and in neither case could any reasonable doubt exist as to its being drug effect.

In some cases I have known a certain disturbance of the bowels to set in after a dose of *Lemna*, but this effect of the remedy is not sufficiently pronounced to be able to say much about it. Still it is interesting to narrate one or two experiences, especially as in the first of these, at all events, the concomitants were interesting.

3. In a married lady, aged about twenty-six, for whom I prescribed *Lemna m.* θA on Saturday afternoon, November 12, 1892, and in whom there existed a good deal of catarrhal pharyngitis, due to high up post-nasal ulceration, and who suffered from a dry feeling at the top of the throat with flatulence, and some pain in the bowels toward the evening, described as "twisting" pain, and in whom the nose was blocked on the right side, but without any visible polypus, and in whom the heart was easily disturbed, causing dyspnœa, the bowels being slightly confined.

Two weeks subsequently she stated that after the dose of *Lemna* the nose felt less blocked, and she felt better in every respect; but that on the Tuesday following diarrhœa set in, which began with twisting pains in the bowels and went on to sickness; continual watery stools. The least chill or nervousness, I must say, upsets her in this way; and she was subject to the same the last two catamenial periods. She still wakes with her throat dry and tongue coated. *Borax* 2x was then (November 25) given without any noticeable effect, and on the 9th of December *Lemna minor* θA was again prescribed for the following symptoms:

Mouth sore after talking or singing, and dry in the morning; tongue coated.

On the 23d of December, reported herself much better; tongue not so coated; heart less disturbed; no indigestion or diarrhœa.

Nose not perfectly clear, but no unpleasant smell or taste as she used to have, and throat no longer dry or uncomfortable. Instead of waking up with a dirty mouth, it feels clean and her taste pure.

4. A man, aged forty-seven, who suffered from old-standing vascular deafness and who specially complained of snoring a great deal, was given *Lemna minor*, and next day a rumbling and disturbance in the bowels set in and he felt as if he had taken medicine of a searching character. This lasted

for three days, bowels acting during this time freely with much heat in the passage (anus); but was not bilious, nor were the motions diarrhœic; the snoring went away, and he ceased to dream unpleasantly when asleep. Hearing, too, seemed somewhat improved.

5. In another case, after a similar dose, diarrhœa came on next day, with pains across the bowels as from flatus; worse after eating, and a very putrid taste with an improvement at the same time in a stuffiness of the nose from which he was suffering.

6. Crusts form in the right nostril and pain like a string extends from the right nostril to the ear of the same side and right ear is deaf. (In a woman, aged twenty-six, great relief.)

It is with great pleasure that I have now to bring forward, not my own observations, but those of two valued colleagues. Dr. J. H. Clarke sends me the following:

Lemna minor, CASE I. A lady, aged forty-seven, two years previously met with an accident; a sign board fell on her head when out walking in the street. Seven days after that was taken with sneezing attacks, suffered from nasal catarrh with little intermission until March, 1893, when she came under my care. *Psorinum* 30 soon put a different complexion on the case, and she became so far relieved of her trouble (which has made her life almost unbearable, as she never dared make an appointment for fear of an attack coming on) that she discontinued treatment. Last Christmas a sharp attack of influenza brought back the catarrh, and this time it proved less amenable to treatment.

Fears of polypus distressed the patient, though I could not discover any.

However, she again made progress, but scarcely as rapid as I could have wished, when I thought of giving her *Lemna* on indications given by Dr. Cooper.

On February 15, 1894, I gave it in the 3x, one tablet four times a day.

February 22, very much better; has felt freer in the head than at any time during the last ten years; has felt very much better generally; spirits braced up.

She steadily progressed to cure, and by March 15th could endure the smell of strong scented flowers, which before was impossible.

CASE II. Captain B., aged forty-four, consulted me on February 29, 1894, for violent neuralgia on the right side of the neck, the part being exquisitely sensitive to touch. He had cough and cold for a month. On getting up in the morning he filled two pocket handkerchiefs with yellow deflusion before he got his nose clear. I gave him *Bell.* 12 to take till the neuralgia was better, and then told him to take *Lemna* 3x gtt. j. three times a day.

On March 9th he reported that the *Bell.* speedily took away the neuralgia, and that then the *Lemna* cleared off the catarrh in a most astonishing fashion. He never had a medicine to act so magically before.

30 Clarges street, Piccadilly, W., April 21, 1894.

The next communication that I have to bring forward is one from Dr. J. C. Burnett:

Dr. Cooper told me that he had relieved a case of nasal polypus with *Lemna minor*, and having several cases of the kind that had long been under my observation I thought it my duty to give them the benefit of *Lemna*.

CASE I. A gentleman of sixty years of age, with nasal polypus only moderately developed, yet of many years' duration, was much troubled by the chronic nasal obstruction which was markedly worse in wet weather.

I gave him *Lemna* 3x, five drops in water, night and morning. Returning in a month, he exclaimed: "That is the best tonic I have ever taken; I have never taken any medicine in my life that has done me so much good. I feel quite comfortable in my nose and can breathe through it quite well."

CASE II. A lady, about forty-five years of age, mother of a large family and whom I had formerly cured of an uterine tumor, was so troubled with nasal polypi that her life was very distressful; moreover, the polypi had swelled so much that they hung out of the nostrils and compelled the patient to remain within doors. This was notably the case in wet weather. Why not have them removed chirurgically?

"Oh, I have had them operated on over and over again, but it's no good; they only come again worse than ever."

I have tried many things to cure these polypi, but in vain; they would get temporarily better, but the first rainy weather brought them back worse than ever; hence Dr. Cooper's recommendation of *Lemna* is very welcome to me.

I ordered, as in the last case, with the result that the polypi very greatly diminished in size, and the patient could again take her place in society.

I have used *Lemna* in many other similar cases, and with the like result. In no case is the polypus really cured, but greatly diminished in size, and the patient rendered relatively comfortable. Clearly the *Lemna* does not either kill, cure or otherwise get rid of the polypi, but it rids them of much of their succulence and thus reduces their volume, and also diminishes the influence of wet weather to which such patients are so prone. And this is no small boon; is itself in every way superior to any operative interference. The tincture I made use of was made by Dr. Alfred Heath. The first prescription only being of Dr. Cooper's own make. Both acted alike well.

86 Wimpole street, June 4, 1894.

From these remarks of Dr. J. H. Clarke and Dr. J. Compton Burnett, as well as from my own, I think there can be no doubt, whatever, that the *Lemna* exercises a powerful influence upon the Schneiderian mucous membrane. How far it is capable by its specific action of removing large groups of polypi remains, as yet, an open question.

My own experience of the treatment of nasal polypi is that we have very few remedies that can at all be depended upon for giving even temporary relief. Even from *Calcarea carbonica* and *Teucrium marum verum* I have not had the effects that some practitioners testify to their possessing.

Lemna has so far given relief in my hands to cases of nasal polypi and to cases where the nostrils were plugged by swollen turbinates and other causes in a matter far surpassing the effect I have obtained from any other remedy.

In saying this I do not at all wish it to be understood that we have in it a specific for all such cases.

We must remember that the symptoms in all such obscure diseases must be our guide for the selection of our remedy, and that, therefore, the important point is to work out the specific indications for the drug as we learn them from clinical observation, in the hope that on some future occasion pathogenesis may render these still more certain.

The indications that I myself have noticed as belonging to *Lemna* are either a putrid smell in the nose or a loss of all sense of smell and a putrid taste in the mouth, especially on rising in the morning, with a general foulness of the mouth, due apparently to the dropping down of impure material from the post-nasal region. Along with this there sometimes seems to prevail a disposition to "noisy diarrhœa."

Dr. Burnett has noticed that *Lemna* patients have their nasal symptoms aggravated in damp and rainy weather, and I have to some extent confirmed this observation.

I hope on some future occasion to return to the subject of *Lemna*; it is in every way well worthy of being prosecuted further.

Thus, for example, a lady patient, æt. fifty-eight, suffering from pains flitting about her head and legs, with pains in her eyes during heavy rain, and in whom drowsiness by day and restless sleep at night existed, had all these symptoms removed by a single dose of *Lemna*, and the pallid, dullish, sickly look in her face changed to a complexion that was natural and healthy.

The truth would seem to be that *Lemna's* symptoms are specially aggravated in heavy rains; *Calendula's*, when heavy clouds are about; *Rhododendron's*, in thunder storms, and *Dulcamara's*, in damp surroundings and in foggy weather.

(In 1895 Dr. Thomas L. Shearer contributed the following concerning the remedy to the *Homœopathic Eye, Ear and Throat Journal*):

Lemna minor where the crusts and the muco-purulent discharge are very abundant with fetor (in rhinitis atrophics). Its action is wonderful, but it must not be administered in too low a dilution, as it then produces a sensation of intense dryness in the pharynx and the larynx. Possibly if it were exhibited in a much higher dilution it would be applicable to cases which have only a slight amount of discharge. It seems best to stop the remedy as soon as its action upon the secretions is marked, and then to wait a while before returning to its further employment. Dr. Cooper, of London, was, I believe, the first to investigate the action of *Lemna minor* upon the upper air passages, but I do not think that he had tried it in cases of atrophic rhinitis. There is a great future for this new addition to our therapeutic resources, and it certainly deserves further investigation. It modifies the secretions to such an extent that we can more readily improve the condition of the nasal chambers with the aid of local measures. Whether it has the power to prevent or even retard the actual process of atrophy remains to be seen.

LEVICO.

PREPARATION.—Dilutions made from the mineral water or triturations from the residue obtained by evaporation of the water.

(Dr. Burnett has called the attention of the profession to this water in his books. The following concerning its constituents is from *The Therapist*, a London journal):

Of all mineral waters those of Levico are distinguished, not only by their contents of these three elements, arsenic, iron and copper, but they are remarkable for the state of combination in which they occur. Situated in South Tyrol, on the confines of Italy, Levico has for many years been a favorite sanitorium of the Italian medical profession for their nervous and skin patients. Of late years Levico water has also been increasingly recognized by the German and Austrian faculty, among whom Bamberger, Billroth, Hebra, Nussbaum, and others testify to the extraordinary remedial activity of the waters, favoring assimilation, increasing nutrition, and in chronic and dyscratic skin diseases functioning as antiseptic or astringent.

Merely as an internal medication *Levico* water has, however, proved so satisfactory that it is a recognized member of the pharmacopœia in many German and Austrian hospitals and clinics. Thus Professor Nussbaum, of Munich, writes that '*Levico* water is given in my orthopædic institute in doses of two or three ounces to scrofulous and anæmic children. The water is well tolerated, and in spite of the smallness of the dose the result is, in many cases, very evident.' Professor Eulenberg, of Berlin, finds *Levico* water especially satisfactory in chorea minor in children and at the age of puberty, as well as for hysterical neuralgia and spasms. A very copious testimony of like nature has been borne respecting *Levico* water.

LATHYRUS SATIVUS.

NAT. ORD., Leguminosæ.
COMMON NAMES, Wild Vetch. Chick pea.
PREPARATION.—Trituration of the dried pea.

(Dr. W. A. Dewey contributed the following paper concerning this remedy to the *Medical Century*, 1899):

HISTORY AND DESCRIPTION OF EFFECTS,

The *Lathyrus* is a vetch, and a member of the leguminosæ family growing in India.

This remedy, which produces a perfect picture of certain spinal affections, has been known for over a century. In *Christison's Toxicology* it is stated that it causes paraplegia, dragging gait, turning-in of the toes, stiffness and semi-flexion of the knee-joints.

The attention of the homœopathic profession was directed to the drug as a possible remedy in paraplegia, in the *British Journal of Homœopathy*, Vol. III. Here is found an account of a wheat famine in India, where the peas of the plant were substituted for wheat and used as a food. Those who subsisted on it were taken, even during sleep, with sudden paralysis of the lower limbs; this occurred without warning, in young men more than in young women, and was never recovered from. Another observer records fifty cases who had eaten the *Lathyrus* bread and all stated that they became paralytic during the wet season of the country, that they went to bed quite well and awoke with stiff legs, unsteady gait, and aching, but no severe pain. The upper extremities were free.

Another who saw the disease in Algeria and described the symptoms found in ten cases observed that they came on suddenly, in damp weather, with some pains in the loins, trembling, motor paralysis and exaggerated reflexes. He attributed these phenomena to an acute transverse myelitis with degenerative changes in the cord.

A German writer states that the drug produces disturbances of nutrition of the muscles of the lower extremities, paresis, and that the muscles of the trunk and neck and face remain unaffected. Sensation remains normal. It seems to produce a sclerosis of the pyramidal tracts of the cord.

In animals the same condition is found; namely, paralysis of the hind legs. Pigs drag their hind legs and horses give out.

AGGRAVATED SYMPTOMATOLOGY.

From all the sources which I have been able to find, the following seem to be the symptoms caused by the drug:

Sudden loss of power in the lower extremities, from the waist down.

Tremulous, tottering gait.

Great exaggeration of the reflexes.

Stiffness and lameness of the ankles and knees.

Excessive rigidity of the legs; flexion difficult; spastic gait, the legs becoming interlocked, and walking is difficult or impossible.

Sudden onset of the trouble, and apparent aggravation in cold and damp weather.

Emaciation of the gluteal muscles also observed.

Those having taken it walked on the metatarso-phalangeal articulation, the heel not touching the ground.

Impossible to stand steady; swayed from side to side, but closing the eyes had no effect. This with the exaggerated reflexes would exclude its use in locomotor ataxia.

Debility and tremors of the legs.

Rigidity of the adductors of the thighs.

Staggering gait, with eyes fixed on the floor.

Could not extend or cross the legs when sitting.

Sensibility unimpaired.

CORRESPONDENCE TO SPINAL DISORDERS.

From these symptoms it will be seen that the effects of the drug correspond to many spinal symptoms, but more especially to what is known as spastic paraplegia. Indeed, Struempel asserts that it produces a perfect picture of this disease.

It is not so often that such a perfect picture of a disease can be had as in this instance. The disease itself is easily recognized by the stiff, spastic gait; the spasm of the adductors, causing the knees to strike each other, or to become locked, causing the patient to fall; the shuffling of the feet; the excessive muscular rigidity and the other well-known symptoms of paraplegia.

Therefore, reasoning from our law we would expect the drug to be of service in such cases, and although our pathogenesis of it is coarse we may be permitted to apply it to a disease whose symptomatology is of the coarse order; for it is often difficult to elicit any fine and characteristic symptoms in diseases like ataxic and spastic paraplegia.

It has been recognized as a remedy by but few of our writers on nervous diseases. O'Connor finds that marked benefit follows its use in old cases of myelitis with marked spastic symptoms. Bartlett, in *Goodno's Practice*, recommends it in excessive knee-jerk and rigidity. Hart speaks of it as a remedy in locomotor ataxia, but the absence of sensory symptoms and the presence of exaggerated reflexes would seem to contra-indicate it in this disease. He also speaks of it in spinal anemia, giving as symptoms: "Numbness, followed by pain in the lower extremities; sensation of a band around the body; unable to step or distinguish one limb from another"— symptoms which I am unable to find that the remedy produced. Elliott also speaks of it.

CLINICAL RÉSUMÉ.

The clinical record of *Lathyrus*, though very meagre, gives great hope that it may prove useful in numerous cases of bed-ridden paraplegiacs and in infantile spinal paralysis, as well as in certain forms of myelitis.

The following is a résumé of all that I can find published:

I. Case of spinal paraplegia, relieved.

II. A case of multiple sclerosis in a young man of twenty-eight who had been ill seven years and unable to walk for six years was greatly benefited by *Lathyrus* 3x.

III. Case of paraplegia, could walk after taking the remedy for some time.

IV. Case of paraplegia, no improvement.

V. Rheumatic paralysis, with stiff knees, could walk after use of *Lathyrus*. (Clark *Homœopathic World*.)

VI. In a case of a clerk with loss of power of the lower limbs, reflexes exaggerated, knee-jerk violent, locomotion difficult and unsteady, probably a case of transverse myelitis, *Lathyrus* 3x, night and morning, gave most satisfactory results. The patient could walk a mile without assistance. (Simpson, *Homœopathic Review*.)

VII. In a man aged fifty-two who had been unable to walk for six years, the paraplegia coming on after a "stroke" from exposure to wet, *Lathyrus* 3x practically cured in eight months. He had been tied to a chair for six, and at the time he stopped treatment he was walking four miles daily. (Blake, *Homœopathic Review.*)

From the fact that the *Lathyrus* disease occurs frequently in certain mountainous regions of Asia it has been remarked that it is akin to Beri-Beri, which has been traced to eating the *Lathyrus* bread.

LIATRIS SPICATA.

NAT. ORD., Compositæ.
COMMON NAMES, Dense Button-Snake-root. Gay Feather. Devil's Bit.
PREPARATION.—The root is pounded to a pulp and macerated in two parts by weight of alcohol.

(The following, by Dr. T. C. Duncan, was called forth by the publication of an item in *Eclectic Medical Journal*, stating that twice during the past year *Liatris* had given good results in dropsy; in one case, on the second day, the patient had passed a gallon and a half of urine. Dr. Duncan's paper was published in the *Homœopathic Recorder* for 1898):

Any new remedy that promises relief in dropsy will be hailed with pleasure by the profession. Happening into a pharmacy soon after receiving the January *Recorder*, a physician rushed in and inquired for "that new remedy for dropsy—that got rid of 'a gallon and a half of urine in one day.' Have a bad case cardiac dropsy. Want to try it. How do you give it?" He could not get it. "Get me some," was his order. "There is the article, be sure to get the right thing, *Liatris*!"

Liatris spicata is the familiar "button-snake-root" that I used to dig every fall for our old family physician (who called himself a "botanic physician") and who gave it for indigestion. It is also called "colic root" and "devil's bit," because a piece is missing from each tuber as a rule, just as if bitten out. *Kost's Medicine* (my first medical work) describes it as follows: "Root perennial, tuberous, ovate, abrupt, beset around the base with many fine fibers; it is aromatic. Stem round, about three feet high, bearing a spike of scaly purple-colored blossoms, bearing in the aggregate a resemblance to an acorn. The leaves are linear or sword-shaped, somewhat resembling the leaves of young corn. It is found in prairies and open woods in the western States."

"The *Liatris* is an aromatic stimulant, diaphoretic, diuretic, anodyne and carminitive. It is particularly useful in colic, backache and flatulency."

It is interesting to know that it has had clinically a good effect in dropsy, (1) due to liver and splenic enlargement, also (2) where the kidneys were involved. In the second case referred to, "*Apocynum can., Aralia, Digitalis, et al.*" had been given, but the kidneys failed to respond until the *Liatris* "was given in infusion," then "on the *second* day the patient passed *a gallon and a half of urine*"—equal to 192 ounces of urine! In the first case the *Liatris* was followed by *Ferrum carb*.

Whether it will prove equally efficient in cardiac dropsy only time will tell. I hope that the readers of the *Recorder* will report results, whether favorable or otherwise. The dose that Dr. Bradley gave was about a pint, drank during the course of the day, containing about half an ounce of the root. The tincture will be more convenient, and it is a question if the dilutions will not be equally efficient. Try the third, and then go up or down the scale as the case seems to demand. This drug should be proved. It is harmless. If any young physician will volunteer I will gladly direct him.

Infusion of *Digitalis* (English leaves) is a favorite prescription with some physicians in cases of cardiac dropsy, but I have not found that form any more efficient than the dilution, except in cases where alcohol had been a cause, then *Strophanthus* or *Arsenicum* had a better effect.

LOLIUM TEMULENTUM.

NAT. ORD., Gramineæ.
COMMON NAMES, Darnel. (G.) Taumellolch.
PREPARATION.—Trituration of the dried seeds.

(The following concerning this little used drug was reported by Dr. Bonino, an Italian physician, translated by Dr. Mossa and published in the *Allgemeine Hom. Zeitung*, July, 1898. The use of the drug by Dr. Bonino was truly homœopathic for the short proving of it. Allen's *Encyclopædia* reports trembling of the limbs and hand so great that "he could not hold a glass of water.")

A carpenter, aged twenty-nine years, had been suffering ever since his eighteenth year of trembling in both hands, especially in the morning; of late also his legs began to tremble. It is remarkable that both his father and his brother were subject to the same ailment, while no definite cause could be indicated. He was first given *Mercurius vivus*, then *Agaricus*, which brought a partial but only transitory improvement. Finally I prescribed *Lolium tem.*, which in a short time effected a cure.

(On this Dr. Mossa comments as follows):

The pathogenetic effects of this remedy which has not yet been proved at all are only known to some degree from its effects when it has been mixed with grain and baked into bread. It has caused chest troubles, *vertigo* (thence the name darnel-grass, in German *Taumellolch*), *trembling*, paralysis with anguish and distress, vomiting, failing of the memory, blindness, headache, epileptic attacks, deep sleep and insanity. The good success obtained by its use in the case given above shows what curative effects may be expected from it in severe affections of the brain or spinal marrow. An Italian physician, Fantoni, has tried it in cephalalgia, meningitis rheumatica and in ischias.

LYCOPUS VIRGINICUS.

NAT. ORD., Labiatæ.
COMMON NAME, Bugle Weed.
PREPARATION.—Tincture of the whole plant by macerating one part by
weight of the fresh plant in two parts by weight of alcohol.

(Although a well-known remedy, the following concerning it may not be
amiss here; it is from the *Homœopathic World*, 1889, by Dr. Proell):

Lycopus Virginicus seems to be a specific for bringing back an old (but long
disappeared) hæmorrhoidal flux in persons with light eyes. I gave, a week
ago, the first decimal dilution to a gentleman (sixty years) for noise and
throbbing in the head during the night (which prevented the quietness of
sleep); because neither *Cactus* (which helped quickly when he had blood-
spitting) nor *Kalmia*, nor *Gelsemium* helped radically. The night after taking
Lycopus, he was a little better, and in the forenoon came a bleeding from the
rectum (about three tablespoonfuls after defecation) with great general
relief. There was chronic catarrhus bronchialis. Two days afterwards, I gave
an elderly lady (sixty years), who had glycosuria, cataract of the left eye, and
every third night was very restless, *Lycopus Virginicus* 1 decimal dilution, one
drop in the evening. The following night was excellent, and in the morning
came an abundant bleeding from the rectum, with great relief. Both patients
are tall, very irritable, have weak innervation of the heart, without decided
organic disease of the heart; both are hypochondriacs; have light eyes; noise
in the left ear. Both had, years ago, hæmorrhoidal flux, which stopped
suddenly.

MALARIA OFFICINALIS.

PREPARATION.—It is prepared in three degrees of strength:

No. I. Is the water that stood on decomposed vegetable matter for one week at a temperature of 90° F.

No. II. Is the water that decomposed vegetable matter for two weeks.

No. III. Is the water that decomposed vegetable matter for three weeks.

(The following is an abstract of a paper on this peculiar remedy, by Dr. G. W. Bowen, that appeared in the Transactions of the Indiana Institute of Homœopathy, 1895):

In the summer of 1862 vegetable matter of different forms was decomposed in my office in glass jars, and malaria was freely generated. Persons were hired to inhale the gas evolved in its different stages of decomposition, and a careful observation of its effects on them was made that gave me a clue to its future use, and the only reliable guide for combatting its effect when acquired naturally.

Not only did the gaseous form demonstrate, but subsequent use of the liquid product proved it capable of producing not only the three leading types that the past years had made me conversant with, but also others of a minor grade yet of unsuspected parentage.

The miser made delight of added gain, Was like a pebble on the shore again,

In comparison to the satisfactory consolation that came as a realization of the comprehension of the producing cause. Henceforth the battle need not be carried on mid the gloom of the night.

The decomposition of the vegetable matter passed through three stages or degrees. The first gave off gases freely, yet of not so offensive odor as later. After ten days or two weeks the expense of securing inhalers was more than doubled, even for one moment of time. After three or four weeks not much gas was generated, for it seemed only capable of lying still and sending its fearful odor heavenward. Inhalation of the gases evolved produced for the first week or ten days a headache, nausea, distress in the stomach, coated the tongue white, and this in from one to two hours time generally; and there, if not carried too far, would generally pass off in two or three days. Inhalations after ten days or two weeks did not produce results in less than twelve or twenty-four hours, according to time and amount inhaled. Then there was fearful headache, nausea, aversion to food, distress through the hypochondriac region, first in the spleen, the liver and stomach, and on the third day chills that would doubtless have continued on indefinitely if not interfered with.

After decomposition had gone on for three or four weeks it was ascetic and simply fetid to a fearful degree, and no results except nausea were apparent in any one exposed to it in less than three or four days. The first was extreme lassitude and loss of appetite, and apparently a continued fever, with an unlimited amount of pains and aches and a lassitude that limited locomotion.

Three vials of the watery tincture were saved, one each from the various stages of decomposition, and from these an attempt was made to make provings and find out what were the reliable antidotes to them, and thus be able to cope with my invisible foe in my daily avocation. Their provings were not carried far enough, or continued long enough to be justified in placing them in our Materia Medica, but are ample to aid and guide the future steps that ought to be taken. Its discontinuance was rendered rather necessary by my enthusiasm that led too far in a few cases, but the antidotal effects of certain remedies amply compensated me for my financial and reputational loss.

Bilious colic, nausea, cramps, diarrhœa and headaches were readily secured from a few drops of the first vial, in many cases, while the second vial gave me a large number of cases where the liver, spleen, stomach and kidneys were apparently seriously involved, and not them alone, but fair types of intermittent fever with its attendant shakes, some daily, some tertian.

With the third vial trouble came, as it did reduce many that had been able to be up and around to their beds, and unmistakably cause them to get worse, and cause them to degenerate into a typhoidal or semi-paralytic condition. In a few cases I was deprived the liberty of finding my antidotes and helping them out of the dilemma.

(Among the experiments made with these strange tinctures, if they may be so called, was the following, which is strangely confirmatory of a speculation advanced by several old physicians that consumptives are benefited, or even cured, by being exposed to malaria):

It was a lady, the last of a family of five, all others had died of consumption, and three in her preceding generation of the same disease. I doubted the probability of saving her, yet *theoretically* decided that as the primitive action of malaria was, first, the spleen, next the liver and stomach, that I would develop an artificial or drug disease there, in hopes that her chest would be relieved and doubtless be benefited. She was given the tincture from second vial, and on the fifth day she had a fairly perceptible chill, and a harder one the sixth and seventh. On the eighth I saw her shake for one hour, and her fever lasted over six hours. Out of pity my drug was neutralized and her health was restored, with no more cough distress in her lungs or heart. She was cured of her tendency and certainty of dying with consumption. She remained well for twelve years when she was lost to my call.

(In his search for remedies, or antidotes, for the malarial poisons, Dr. Bowen was disappointed in *Eupatorium perf.* In his experience the following remedies are best):

For the first or primitive effects, the remedies that did act most promptly and effectually were *Nux vomica* and *Bryonia*, thus calling to mind the effect of those remedies that experience had led me to use in the attacks that come in the summer, that are usually designated as of a bilious nature.

In the secondary form, or where my malaria seemed to be the result of the decomposition of the material or vegetable fiber, its effects were more permeating, as different symptoms were developed by it. Then a change of remedies (or chemical antidotes, if you please), became necessary, and far the best results were secured by the use of *Bryonia* and *Arsenicum. China* did not act well or give any reasonable satisfaction.

Prior and later experience give ample satisfactory proof of the utility of the use of *Arsenicum* in all types of an intermittent nature, yet not to discredit the fact that other remedies can and will cure this form. But that a pernicious case can, or will, be as readily restored by any other remedy, I reserve to myself the liberty to doubt. Opportunities and time have demonstrated that these two remedies are able to restore the system and remedy a majority of the diseases that are wont to make their advent in the early autumn or late in the spring.

Later, after the total decomposition of my vegetable matter had taken place, and it almost seemed to possess a demoniacal potency or power to undermine the humblest human form, then to my surprise *Bryonia* seemed to hold prestige and give splendid results, but needed a different assistant, one that could and would permeate the muscular system, yet slowly, and for this *Rhus tox* was called into requisition, and from that day to this it has not been the means of causing me a single disappointment.

(Again, and as a last quotation from this interesting paper, we quote):

Many years of observation have demonstrated one more important fact in relation to the means that will render the system less liable to its absorption, at least to that extent that it will give evidence of its presence, and that is, by the liberal use of coffee.

(In 1897 Dr. Bowen sent the following to the *Homœopathic Recorder* concerning *Malaria off.*):

Messrs. Boericke & Tafel prepared me a new supply of it, and I have used so far only one form of it and in the one attenuation.

It was prepared in three degrees of strength:

No. I is the *water* that stood on decomposed vegetable matter for one week at a temperature of 90 degrees.

No. II is the *water* that decomposed vegetable matter for two weeks.

No. III is the *water* that decomposed vegetable matter for *three* weeks, and it is fearfully offensive.

I have only used the No. II, or that that had only partially decomposed the vegetable fibres.

In preparing it for use I put *ten drops* of the water to ninety drops of alcohol and then medicated my pellets (No. 30), and it does not soften them up. This is the only form I have used it in, and give from three to ten of these pills for a dose two, three or four hours apart.

I have been confined to my home for three months this year, and hence will only report a few of the most marked cases.

CASE I. Mrs. R., aged 45, weighing 245 pounds, could scarcely walk or get into a buggy for two years, from the effects of rheumatism in her back and limbs. I gave her last March two drams of No. 30 pills medicated with the first decimal, or No. 2 preparation, with orders to take ten pills three or four times a day. In *one week* she could walk as well as ever and has no rheumatism or lameness since.

CASE II. Mr. S., foreman in a large saw mill, has been afflicted with rheumatism for years. He came to me in April with a stiff neck and his right arm and shoulder helpless and painful. He wished me to keep it from his chest and heart. I gave him two drams No. 30 pellets, first decimal, and a vial of *neutral* globules, with orders to take two hours apart, changing, when better, three hours apart. In three days he was better and could turn his neck and use his arm fairly well. One week later gave him two drams more of *Malaria*, to be taken six hours apart. He has not had any rheumatic troubles since that time.

CASE III. Mr. C., proprietor of two large saw mills, one in Arkansas, where he passes part of his time (and frequently gets wet), has been afflicted with what some doctors called gout. I found it was of a rheumatic nature (caused from malaria) and made worse by *Quinine* and external applications. I gave him *Malaria*, two drams, No. 30 pills. In three days he assured me he was better and did not have half as many pains or aches. He took only four drachms, at from three to six hours apart, and has not had any rheumatic or gouty pains since. I saw him last week and he says he is fully ten years younger than he was last spring.

CASE IV. I was called to see I. S., aged 55, a veteran and pensioner of the last war. He was poor and bronzed in color. Had not been able to walk for years. After repairing his heart, chest, stomach and curing his piles and regulating his bowels he was content, yet he could not walk. Being assured that his back had been injured while in the army, and as his limbs would not move at his will and he could not walk alone or get out of a chair, I gave him for a week *Ruta graveolens* and *Rhus tox.*, of each the first cent., three hours apart. This enabled him to get up and down two steps alone to the kitchen. Then, concluding his trouble was due to rheumatism, and that was caused by malaria, I gave him two drams of No. 30 pellets of No. 2 form of *Malaria*, first decimal, with orders to take ten pills three or four times a day. In one week he rode to my house and came up and down steps alone. I gave him two drams more and in five days he came to my office, having walked nearly three miles that morning alone. I need not say I was deeply surprised and could hardly believe it was all due to *Malaria*. It certainly was, as nothing else was taken or applied. He has gained flesh and seems to be at least ten years younger than he was.

These are a few of the surprising results that have been obtained from *Malaria* this year. I much wish that others would try it and help to obtain its proper place as a medicine and healer when used where it should be given.

(Dr. W. A. Yingling contributed the following to the same journal):

On the day I received from Boericke & Tafel *Malaria off.* 30, I was foolishly led to try Hahnemann's inhalation. The thought just occurred to me on the spur of the moment, and without stopping to think I took three strong inhalations, with both sorrow and a proving resulting. None of the symptoms were distressing, yet marked and clear cut. The remedy commenced its work very promptly and in the order following:

Aching in both elbows.

A kind of slight concentration of feeling at root of nose, and just above, as though I should have a severe cold, similar to that complained of by hay-fever patients.

Aching in the wrists.

A tired ache in the hands.

A tired ache in the knees, and for a distance above and below.

A feeling as though I should become dizzy.

Pain in top of left instep.

A tired feeling in wrists.

Aching in an old (cured) bunion on left foot.

Sensation on point of tongue as though a few specks of spice or pepper were there.

Itching on right cheek over molar bone; ameliorated by slight rubbing or scratching.

When leaning face on left hand, elbow on the table, perceptible feeling of the heart beats through upper body and neck.

Slight itching on various parts of the face and extremities; ameliorated by slight rubbing.

Sense of heat in the abdomen.

Chilly sensation in left forearm. Soon followed by chilly feeling in hands and fingers; feet are cold with sensation as if chilliness was about to creep up the legs. A few moments later knees feel cold. A sense of coldness ascending over body from the legs.

Arms feel tired.

Belching several times, easy; no taste.

A drawing pain in right external ear.

Lumbar back feels tired as though it would ache.

Neck feels tired, with slight cracking in upper part on moving the head.

Shallow breathing which seems from languor, with a desire to take a deep inspiration occasionally.

A kind of tired feeling through abdomen and chest.

A general sense of weariness.

A feeling about head as though I would become dizzy.

Pain in upper left teeth.

A sensation as though I would have a very loose stool (passed away without a stool).

Feeling rather stupid and sleepy.

A sensation in the spleen as though it would ache.

Saliva more profuse than usual; keeps me swallowing often.

Pain in abdomen to right of navel.

Dull aching through forehead.

Face feels warm as if flushed, also head; becomes general over body, as if feverish.

Aching across upper sacral region.

Legs very weary from short walk.

Pain at upper part of right ilium.

General sense of weariness from a very short walk, especially through pelvis, sacral region and upper thighs. I feel strongly inclined to lie down and rest.

Qualmishness at stomach, as though I should become nauseated.

General sense of malaise and weariness becoming quite marked.

Aching above inner angle of right eye.

A kind of simmering all through the body.

Felt impelled to lie down, and on falling to sleep a sense of waving dizziness passes all over me, preventing sleep.

At times I feel as though I should become cold or have a chill, then I feel as though I should become feverish or hot, though neither is very marked.

Eyes feel heavy and sleepy.

Uneasiness in lower abdomen.

Gaping, yawning and desire to stretch.

Legs are restless; feel like stretching and moving them.

I feel very much as I did one time before having the ague, twenty-five years ago.

Odor from cooking is pleasing, but I have no desire for dinner. Yet when I sit down I eat a good dinner with relish.

Dizziness on rising from a reclining position.

Feel generally better after eating dinner.

Aching in the occiput.

During the afternoon leg weary.

Unusual hearty appetite for supper (the good appetite keeps with me for some days).

A good night's rest following, and have felt much brighter and generally better ever since the first day. (Healing.)

I have no doubt had I repeated the inhalations several times I should have been very sick. It is not necessary to push a proving to extremes. I think Hahnemann did not as a rule. If I were strong I should push this proving, but I dare not. Who will take it up?

(Apropos of the foregoing Dr. G. Hering, of England, made the following suggestions which hint at a possible use of the remedy in tuberculosis):

What curious discoveries are made by the observant! Witness the following remarks of Dr. Casanova, as recorded in the *Homœopathic Review* of over thirty years ago:

"I know several localities in South America, Africa and Spain where the marsh miasma has unquestionably arrested and cured that fatal scourge of the human race, phthisis pulmonalis, without any other treatment or restriction in food or drink. And why should not the climate of the fen lands of Lincolnshire, in the neighborhood of Spalding, prove as curative an agent for this disease as the climate of so many foreign regions where patients go and die, deprived of all the comforts of a home? Penzance, among the British localities, is reported to be superior to nine-tenths of the places to which patients are sent. Penzance, then, and Spalding should be particularly studied by medical men and recommended to consumptive individuals who wish to enjoy the benefits and advantages of a national place of relief, if not of cure."

Upon reading this I began to reflect upon the limitless nature of science. We never seem to find either beginning or end to it. Circles within circles, and no one can tell what communications there are between those circles. We cannot trace them. We are lost in infinity.

Miasmatic places are the most healthy places—for some of us at least.

Now, I think of it, I find I can give some support to this statement of Dr. Casanova. I was once on board a Liverpool steamer which put into Aspinwall, on the swampy Isthmus of Panama, for nine days. Upon our return home several of the sailors, otherwise healthy fellows, were prostrated by what was called Panama fever, whilst I myself, who had formerly suffered from tubercular disease of the lungs, was totally unaffected.

MULLEIN OIL.

PREPARATION.—Fill a bottle with the blossoms from the Verbascum thapsus, cork tight, and hang in the sun for four or five weeks. By that time there will be an oily liquid distilled. Mix with ten per cent. of alcohol.

(Dr. A. M. Cushing introduced this now rather well-known remedy to the medical profession in 1884. He writes of it as follows):

The history of it is this: My father's house was the home for all poor tramps, as well as ministers, etc. He fell into the river, got water in his ears and was quite deaf for months. A blind man called, heard loud conversation, asked the cause, etc., then said for kindness received he would tell us how to make something that would surely cure him, and it was worth a thousand dollars in New York city. We made the oil, put it in his ears at night, and he was well in the morning. For years we kept a bottle of it, and it travelled all around the towns and did wonders. That was when I was a youngster. When I studied medicine, or when I was practicing, I wanted to know if it was homœopathic, and made a proving, and developed the symptoms of almost constant but slight involuntary urination, keeping my pants wet.

I did not make any this past season, and have divided till I have but a little, half-and-half alcohol, left. I could spare a little of that, and next season, if I live, will try and make a quantity.

(The next item is from a letter of Dr. H. C. Houghton's, of New York, addressed to Boericke & Tafel.)

I have been much interested in the clinical study of this remedy—new, yet not new—but I have not succeeded in demonstrating what the symptom—deafness means in this case. Dr. Cushing does not claim to be an expert in this department, so time must help us out, and I am anxious to learn all I can of its effects on the ear.

In an old note-book of Dr. Hering's, *Hearing and Ears*, copied for me with the author's permission by my friend Dr. C. R. Norton, I noticed the following: "In Germany, flowers of Verbascum thapsus put in a dark-colored bottle, hung up in the sunlight, give in two or three weeks an oily fluid which has cured many old people and children." This method is impracticable, the amount produced being so small. Verbascum prepared in olive oil or fluid petroleum has the same effect as any oil; excellent in chronic disease of the integument; negative in middle ear disease. When your house brought out *Mullein oil* under Dr. Cushing's direction, I took it up again, and have prescribed it in a large number of cases. In chronic dermatitis of the external meatus and drum-head, or exfoliation after furuncle, it is excellent; in chronic catarrhal inflammation of the tympanum I have not been able to see any effect, but in chronic suppurative disease of the tympanum, or in accumulations of detritus in cases of perforation, scarred drum-heads, etc., it acts to dislodge accumulations, free the ossicula from pressure, and thereby improves the hearing; this process goes on for months till the tympanum has thrown out an amount of *débris* that is surprising. In a few cases it has caused soreness and increased muco-purulent discharge, due, I think, to excessive use.

My experience with it in chronic catarrh of the tympanum coincides with that of my friend, H. P. Bellows, M. D., of Boston, as published by him, but I purpose to continue the study of the drug, and hope for better results. In sub-acute or chronic disease after suppuration its effect is very gratifying; it aids exfoliation and checks irritation from exfoliated material.

I am able to confirm the symptoms noted of its effects in nocturnal enuresis in many instances. There is one effect I have not seen noticed by any observers: relief of night cough. More than ten years ago, Dr. H. A. Tucker, Brooklyn, N. Y., told me of a *Glycerole of Mullein* made by macerating the plant in Jamaica rum for two or three weeks, expressing it and adding to this product an equal quantity of glycerine. This led me to the use of the fluid extract of the plant, glycerine and water, equal parts, as a mollifier in cases where patients would resort to some popular remedy containing opium or similar opiate. The same effect can be produced by drop doses of *Mullein oil*, the teasing cough which comes on lying down, preventing the sleep usually yielding to a few doses.

(Dr. J. C. Wentz contributed the following bit of folk-lore):

The application of *Mullein oil* is of more general application than anything I have found in print. I report to you some cases:

CASE I.—Mertie B., aged sixteen. Called to see her May 20, 1888. Found her suffering great pain in right ear. Parotid gland very much enlarged and painful. The right side of the head and face much swollen. Pulse about 100; tongue coated.

Treatment.—Mullein oil in the ear, and used as a liniment twice daily on the swollen parts. For the fever, *Aconite*. Great improvement during the first twenty-four hours, and on the 23d found the case convalescent.

CASE II.—Carrie H., aged twenty-two. Her second child four weeks old. Called November 15, 1888. Right breast inflamed and sore. Two weeks previous it had been lanced by another physician, a little above the nipple, but now a place a little below and to the left of the nipple gives evidence of forming pus. I told her that in my judgment it had gone too far to check it then.

Treatment.—*Mullein oil,* one-half ounce in four ounces of water. Wet cloths and apply. The inflammation and soreness disappeared in one week, and by the use of the same remedy occasionally has entirely recovered without breaking. Her husband, when he paid me, said: "Well you have done better than any of the rest of the doctors."

CASE III.—Linford S., aged sixty-four. Called to see him September 20, 1888. Has just recovered from typhoid fever, but is able to be around. Taken with inflammation of the right testicle. Swollen to the size of a goose egg, and much pain. Red and shining appearance of the skin. Cause unknown, unless it was in connection with chronic enlargement of prostate gland.

Treatment.—*Mullein oil* applied twice daily as a liniment. *Mercurius sol.* internally. In three days the soreness and pain had entirely disappeared, but the enlargement continued several days. He walked around with ease three or four days before swelling had diminished any.

CASE IV.—F. C., aged thirty. Called November 16, 1888. Found inflammation of left kidney and of left testicle. Had been under treatment by another doctor and had recovered partially, but relapsed. Suffering much with pain in testicle, which ran up the spermatic cord and through to the left kidney.

Treatment.—*Cantharis* and *Aconite,* as there was some fever. *Mullein oil* applied to the testicle. Rapid improvement during the first twenty-four hours, and made a quick recovery.

I have also cured a case of chronic inflammation of the eyes, and a case of chilblains from which the patient had suffered, during the winter, for about six years. * * *

Every drug has its exact range. This one being new to the profession, we are just learning what it will do. In all these cases the *Mullein oil* has had an outward application twice daily.

A short time ago I was in Dodge city and was talking with a friend about the use of various remedies in veterinary practice, and amongst them I mentioned an almost instant cure of earache in a boy and also the same in a cat by the use of *Mullein oil.* He said: "Why do you homœopaths use that? I used to have the well sweep full of bottles of mullein blossoms when I was a boy. We used the oil as a dressing for burns, and it was the best thing we could get." He also related to me the following case, which is of interest and may prove of great value: An old neighbor, a Mr. Kemmis, had spent a large amount of money treating with various physicians for what they pronounced a rose cancer and without any relief. An Indian squaw told him to use *Mullein oil*. He distilled it (as it is now prepared, by sun exposure), and for a short time bathed the cancer with the oil. The growth of the cancer was permanently checked, but was not healed. Mr. K. lived, perhaps, forty years after the treatment was used, and the cancer never again bothered him.

MUCUNA URENS.

NAT. ORD., Leguminosæ.
COMMON NAME, Horse-eye.
PREPARATION.—The pulverized bean is macerated in five times its weight of alcohol.

(Delgado Palacios, of Venezuela, in 1897, wrote Messrs. Boericke & Tafel concerning this remedy):

Reading the list of remedies of your "Physicians' Price Current," I was very much astonished to meet with the name *Dolichos pruriens*, which the greater and modern authorities in botanical matters consider an identical plant with *Mucuna urens*.

You will meet the botanical description of *Mucuna urens* and *altissima* (two varieties) in the Flora of West Indian Islands, by A. H. R. Grisebach, p. 198 (Grisebach regards *Mucuna* and *Dolichos* as two different genus).

If one consider that there is a discussion upon this subject, and on the other hand that the mother tincture you possess is that which is made with the hair on the epidermis of the pod (*North American Journal of Homœopathy, vol. 1, p. 209. Allgemeine Homœopathische Zeitung, vol. 53, p. 135. Oehme, Hale's Amerikanische Heilmittel, p. 242*), while the tincture which we employ is made with the pulverized bean (1:5 alcohol) enclosed in the pod of a special plant which grows in the calid regions of Venezuela I believe you must try the same tincture we use and the success will be that which we obtain.

I have used my tincture of *Mucuna urens* extensively in a great number of hæmorrhoids and with the most satisfactory results. It seems that the characteristic symptom or key-note is a sensation of burning. The hæmorrhoids may be or not in a great stage of development, there may be more or less blood, etc.

One can consider the *Mucuna urens* as a specific against the hæmorrhoidal diathesis. The diseases of other organs, depending upon that cause, liver, uterus (hæmorrhage) and intestinal affections, yield admirably to its use.

I have been treating recently a remarkable case of chronic ingurgitation of a testicle, small and frequent hæmaturias, and other intestinal troubles with a prominent symptom, the hæmorrhoidal state, which led me to use *Mucuna*, and in a few months I have obtained a perfect success.

The experiences have taught me, and I have the conviction that this tincture is a more perfect remedy for the cure of hæmorrhoids than any other remedy known. I rely upon it more faithfully than I do upon *Hamamelis, Æsculus,* etc.

Its pathogenetics are not known.

I frequently use the mother tincture in the hæmorrhoids, one drop daily. I seldom use the lower dilutions. *Mucuna* may be used also, and with success, as an ointment.

The beans are very difficult to obtain; the plant has a single yearly crop.

NAPHTHALIN.

ORIGIN—A chemical compound procured from coal, alcohol, ether vapor, etc.

PREPARATION.—Trituration of the pure naphthalin.

(Two clinical cases illustrating the use of *Naphthalin*. The first is by Dr. W. L. Hartman, in Transaction of the Homœopathic Medical Society of New York, 1896.)

In treating children we are often disappointed in our results; in making prescriptions we think we have just the right thing in the right place, but when we come to see our case again we are confronted with the same condition that we had before. We may say the same in adults, but not so often. In whooping cough in the very young who are unable to tell us how they feel we must rely on what the mother may tell us; but how often do we find mothers who cannot tell their own symptoms, let alone those of their children? Now, what do we do? Sit and look wise and guess at our prescriptions while we hear the little fellow coughing, in fact trying to cough his head off and at the same time lose his breath.

Well, now while you are thinking and looking wise in this case, just think of *Naphthalin* and give a tablet triturate of the 1x every two hours, and when you are consulted the next time you will not be annoyed with the dreadful choking spell. Now in prescribing this remedy it is not necessary to wait until the child chokes to death with the cough, but give it from the first and you will be surprised how it will cut the disease short. I do not know as I have ever given this remedy without receiving benefit, and in many cases it was unnecessary to give any other remedy to cure the case; if it is, *Drosera* will follow best.

The grand characteristic of this remedy is long and continued paroxysms of coughing, unable to get a respiration, sometimes so violent as to cause perspiration.

This remedy is not only good in whooping cough, but in any condition where you get the above symptoms *Naphthalin* will cure your case just the same. Now my experience with this remedy where I have prescribed above the 1x has been very unsatisfactory, so, of late, I only use the one potency.

(The other by Dr. W. A. Weaver in *Hahnemannian Monthly*, 1898.)

My experience with *Naphthalin* in whooping cough is as yet limited, but the results obtained have very much exceeded other remedies and I wish to cite a few cases in which the alleviation of the symptoms was soon appreciable.

CASE I.—Francis——, a boy of 9 months, with a severe bronchitis as a complication. The breathing was labored. The respiratory murmur was feeble and a large number of sibilant and sonorous râles were heard, when I was called to see the case. The child had become emaciated, had a cyanotic appearance, was unable to retain food for any length of time, because of the frequent paroxysms accompanied by vomiting, and was very much exhausted. Later, the moist râles became very prominent over the entire chest. The paroxysms were of great length, and accompanying was a free discharge of thick, tenacious mucus from the nose and mouth. Many of the favorite remedies employed in this disease were prescribed, but with little effect. *Naphthalin* was then given, four or five drops of the tincture in one-half glass of water. In a short time the paroxysms were lessened in severity and frequency, the expectoration was freer, the number of râles were lessened, and shortly convalescence was well established.

CASE II.—John——, 3-1/2 years, with an accompanying bronchitis. Symptoms worse at night. Paroxysms very long and severe; would hold his head to relieve the pain from coughing. Great difficulty experienced in breathing. A number of râles heard over portion of the chest, with little expectoration. After *Naphthalin* had been given for a short time improvement began, and terminated without further complications.

CASE III.—Patrick——, a man 23 years of age, large physique and healthy appearance, contracted pertussis from other members of the family, and, although not accompanied by the whoop, the paroxysms were very severe. They were not frequent during the day but many during the night. He would wake the entire house by coughing and would become purple in the face. He had been suffering a week or two before I saw him. I prescribed *Drosera*, *Corrallium rub.*, *Ipecac* and *Hyoscyamus*, without appreciable improvement. He gradually grew worse until *Naphthalin* 1x in pellets was given. The spasmodic condition was relieved very shortly, and although the cough remained for a short time it never became severe and soon entirely disappeared.

NARCISSUS.

NAT. ORD., Amaryllidaceæ.
COMMON NAME, Daffodil.
PREPARATION.—The young buds, stems and leaves are macerated in two times their weight of alcohol.

(The following is from the *Homœopathic Recorder* for May, 1899):

"Agricola," one of the *Homœopathic World's* oldest contributors, has the following to say of this very old, yet little known, remedy. After stating how he prepared it, he continues as follows:

"A case of bronchitis (a *continuous* cough) has from *Narcissus* 1-3x obtained such *prompt* marked relief, where a most varied selection of the standard remedies had hitherto failed, as to induce me to write these few lines in hope that as this beautiful flower is about to be found in most cottage gardens the prevalent bronchitis, whooping and other coughs may meet with prompt cures. Dr. Chargé's work, *Maladies de la Respiration*, quotes the great Laennec, M. D., as an authority *in re Narcissus*."

There is no proving whatever of this drug, although in the *Encyclopædia* (Allen) a case of poisoning from the bulbs eaten as a salad is given; but the remedy as prescribed by Agricola was prepared from the young buds, stems and leaves, so the case in the *Encyclopædia* is not apropos, nor is the old tincture from the bulbs of use.

The name of the plant, *Narcissus*, is not from that of the fabled youth who fell in love with his own image reflected in the water, but is from the Greek *Narkao*, "to be numb," on account of the narcotic properties of the drug. The classic Asphodel and the Narcissus are the same, from which it may be seen that the plant dates back as far as man's records go. Fernie, in his excellent *Herbal Simples*, from which we gather the preceding, also says: "An extract of the bulbs applied to open wounds has produced staggering numbness of the whole nervous system and paralysis of the heart. Socrates called this plant the 'Chaplet of the Infernal Gods,' because of its narcotic effects."

Fernie also says that a decoction of the dried flowers is emetic, and when sweetened will, as an emetic, serve most usefully for relieving the congestive bronchial catarrh of children. "Agricola's" experience, quoted above, however, seems to disprove the notion that the beneficial action in bronchial catarrh is the result of the emetic properties of the drug, but demonstrates rather that it is peculiarly homœopathic to this malady and long-continued coughs, especially of nervous origin, as may be inferred from the following, the concluding paragraph in Fernie's section on the *Narcissus*:

"The medicinal influence of the Daffodil on the nervous system has led to giving its flowers and its bulb for hysterical affections, and even epilepsy, with benefit."

The *National Dispensatory* says practically the same, *i.e.*, "The emetic action of *Narcissus* has been used to break up intermittent fever and relieve bronchial catarrh with congestion or obstruction of the air tubes. Like *Ipecacuanha*, it has also been prescribed in dysentery, especially of the epidemic form. Its influence upon the nervous system, is attested by the vogue it has enjoyed in hysteria, chorea, whooping cough and even epilepsy."

It is still the emetic action that is looked to here, but any good homœopath will see beyond that, in Agricola's experience, and perceive a strong homœopathic action in the drug to the conditions named, for if it were the emetic action only that is efficacious then, certainly, one emetic would do as well as another, but there is something more, and the curative action can be obtained from homœopathic doses without the emetic action. The tincture should not be prepared from the bulb, as has been the case in the past, but from the fresh buds and leaves. From such a preparation considerable benefit in obstinate bronchial coughs should be confidently expected.

NEGUNDO.

NAT. ORD., Sapindaceæ.
COMMON NAMES, Box Elder. Ash-leaved Maple.
PREPARATION.—The bark of the root is macerated in twice its weight of alcohol.

(In the *California Medical Journal*, 1898, Dr. O. S. Laws, of Los Angeles, California, writes of a new "pile" remedy, *Negundo*):

I suggested that we have a "Symposium," in Our Journal, on single remedies. They are the backbone of whatever science there is in therapeutics, and should be kept in view. As a starter I offer one that is entirely new to the medical fraternity, as I cannot find it in any medical work.

In botanical language it is known as Negundium Americanum. The common name is "box elder." It is a native of Kansas. It is a distant relative of the Acer family. I had just fairly begun to test its value when I left Kansas for California, and not finding it here, except as a shade tree on the sidewalks, I cannot get any of the root bark, which is the part used. From the short experience I had with it I conclude it is the best internal remedy we have for hemorrhoids. I have used *Colinsonia* and *Æsculus* without ever being impressed with their prompt action. But *Negundo* goes at it as *Colocynth* does in its specialty, so that the victim who has been writhing with an engorged rectum "will arise up and call you blessed." So you see this is not only a single remedy, but a "fundamental" one. The bark of the root in the yearling plants is what I prefer.

Recent cases of hemorrhoids can be completely cured in this way, and the old hard cases temporarily relieved. So, gentlemen of the medical profession, I hereby introduce to you my friend *Negundo*.

ONOSMODIUM VIRGINIANUM.

NAT. ORD., Borraginaceæ.
COMMON NAME, False Cromwell.
PREPARATION.—The entire plant with root is macerated in twice its weight of alcohol.

(This paper was prepared by Dr. W. A. Vingling for the Kansas State Homœopathic Society, and reprinted in *Homœopathic Physician* for July, 1893).

To the homœopathic physician a new remedy, well proven, is an acquisition of greater importance than honor or wealth, for his sole duty being to relieve the sufferings of humanity, he acquires a new tool with which to accomplish his work. To the degree that the new remedy has peculiar characteristics its value is enhanced, to the extent that the pathogenetic effects are different from every other drug its usefulness becomes the more apparent. Generalities constitute a poor basis upon which to prescribe. Peculiarities, the unusual symptoms, give certainly an assurance in every prescription.

We have in *Onosmodium* a remedy with some peculiarities, and occupying a sphere unique, a curative range differing from that of every other drug. The remedy holds within its grasp the power to restore peace to the disrupted family, and to prevent the truant husband seeking the sweets of "stolen waters" by restoring the wife to the enjoyable performance of her wifely functions, and thus gratifying the dissatisfied husband. This generation of one-child families, Malthusian, with the long train of misery entailed upon the licensed family, adultery consequent upon preventive measures, *malum in se*, has its remedy in *Onosmodium* to a very large extent.

We pass to consider the more important pathogenesis of the remedy in regular course. A great part of this paper is necessarily based upon the notes of the original author, Dr. W. E. Green, with some isolated symptoms from the journals and my own experience.

We find marked in the mental sphere a DROWSINESS OF MIND and CONFUSION OF THOUGHT, DULNESS OF INTELLIGENCE, a DAZED feeling of the mind. The party wants to think and not move, so absorbed in thought as to forget all else and where she is. There is a *complete listlessness and apathy* of the mind; she cannot *concentrate* her thoughts. From this want of concentration there follows an impairment of the memory, *she cannot remember what is said.* In conversation she will forget the subject, will begin a new one, and then suddenly change to another. There is great *confusion of ideas*. This listlessness is so great as to cause forgetfulness of what one is reading, or that one is reading at all: the book drops in vague and listless thought. The time passes too slowly, and minutes seem like hours. There is great irritability of temper.

There is a continuous and ever-present feeling of heaviness of the head. PAINS IN THE LEFT SIDE OF THE HEAD and *over the left eye*, extending round the left side to the back of the head and neck, greatly aggravated by moving or jarring. Intense pain driving her to bed; relieved by sleep, but soon returning after waking. There is a constant dull headache, chiefly centered over the left eye and in the left temple; always worse in the dark and when lying down. Here we have a contradictory symptom—always worse lying down. The general symptoms are ameliorated by lying down. This peculiar feature is also seen in some of the polycrests. *Bryonia alb.* has a "pain and pressure in the shoulder when at rest." *Rhus tox.* has a "stiff neck, with painful tension when moving;" *Arsenicum alb.* has a headache relieved by cold water.

Onosmodium has a DULL, HEAVY PAIN IN THE occiput pressing upward WITH A DIZZY SENSATION. Pain changing from the right frontal eminence to the left and remaining there. Darting and throbbing in the left temple. A dull pain in the mastoid process. She cannot bear to move. A sense of fullness in the head. Relieved by eating and sleep.

The eyes are HEAVY AND DULL; the eyes feel as though one had lost a great deal of sleep. The lids are heavy. The eyeballs have a *dull, heavy pain with soreness*. A sensation of the eyes being very wide open, with a desire to look at distinct objects, it being disagreeable to look at near objects. Distant objects look very large. *Picric acid* patients can only see clearly at very close range, often at only five inches from the eye; *Natrum sulph.* has impairment of vision for distant objects. With *Onosmodium* the ocular muscles feel tense, tired, and drawn. Pains in and over left eye. Pain in upper portion of left orbit, with a feeling of expansion. The vision is impaired and blurred.

The hearing is impaired. There is a stuffed-full feeling in the ears as after catching cold. Singing in the ears as from quinine, but very slight.

The NOSE FEELS DRY. There is a stuffed feeling in the posterior nares. The discharge from the posterior nose is whitish and sticky, producing a constant hawking. Constant sneezing in the morning; sneezing when first getting up. The bones of the nose pain.

Flushed face, with relief from headache. That dry feeling of the nose is also present in the mouth and lips. Bitter, clammy taste in the mouth. Saliva is very scant, with the dry feeling in the mouth; cold water relieves. Sore throat. It hurts to swallow or speak. That dryness follows down the *throat* and *pharynx*, and is accompanied with *severe soreness*. Raw, scraping feeling in the throat. When swallowing the pharynx feels constricted. All the throat symptoms are relieved by cold drinks and by eating. The voice is husky. The chest feels sore.

Morning sickness like that of pregnancy. Distaste for water, yet there is a *craving for ice water and cold drinks; wants to drink often*. The abdomen *feels bloated* and distended, which is relieved by undressing. The pains in the lower part of the abdomen are also relieved by undressing or by lying on the back. This amelioration from undressing is observed to run through all the symptoms of the drug. A constant feeling as though diarrhœa would come on.

The stools are yellow, mushy, or greenish-yellow, stringy, mushy, with tenesmus. Also, slimy, bloody, stringy stool, with tenesmus. The provers were hurried out of bed in the morning to stool.

The urine is scanty, highly colored, dark straw and brown, very acid, and of high specific gravity. The desire is seldom, or else frequent, with scanty flow.

In regard to the sexual organs we quote from that racy writer, Dr. S. A. Jones, who says: "*Onosmodium Virginianum* in its primary action seems directly opposite to *Picric acid*. Perhaps provings of it with smaller doses will oblige me to change this *dictum*. If they do not, then *Onosmodium* will occupy the singular position of a remedy that *primarily depresses the sexual appetite*. If this should ultimately prove to be the case, it will invest this remedy with an unmistakable significance to physicians who are practicing at the *tail end* of the nineteenth century, for, from our habits of life, it is the *end* that is showing signs of distress. In estimating the validity of this suggestion, the reader will bear in mind Hahnemann's *dictum* that *only the primary symptoms of a drug afford the indications for its therapeutical application*. This is a canon of Hahnemannian Homœopathy, and it *is true as regards the infinitesimal dose*. Then, this being true (for I will not stop to discuss it), *Picric acid* will be indicated for the *initial stage* of sexual debility and *Onosmodium* for the *fully developed consequences* of sexual abuse; and this, because the said 'initial stage' is characterized by erethism while the ulterior consequences are denoted by atony asthenia. The erethism of sexual debility is plainly evinced in *Picric acid*, and the ultimate asthenia is as really discovered in *Onosmodium Virginianum*."

In the male we find diminished sexual desire. Cold feeling in the glans penis. Nocturnal emissions. Too speedy emissions. Deficient erections with diminished pleasure.

In the female we find SEVERE UTERINE PAINS. BEARING-DOWN PAINS IN THE UTERINE REGION. Uterine cramps. *Soreness in region of uterus*, increased by *pressure* of the hand or of the clothing; had to remove the corset. Return of old uterine pains. Dull, heavy aching, and slowly pulsating pains in the ovaries. Pains pass from one ovary to the other and leave a soreness which remains till the pain returns. Ovarian pains increased by pressure. SEXUAL DESIRE COMPLETELY DESTROYED. This symptom I have verified a number of times, and in every case the parties prevented conception. The uterine pains are all better when undressed or lying on the back. Constant feeling as though the menses would appear. Menses early and profuse, but otherwise normal so far as known. Leucorrhœa light yellowish, slightly offensive and excoriating; profuse, running down the legs. Itching of the vulva aggravated by scratching and from the leucorrhœal discharge. Aching in both breasts, but worse in the left. Breasts feel swollen and engorged. Left breast feels bruised and painful on pressure. Nipples itch. In one case where this remedy was given for dryness of the nose and throat, the diminutive almost absent, breasts were restored to their pristine glory, and resulted in the displacement of the cotton batting pads to the exceeding joy and delight of the proud woman.

Pains in the neck, running back from the forehead. *Dull aching in the neck*. Bearing down pain in the lumbar region. Dull, aching pain in the lumbar region. In the female provers there was produced a pain over the crest of the left ilium. TIRED, WEARY AND NUMB FEELING IN THE LEGS AND POPLITEAL SPACES. FEELING OF NUMBNESS, MOSTLY BELOW THE KNEES. The legs feel as if they were partially anæsthetized. The tendons and joints of the knees have a dull, aching pain. Tremulousness of the legs. DISTURBANCE OF THE GAIT IN WALKING, WITH A SENSE OF INSECURITY IN STEP. STAGGERING GAIT, *he cannot keep in the walk*. The sidewalks seem too high; he must step high which jars him and greatly aggravates the headache. Dull, heavy pain in the instep of the left foot. Numb, tingling pain in the outer side of both little toes. THE LEGS FEEL TIRED, *as though they would not sustain the weight of the body*. Sensation of formication in the calves of the legs. Ankles swollen.

Pain in the left scapular region, confined to a small spot. *Fluoric acid* and *Lilium tig.* have pain confined to a small spot in any location, while *Oxalic acid* has a pain confined to small longitudinal spots. *Magnesia phos.* has a sharp burning pain, about an inch in diameter, under the border of the left scapula, as from a hot iron (see also *Phos.*); with *Onosmodium* there is a dull, aching pain in the biceps muscle, also a pain of like nature in the elbow joint and wrists. *The arms and hands feel tired and weak*; they tremble. Inability to co-ordinate the muscular movements of the arms. Pain in the phalangeal articulation.

The aggravations are generally from motion or jarring; from pressure or tightness of clothing.

The ameliorations are peculiar and marked. Better when quiet, *when lying down on the back, when undressed,* when in the open air, from sleep, *from cold drinks, from eating.*

In the generalities we find great MUSCULAR WEAKNESS OR PROSTRATION AND TIRED FEELING OVER THE ENTIRE BODY. A feeling as though one had just gotten up from a severe spell of sickness. Nervous trembling as if from hunger. The least exertion produces a tremulousness. *The muscles feel treacherous and unsteady as though one did not dare to trust them.* A desire to change position without any definite cause or reason, and without any change for the better or worse. Later in the proving there was a desire to lie down and be quiet, with a drowsy, sleepy feeling. *A sensation as if a chill would come on;* a tired, aching, stretching, gaping, disagreeable feeling. All sensations are worse in the left side.

In my own experience I have used the remedy from the mother tincture up. I got no results from the tincture. Hardly any from the 30th, but a marked, decided, and very rapid action from the CM. I use nothing lower than the CM, and prefer the higher.

ORIGANUM MAJORANA.

NAT. ORD., Labiatæ.

COMMON NAME, Sweet Marjoram.

PREPARATION.—The whole plant without the root, gathered when in flower, is macerated in two times its weight of alcohol.

(A treatise on the "Sexual Passion," by the late Dr. Gallavardin, Lyons, France, contains this item on *Origanum*):

The person who discovered a remedy that in a certain sense may be considered as a specific against sexual passion was a clergyman of Mizza, the founder of an orphan asylum. This remedy is *Origanum majorana* (or common marjoram), which proves effective in masturbation and in excessively-aroused sexual impulses. The author uses it in the 4th dilution, as he has not found the higher potencies effective. He dissolves five or six globules of this dilution in four teaspoonfuls of fresh water, and the young masturbator takes of this every two days, a quarter of an hour before the meal, one teaspoonful. If the cure is not accomplished eight days after this solution is used up, the same dose is repeated in the same way. When desired, this remedy can be used, according to the author, without the knowledge of the patient, by pouring a teaspoonful into the soup, milk or chocolate.

The effect frequently appears very rapidly, but sometimes it does not appear.

OXYTROPIS LAMBERTI.

NAT. ORD., Leguminosæ.
COMMON NAMES, "Loco" Weed. Rattle Weed.
PREPARATION.—The whole plant without the root is macerated in two times its weight of alcohol.

(The following proving of the "loco weed" was conducted by the late Dr. W. S. Gee, of Chicago, in 1887):

OXYTROPIS LAMBERTI, Pursh.—*Commonly taller, as well as larger*, than other varieties (the scapes often a foot or more high); silky,—and mostly silvery-pubescent, sometimes glabrate in age; leaflets from oblong-lanceolate to linear (4 to 16 inches long); *spike, sometimes short-oblong and densely flowered*, at least when young; *often elongated and sparsely flowered; flowers mostly large* (often an inch long, but sometimes much smaller), variously colored; pod, either narrowly or broadly oblong, *sericeous pubescent, firm-coriaceous*, half-inch or more long, *imperfectly two-celled.* Includes O. *Campestris* of Hook, Fl. Bor. Am., in part. Common along the Great Plains from Saskatchewan and Minnesota to New Mexico, Texas, etc., and in the foot-hills.—From Coulter's *Manual of the Botany of the Rocky Mountain Region.*

It is one of the poisonous members of that family. It is found in California and New Mexico.

It is a perennial plant, with herbaceous or slightly shrubby stems, the foliage remaining green during winter when grass is scarce, and so attracting animals that would otherwise probably instinctively shun it. The plants do not appear to be equally poisonous at all seasons or in all localities, and it has been doubted whether the active properties they possess are due to a normal constituent of the plant. No medical use has ever been made of these plants, although their poisonous character has often led to the suggestion that they might be found valuable. No physiological study has been made of the action of the poison, and no complete chemical analysis has as yet appeared.

The stockmen speak of it as causing intoxication in the animals which eat it, and a prominent symptom is the "loco" condition, in which the power of co-ordination is lost or greatly limited. They cannot readily readjust for changes in gait, etc. A horse travels on level ground, but finds great difficulty in changing to pass over an elevation or depression, or, when going up hill, he has great difficulty in starting down hill; it is difficult, when he is still, to impress him that he must go, and as difficult to stop him when desired. The same rule applies to eating and other necessaries. Such a horse is said to be "locoed." Professor Hawkes procured specimens from which Boericke & Tafel made a tincture. To further test the merits of the remedy, the students of the class at Hahnemann Medical College of Chicago kindly participated in a proving.

Professor Hawkes received some reports from his group, but has mislaid his papers, and he is unable to give in detail the symptoms produced. He stated, however, that the principal action corroborated that given above.

During 1886-'87 term I made another attempt, and a few reports were received. The remedy was given by number, that the prover should not know what he took, nor the strength of it. Some were given the θ, others 1xd , 2xd , 3xd , 12x powders, 30x powders, and some higher.

A few reported "no effect" from the θ. The following includes the report from five persons:

1. (Mr. S. P. F., 10 drops of θ.) 2. (Mrs. W., 10 drops of 3xd repeated.) 3. (Mr. G. H. A., 15 drops of 3xd .) 4. (Mrs. P., powders of 12x repeated.) 5. (Mrs. L., powders of 30x.) 6. (Mrs. L., powders of 12x.)

SYMPTOMATOLOGY.

Mind.—Great mental depression,1 ,3 . Cannot think or concentrate his thoughts,1 ,3 . Very forgetful of familiar words and names,3 . No life,1 . Disinclination to talk or study,3 . Wants to be alone,3 . Is better satisfied to sit down and do nothing,3 . Feels perfectly despondent,3 . A feeling as if I would lose consciousness,3 . All symptoms worse when thinking of them,1 ,3 .

Sensorium.—Strange sensation about the head,4 . A feeling as if I would lose consciousness, or as if I would fall when standing,5 . Sense of fulness of the head, and of instability, when standing or sitting,6 .

Head.—The head has a feeling of great pressure, especially on moving the eyeballs,4 . Head hot,6 . Was unable to move around on account of this strange, uncertain feeling of numbness, with prickling sensation in left arm and hand,4 . Full, uncomfortable feeling in the head,5 . Slight headache in vertex and occiput in forenoon, over the eyeballs about noon,1 . Pain in the helix of the ear for two or three minutes, then pain commenced between the eyes and went in a straight line up over the head and down to the base of the brain,2 . Pain across the base of the brain,2 ("gone in a minute or two"). Dulness in frontal region, must lie down,4 . Pain in occipital region is constant since 1 P.M.; heavy ache, as if a weight were attached to the lower edge, pulling it back, but pain does not extend down the back,2 ; all stop at 3 P.M.,2 . A pressing headache from 2 to 5 P.M.,3 (on 2d day). Awoke with slight pressing pain in forehead, which increased gradually until about 2 P.M., and then gradually decreased,3 . Pain, dull and heavy, in the head, with sense of pressure,4 . Head very sensitive, < on the side on which I lie,3 . Pressure upon the head disappearing after sleep,4 . Dull, heavy feeling in the head, with uncertain gait and walk, so that she was obliged to lie down, when she fell into a deep sleep and woke up with the metallic taste.

Eyes.—Feel dull and heavy, blurred, pupils dilated,3 ,4 . When reading, it seems as if a light were reflected from a bright copper plate seen at the left side, as if the light were at the end of the room,6 . Pain in the eyeball,4 . Pain over the right eye,6 .

Ears.—Roaring sound in the ears,3 .

Nose.—Very dry; scabs form in the nose,3 . Frequent violent sneezing, with fluent coryza in the evening,1 . Nose feels as if sunburnt; red and shining, especially on alæ,1 . Feeling of pressure over the bridge of the nose,1 . Fluent coryza, somewhat bloody,1 .

Mouth.—Very dry, especially in the morning,3 . Metallic taste in the mouth, strongly marked,1 . Gumboil on left lower maxillary; profuse saliva,1 . Pain in left lower maxillary,1 . Tenderness of all the molars,1 .

Throat.—Slight inflammation of the pharynx, a "husky" feeling,1 . Dry and sore,3 .

Eating and Drinking.—Appetite gradually increasing,1 .

Appetite good; symptoms, < after eating, > after an hour,2 . Loss of appetite,6 (unusual).

Nausea and Vomiting.—Eructations, as after taking soda-water (after each powder), with colicky pains,5 , and looseness of the bowels (constipated before taking the remedy),5 . Eructations, empty, frequent,1 . Slight nausea, all day at intervals,2 (first day). A very tired, languid feeling all forenoon, accompanied by nausea on lying down, passing away on getting up, and returning on lying down again (not at night).

Stomach.—Tenderness in the epigastric region,1 . A kind of pressing soreness,3 . Cold during the chill,2 .

Abdomen.—Sharp, lancinating pains all through the abdomen, early in the evening,5 (observed but once). Sharp pain, running from right to left across the bowels, for several minutes, followed by a very strong desire to go to stool; entire relief after stool; slight griping pain in the region of the umbilicus, working down at 8 P.M., followed at 10 P.M. by discharge of flatus; full feeling in abdomen, causing short breathing after lying down in bed,1 .

Stool.—Symptoms marked and constant. Fæces of the consistency of mush, which slips through the sphincters in little lumps, very similar to lumps of jelly,3 . Stools dark brown, or like jelly,3 . Urgent desire for stool, sometimes removed by passing wind; quantity normal,3 . Sore feeling in the rectum,3 . Crawling sensation in rectum as if little worms were there,3 . Stool inclined to be hard; unsatisfied feeling, as though not done,1 . Stool solid at first, then diarrhœa,1 . Movement of the bowels at an unusual time,2 (6:30 P.M., had moved the morning of same day). Sharp pain from right to left across the bowels, followed by very strong desire for stool,2 . Stool, first hard, then loose,2 . Entire relief from pain after stool,2 .

Urine.—Symptoms very marked,3 . Characterized from the first by a very profuse flow of clear, or almost colorless urine, nearly the color of water,3 . Three to four times the normal quantity,3 ,1 ,4 ,2 . When thinking of urinating I had to go at once,3 . No sediment whatever,3 ,1 . Pain in the kidneys, hardest in right, with some tenderness,1 . At the expiration of every two or three hours after stopping the remedy, there was an enormous flow of pale, straw-colored urine, and with this would gradually disappear the metallic taste which was so marked,4 . Free urination, dark in color, no distress,2 . Urine scanty, and looked like that of a child troubled with worms, light red-colored stain on bottom of vessel,2 (second day). Awoke with a heavy pain in the kidneys,2 (third day). Urine clear on passing, but becomes as above described on standing,2 (third day). During day urine scanty, with considerable irritation, as if the muscles of the bladder were contracting, > moving about,2 .

Male Sexual Organs.—From being naturally of a passionate nature, the *desire* and *ability* diminished to impotence,3 . No sexual desire or ability,3 . Bruised feeling in the testicles, beginning in the right and extending to the left—came on after going to bed,1 . Occasional pain, of short duration, in glans penis,1 . Pain in testicles, worse with extension along spermatic cord and down thighs,1 (third day).

Sexual Organs, Female.—At 1.30 P.M., felt a pain in left ovary, like something grasping or holding tightly for about an hour, then disappeared,2 .

Larynx.—Slight accumulation of mucus in the larynx, hard to cough it up,2 .

Breathing.—Short and quick breathing from the full feeling in the abdomen,1 . Hard breathing, as though lungs and bronchi were closing as the chill passes off.

Cough.—A dry cough, from any little exercise,3 (eleventh day). A short, hacking cough, with tightness across the chest,2 (third day).

Lungs.—Oppression at 9 P.M.,1 (first day).

Heart and Pulse.—Palpitation after lying down at night, for 15 to 20 minutes,1 (seventh day). On going to bed, pain, like a wave, over the heart,2 (second day), < lying down. Pulse 84, intermittent,2 (2 P.M. of third day).

Outer Chest.—A warm, tingling sensation over left chest, just under the skin,2 (lasted five minutes).

Neck and Back.—Neck pains. Pain and stiffness of the muscles of the back of the neck.

Upper Extremities.—Stitching pain in right wrist for half an hour, leaving a tired feeling in joint,2 . At 12:30, a sharp, cutting pain running from point of shoulder down front of chest to point of hip bone, going suddenly,2 . Flesh feels as though she had taken a heavy cold,2 . Sharp pain, with coldness, from left shoulder-joint extending down the arm < in shoulder-joint, > sleep; goes away gradually,4 . Prickling sensation in left arm and hand,4 .

Lower Extremities.—Stitching pain in right leg and knee-joint for half an hour, leaving a tired feeling in the joint,2 . Hard pain in the left big toe-joint,2 . Pain inside of left leg from the groin to the knee,2 .

Extremities in General.—Flesh on under side of limbs sore,2 . Sore feeling of all the muscles of the right side of the body,2 . All the pains come and go quickly, but the muscles remain sore and stiff,2 . Frequent fine pains all over the body until 3 P.M., when all disappeared and felt as well as usual,2 .

Position.—All pains better when moving about and when in the cool air,2 . Nausea, heart symptoms and breathing, < lying down,1 ,2 .

Nerves.—At 10 A.M. a very sick, exhausted feeling appeared,2 .

Sleep.—Not very sound,3 . Dreams of a pleasant or lascivious character,3 . Wakes often,2 . On rising feels sad, weary, despondent,3 . Twitching of the muscles on falling asleep roused him,3 (once three or four nights). Dreamed of spiders, bugs,2 (first night), of swimming in water,2 (second night—am not in the habit of dreaming).

Chill.—Chill at 11:40 A.M., beginning in back between shoulders, down over body to feet; stomach feels cold; pains all over body during chill; a peculiar sensation of crawling or contraction of the abdominal muscles, hardest about the navel, lasted about half an hour,2 . As the chill passes off a smarting in the throat and a feeling as though the lungs and bronchi would close up, making breathing very difficult; chill lasted until 1 P.M., followed by perspiration of palms of the hands and soles of the feet; the changeable pains remained until 3 P.M., when all disappeared,2 . No thirst in either stage,2 . Felt badly for three days at same hour as chill,2 . For four weeks on every seventh day had a chill with all the above symptoms; the coldness of the spine was continuous for eight weeks, and was then removed by *Gelsemium*,2 .

(Dr. W. D. Gentry, while at Las Vegas, New Mexico, made the following summary of the action of the remedy. *Homœopathic Recorder*, 1895):

For the present I will only give a few of the leading symptoms produced by the *Loco weed*:

Brain and Mind: Stimulation of mind; pleasant intoxicated feeling. Satisfied indifference to all influences and interests.

Head: Full, warm feeling about the head.

Eyes: Strange feeling of fullness about the eyes, with sight obscured, so that it appears that one is looking through clear water which produces about all of the seven prismatic colors, red, orange, yellow, green, blue, purple and violet.

Paralysis of nerves, and muscles of the eyes, producing amblyopia. Pupils contracted and do not respond to light.

Eyesight lost with feeling as if in consequence of long exposure to strong, arc-electric lights.

Neck and Back: Numb, pithy or woody feeling about and in the spine.

Lower Extremities: Loss of power to control movements of body or limbs.

Swaying, staggering gait.

Reflex action of tendon-patella lost.

General: Weakness and insecurity of all powers of locomotion.

Feeling of intoxication, with almost entire loss of vision.

Amblyopia: sense of touch greatly weakened.

(From the *Kansas City Star.*)

The loco weed of the Western plains is to vegetation what the rattlesnake is to animal life. The name comes from the Spanish and signifies insanity. It is a dusky green and grows in small bunches or handfuls and scatters itself in a sparse and meagre way about the country. It is in short a vegetable nomad and travels about not a little. Localities where it this season flourishes in abundance may not see any of it next year, nor indeed for a number of years to come.

The prime property of the loco is to induce insanity in men or animals who partake of it. Animals—mules, horses, sheep and cattle—avoid it naturally, and under ordinary circumstances never touch it. But in the winter, when an inch or two of snow has covered the grass, these green bunches of loco standing clear and above the snow are tempting bits to animals which are going about half starved at the best. Even then it is not common for them to eat it. Still, some do and it at once creates an appetite in the victim similar in its intense force to the alcohol habit in mankind.

Once started on the downward path of loco a mule will abandon all other forms of food and look for it. In a short time its effects become perfectly apparent. You will see a locoed mule standing out on the shadowless plain with not a living, moving thing in his vicinity. His head is drooping and his eyes are half closed. On the instant he will kick and thresh out his heels in the most warlike way. Under the influence of loco he sees himself surrounded by multitudes of threatening ghosts and is repelling them.

The mind of the animal is completely gone. He cannot be driven or worked because of his utter lack of reason. He will go right or left or turn around in the harness in spite of bits or whip, or will fail to start or stop, and all in a vacant, idiotic way devoid of malice. The victim becomes as thin physically as mentally, and after retrograding four or five months at last dies, the most complete wreck on record. Many gruesome tales are furnished of cruel Spanish and Mexican ladies who, in a jealous fit, have locoed their American admirers through the medium of loco tea. Two or three cases in kind are reported in the Texas lunatic asylum.

ŒNANTHE CROCATA.

PREPARATION.—The fresh root is macerated in two parts by weight of alcohol.

(The following paper on *Œnanthe crocata* was kindly sent to the editor by Dr. W. A. Dewey, of the Ann Arbor University, Michigan):

Œnanthe crocata belongs to the large family of the Umbelliferæ which furnishes us with *Conium* and *Cicuta*. It grows in marshy localities in England and France. In Botanical works of the 16th and 17th centuries it was often confounded with *Cicuta virosa*, an error which has even been made in more recent times, in fact, only one Botanist of the 19th century described the plant with sufficient exactness for its recognition, and that was DeLobel, who published his Botany in 1851. It is one of the largest plants of the family, being 3 to 5 feet high. Our tincture is from the fresh root.

HISTORICAL.—*Œnanthe* was known to Galen and Dioscorides, and numerous citations might be made to show that the drug was used from the earliest times in various affections, affections that nearly every drug was tried in, but it is in the "Cyanosura Materia Medica of Boecler, published in 1729," that we first find a hint as to its true action. "Those who ate much of it were taken with dark vertigos, going from one place to another, swaying, frightened, turning in a circle as Lobilus pretends to have seen."

Hahnemann, in his "Apotheker Lexicon" (Leipzig, 1793), says of the drug: "It is said that the whole plant is poisonous and causes vertigo, stupefaction, loss of force, convulsions, delirium, stiffness, insensibility, falling of the hair, and taken in large quantities will cause death."

He says further: "That, administered with great circumspection, it should prove useful in certain varieties of delirium, vertigos and cramps."

This is interesting coming from Hahnemann at the time when he had discovered the law, but had not as yet given it to the world.

Œnanthe was considered in the last century as one of the most pernicious plants of Europe, especially for cattle, who, having eaten it, can neither vomit nor digest it and they soon die in convulsions; this from the root, however, as they eat the leaves with impunity. It is interesting to note that animals poisoned with it decompose rapidly.

Much of the following study is taken from a series of excellent papers on the drug, which have been appearing for over a year in "Le Journal Belge D'Homœopathie," from the pen of Dr. Ch. DeMoor, of Alost, Belgium.

GENERAL ACTION.—From a very large collection of observations of cases of poisoning with *Œnanthe*, dating from 1556 to the present time and recorded in "Allen's Encyclopædia," the "Cyclopædia of Drug Pathogenesy," and in the article of Dr. DeMoor, above mentioned, we find that *Œnanthe crocata* produces, almost invariably, convulsions of an epileptiform character and which are marked by the following symptoms:

Swollen, livid face, sometimes pale.

Frothing at mouth.

Contraction of chest and oppressed breathing.

Dilated pupils or irregular. Eyeballs turned upward.

Coldness of the extremities.

Pulse weak.

Convulsions are especially severe, at first tonic then clonic.

Locked jaws.

Trembling and twitching of muscles.

Œnanthe also produces a delirium in which the patient becomes as if drunken, there is stupefaction, obscuration of vision and fainting.

The Greek name of the plant signifies "wine flower," and so-called on account of its producing a condition similar to wine drunkenness, and there is a difference, so I have heard, between wine and other beverages in this respect. Hiccoughs are also produced by the drug.

There is also great heat in the throat and stomach and a desire to vomit and to have stool, and a great deal of weakness of the limbs and cardialgia. Like other members of the same family, as *Conium*, it produces very much vertigo, this has always been present in the cases of poisoning with the plant. In a number of cases who had been poisoned by the drug the hair and nails fell out.

HOMŒOPATHIC ACTION AND APPLICABILITY.—The uses of *Œnanthe*, homœopathically, have been taken from the reports above mentioned; the drug has never been proved, and it is doubtful if one could be found who would prove it to the convulsion-producing extremity. All the evidence in all the authorities shows clearly that the drug produces in man all the symptoms of epilepsy, and it is in that disease that clinical testimony is gradually accumulating. Accepting the theory that epilepsy is a disturbance or irritation in the cortex of the brain, it would seem that *Œnanthe crocata*, which produces congestion of the pia mater, would prove a close pathological simillimum to epilepsy. Its usefulness in this disease is unmistakable and only another proof of the truth of the homœopathic law.

Let us review briefly some of the evidence of its action: Dr. S. H. Talcott, in the report of the Middletown Asylum, 1893, notes that Œnanthe possesses a marked power in epilepsy, stating that it makes the attack less frequent, less violent and improves the mental state of the patient. He prescribes it in the tincture, 1 to 6 drops daily.

In the Materia Medica Society of New York its use has been verified several times. Dr. Paige greatly benefited a case with the 3x potency.

Dr. F. H. Fisk reports the cure of a case which had lasted two years, with the tincture. This case during the last month before the doctor took it was having from 6 to 10 attacks daily.

Dr. Garrison, of Easton, Pa., reports a case of reflex uterine or hystero-epilepsy in which the 2x acted promptly.

Allen in his Hand-Book mentions the cure of three cases with the remedy.

Dr. J. Ritchie Horner reports that the remedy greatly modified the attacks in a lady who had had the disease over 20 years, and who, for the two months previous, had had a convulsion daily. He used the 3x.

Dr. J. S. Cooper, of Chillicothe, Ohio, reports the cure of a case of 25 years' standing with the 4x.

Dr. Henderson reports the cure of a case of 9 years' standing, where the patient was almost idiotic; the convulsions were relieved and the mental condition was greatly relieved and improved. In two other cases equally satisfactory results were had.

Dr. D. A. Baldwin, of Englewood, N. J., entirely controlled the convulsions in a young man of 16 with Œnanthe.

Dr. Ord reports a case of petit mal cured with the 3x, and in a South American homœopathic journal a Dr. Rappaz reports the cure of a case of three years' standing with increasing seizures with the remedy in doses ranging from the 6 to the 12.

The late Dr. W. A. Dunn reported a genuine cure of a young girl of 16 who had been epileptic for 7 years, latterly having as many as 4 or 5 attacks during a night. The remedy caused these attacks to entirely disappear. The girl commenced menstruating at 12, so the establishment of the menses had nothing to do with the cure.

Dr. Charles A. Wilson, of San Antonio, Texas, reports a number of cases cured with Œnanthe in the 3x dilution, and the same potency greatly lessened the number of seizures in others.

Dr. Purdon, of the University of Dublin, relates a case of epilepsy cured with this drug in 1 to 6 drop doses several times a day.

Dr. F. E. Howard, in a case which had 3 or 4 attacks a week, gave 5 drops of the tincture every two hours, which caused violent pains in the head, but complete recovery followed on reducing the dose.

Several cases of the cure of epilepsy with Œnanthe in alternation with Silicea or some other drug have been reported, but as the question, "which cured?" comes in they need not be given.

In my own practice I have had some marked results from its action and have seen it modify attacks when everything else failed. In two cases, one a boy of 13 who had had the disease 5 years and who had suffered much of many sphincter-stretching orificialists and "lots of other things," the remedy made a complete cure; the other case was in a man of 30 who had the grand mal, the petit mal and the epileptic vertigo. Œnanthe removed entirely the two former conditions leaving only the latter, and that in a very mild degree. It also greatly improved the mental condition of the patient.

I have several cases under treatment at the present time, and some of them are showing a marked effect from its use. The question of dose I believe to be an important one. I used generally the tincture in water, but latterly I have been using the third, and I believe with better effect than I ever obtained with the tincture, and I am now of the opinion that the lower dilutions, say from the 3 to the 12, will be found more efficacious than the tincture, and the higher potencies will suit certain cases. In order to prescribe the drug with accuracy provings will be necessary to develop its finer symptomatology.

PARAFFINE.

PREPARATION.—The purified Paraffin is triturated in the usual way.

(This proving was made by Dr. Wahle, of Germany, who was the chemist of Hahnemann. He never published it, but gave the manuscript to his son, who in his turn gave it to Dr. Held, now a practicing physician in Rome. Dr. Held at the request of his colleagues translated it into Italian and it appeared in the medical journal, *L'Omiopatia in Italia*, from which this article is translated and slightly condensed. The remedy is used by the homœopaths of Rome and found to be valuable in uterine and other troubles, indicated by the proving. It is particularly serviceable in constipation.)

PROVING OF PARAFFINE.

HEAD.

Weight in the head.

Bruised feeling in the left side of the occiput.

Head heavy and dull; a feeling when leaning forward as if a weight fell toward the forehead.

Pulsation in the head.

Pressing pain in the head, extending from the vertex toward the forehead as if something would come out.

Pricking, stinging in the head, extending to the left temporal bone.

Pain as of a contusion in occiput.

At 9 o'clock in the morning there comes a pain in the left side of the vertex as if a nail were being driven into the head, with extension of the pain to the left lower jaw.

Touching the left side of the head causes pain as if the part were crushed and a feeling as if the whole side of the head were soft and spongy.

Twisting and wrenching in the sinciput so that he must lie down; having lain down a quarter of an hour, and having placed the right hand under the head, there was experienced a feeling of painless shock so that the hand under the head was drawn away and the legs were thrown down from the sofa. Soon afterward occurred severe palpitation of the heart.

Twisting and wrenching in the whole head, as well as the face.

Feeling as of knife stabs under the right temporal bone extending into the right eye and becoming worse on bending over. On the outside of the forehead a pressing pain which seems to thrust inward, passing, in half an hour, into the inside of the head.

Painful pulsation in the forehead, which gradually disappears when lying down, but becomes worse when bending over.

The left side of the head and face suffer most; pains stinging and twisting, often going and returning at the same time.

Twisting in the left side of the head and face; the teeth of the same side ache as if they would fall out.

On touching the vertex the skin pains as if it were suppurating, in the afternoon.

Sticking in the forehead extending into the nose.

The skin of the head feels soft on being touched or as if suppuration was going on underneath it.

Falling out of the hair.

EYES.

Throbbing and sticking over the right eyebrow laterally and from without, extending into the lower jaw and there disappearing.

Stinging pains above the left eye and toward the temple.

Raised spots upon the cornea.

The eyes seem as if there was a veil before them in the morning.

In the morning the eyelids are closed with mucus; dry mucus in the internal angles of the eyes.

Itching in the internal angles of the eyes which ceases a moment on rubbing, but a sore pain remains and very soon the itching returns again.

Pressing pains under the right upper eyelids as if some foreign body had gotten in.

Pain under the upper eyelids as if from the prick of a needle.

The eyelids are red, as after crying.

Pain as of a wound in the external angle of the left eye, in the morning.

Itching of the eyelids, lasting the whole day. Rubbing relieves only for a short time.

A feeling in the eyes as if they had fat in them.

A feeling in the eyes as if they were always moist.

Eyes moist and tearful.

The mucus in the internal angles of the eyes is cold and viscid.

Lachrymation and itching of the eyes in the morning on rising.

In the morning the left eye is closed with mucus and seems to have a veil before it.

A veil before the eyes or they feel as if they contained fat observed on rubbing the eyes.

The eyes are dim, she sees nothing, but feels everything; has sensation as if all the limits were numb for five minutes toward evening.

The eyes are pale; things seem to be seen through a veil. Little black flies are seen before the eyes.

Short vision on account of the many little black flies before the eyes.

On fixing any object for some time the eyes become moist, as if a cold wind was blowing into them, with a gentle itching.

In the open air there seems to be a black veil before the eyes; objects seen seem to be pale, with short vision.

She sees objects as if in a mist.

The white of the eye is full of blood; worse toward the external angle.

FACE.

Itching in the face as from urticaria, smooth red spots come out on the face.

EAR.

Roaring in the right ear like the rumbling of a mill wheel, in the afternoon.

Gurgling in the left ear like the beating of the pulse.

Ringing in both ears, in the morning.

Stinging and twisting in the left ear, with a feeling as if it was stopped up.

The odor of cordials is perceived.

The nose is moist and there is frequent desire to blow it, but without sneezing.

Blood from the nose of a dark red color.

TEETH.

Tearing in the teeth on the right side of the jaw, extending to the ear on the same side. It is not relieved until support is given to the painful cheek.

Stabbing pain in one of the left lower molar teeth.

Twisting in the teeth, with stinging in the ear, which after some hours affects the whole left side of the head and face, down to the lower jaw.

Twisting pain in the lower teeth of the left side, affecting also the temporal region, sleep is rendered thereby impossible.

MOUTH AND THROAT.

In the evening there appeared under the upper lip, upon the gum, a hard painless tumor which broke of itself during the night.

Mouth full of saliva; she was obliged to spit constantly, lasting for twenty-four hours.

Voice hollow and harsh.

Mouth feels sticky.

Dryness of the throat, the fauces are as if they were dried up, but without thirst.

Sense of suffocation in the pharynx.

The mouth is without taste and the appetite fails.

Bitter taste in the mouth.

Tongue slightly coated; dirty-white in color; chill, followed by dry heat with thirst, which is soon followed by sweat, lasting a long time.

STOMACH.

Acid eructations some hours after eating.

A constant feeling of satiety.

Appetite good, but nothing seems to taste as it should.

Inclination to vomit at 9 o'clock in the evening.

After eating, repeated urging to vomit with expulsion of the ingested food.

Disturbance of the stomach with increase of saliva in the mouth as if emesis must occur, with stinging pains in the forehead and cold over the whole body, without thirst or feeling of heat following.

Hunger almost all the time.

Pain across the stomach as if a blow had been received.

The pain persists even after thirty-six hours.

On account of the severe pain in the stomach can only breathe slowly and carefully.

The pains in the stomach extend to the chest, causing oppression thereof, and then pass into the shoulders, with much belching and alternating pains in the throat and in the spine.

Great sensibility of the stomach; cannot draw the vest together.

In walking, a feeling of relaxation in the region of the stomach as if there was a sore in it which was causing pain.

Smoking soon causes pain in the stomach and tobacco is distasteful.

Pain as if from a beating in the region of the stomach; she wished to gape and was obliged to support the region of the stomach with the hand, thereupon arose a fixed pain in the left hypochondrium as if some of the parts were being twisted.

Chill, heat and sweat, frequently alternating. The stomach swells up like a ball and forces itself upwards; hard and very painful to the touch; there is also very little appetite.

When the pains in the stomach subside, those in the teeth also disappear, as if there was a causal relation between the two.

Weight in the stomach as if there was a stone placed upon it, in the morning, evening and after dinner during the time of digestion, that is from half an hour to an hour after meals.

Sometimes there occurs palpitation of the heart in connection with these stomach symptoms, so severe that he is often incapacitated from doing anything whatever.

After breakfast, between nine and ten o'clock, griping and drawing with crawling in the stomach, which extends into the chest and between the shoulders, causing oppression of the chest with a sense of heat.

The face and hands become hot and red and there is hot sweat upon the upper part of the body, especially upon the forehead.

ABDOMEN.

Sense of lassitude in the abdomen which grows less when the parts are supported.

Swelling of the abdomen and nausea as if about to vomit.

Feeling in the abdomen as if he had been disemboweled; he wishes to walk fast which causes the parts to pain severely.

Cutting pains in the abdomen so that he was unable to sleep the whole night.

In the morning at 9 o'clock, colicky pains in the abdomen which ceased after some minutes and a quantity of white mucus issued from the vagina; these attacks are often repeated.

Under the umbilicus, a cutting pain as if caused by a sharp knife, extending down to the genitals.

Colicky pains for some hours internal to the umbilicus with a painful sensation as if a cord was bound around the abdomen above the stomach, lasting ten minutes.

A griping sensation in the region of the umbilicus extending to the spine.

When sitting, spasmodic pains in the lower portion of the abdomen extending into the rectum and coccyx. After long sitting the pains are relieved, but walking makes them worse so that the body must be held in a slightly curved position.

Toward six in the afternoon, griping and cutting internal to the umbilicus with nausea, afterward vomiting of acid water and at the end a little food, with twisting pains in the vertex and temples; dryness of the mouth with much thirst.

Wrenching pains in the calves extending into the toes and preventing sleep the whole night; she does not know where to put her legs.

At 10 o'clock in the evening, without having supped, the abdomen suddenly swelled as if she had eaten to excess; before and during the attack flat and viscid taste in the mouth. She went to bed in this condition and on waking in the morning the attack was entirely gone, the bowels, however, refused to move.

Painless swelling of the abdomen lasting twenty-four hours.

Abdomen hard; tense and swollen with painless rumblings unaccompanied with belching of wind; he goes to bed with these symptoms, but they are gone in the morning.

However, there remains a constrictive pain below the ribs, passing across the stomach with much thirst. Five hours later there occurred alvine discharges; the first was very hard with much tenesmus, so that the whole abdomen was retracted; the last discharges were fluid, abundant and without tenesmus, in consequence of which the swelling of the abdomen went down a little.

The pains disappear, however, with redness of the face, alternating with cold sweat.

Standing and walking soon bring back the symptoms again.

Pressing the arm against the stomach and squeezing it relieved the pain and then she was able to breathe deeply, which she could not do otherwise.

Stomach swollen in the afternoon; went to bed at 10 o'clock and slept one hour, awoke with urging to vomit and soon after threw up acid water and the food taken the preceding day.

Griping in the abdomen, extending down into the rectum, with a feeling as if this organ was ligated; she feels so weak that she has to support herself to keep from falling, with cold sweat in the face, lasting half an hour.

Severe itching in the abdomen which ceases and is always followed by copious white expectoration, with flashes of heat in the face and great weakness.

At first coldness in the feet, then stinging and pressing pains in the right hypochondrium. From here the pains pass to the stomach with swelling of the abdomen; then they extend up the spine to the shoulders.

Spasmodic, stabbing pains, one after the other, in the Mons Veneris, when standing on her feet she has a desire to put one foot over the other.

A spasmodic pain in the left inguinal region as of incarcerated wind, which extends upward across the abdomen, causing a painful spot in the region of the spleen.

STOOL.

Bowels confined for two days and very hard; the evacuation occurs in small pieces.

No evacuation for three days, the abdomen seems very full, as if much had been eaten, with loss of appetite.

Evacuations accompanied with stinging, cutting pains in the rectum which persist more than an hour, with vehement tenesmus.

Obstinate constipation in children is readily cured.

The child has a movement only once in three or four days, accompanied with severe pain in the anus.

Frequent desire for stool without result.

Stools hard but occurring every day.

After going for three days without stool he is obliged to remain an hour before expelling anything and becomes very much fatigued.

Evacuations hard as nuts expelled with much difficulty, with spasmodic pains in the intestines; the feces escape in small pieces.

Chronic constipation with hemorrhoids and continual urging to stool without result.

URINARY ORGANS, ETC.

Often passes much urine.

Frequent desire to pass urine after cramps in the stomach.

Was obliged to urinate three times in the space of four hours, but only a small quantity each time; otherwise she only urinated once during the same length of time and with strangury.

Urine very hot and light colored.

Passes much urine and after a quarter of an hour passes an equally large quantity, although she had drunk but little.

Slight itching and burning in the vulva when not urinating.

Feeling of heat in the vulva.

Very hot urine causing heat at the vulva.

Very hot urine with burning pain at the vulva.

The menstruation appears several days too late.

The blood is black and abundant.

The menstrual blood is reddish-black.

The menstruation comes on six days too soon, when on the feet the blood flows continuously.

During the menstruation she feels cold externally and hot internally and must drink a great deal.

Cutting pains through the body on the second day of the menstruation.

White fluid discharge like milk coming away in drops.

Very profuse white discharge, leaving white and gray spots on the linen, with itching in the abdomen.

The white discharge has a sweetish odor.

A chronic rattling in the throat causes a dry cough.

The whole chest pains as if compressed, and when breathing, sharp stabbing pains traverse the chest, worse on the left side.

Stinging in the chest which prevents him from taking a long breath.

Pain in the region of the diaphragm as if it was inflamed; when gaping, drawing pains under the right ribs, extending as far as the spine; they come and go frequently and are aggravated by respiration.

Stabbing pains one after another in the upper portion of the left breast, worse when breathing, lasting half an hour.

Stinging pains under the false ribs on the left side which grow on lying down, on external pressure and on deep respiration with flashes of heat.

Twisting pains in the left breast.

The nipples pain on touching them, as if they were sore inside.

BACK.

Pains in the spine, extending into the lumbar vertebræ and then into both sides above the crests of the ilia and into the inguinal regions, where a pain as of inflammation is felt.

The dorsal pains are increased by bending.

Pains in the spine as if it had been injured, as bad during repose as when in motion.

Drawing and stinging between the shoulders with oppression of breath.

Drawing pains between the shoulders, extending downward along the spine, toward the liver and upward into the chest; then the respiration becomes oppressed and frequent shooting pains traverse the entire body.

In the left axilla, an electric shock which shakes the whole body, and in all the joints there occurs a trembling, such as might be produced by an electric machine, and which causes each time a sensation of fear.

UPPER EXTREMITIES.

The whole right arm, but principally the axilla, feels as if it had been dislocated by a blow.

Stabbing pain under the right arm toward the breast.

The right arm feels heavy and she cannot lift it well; feels a sensation of numbness as if the clothing was too tight, with turgescence of the veins.

The muscles of the forearm seem to grow large and have a feeling of stiffness.

Wrenching pains in the elbow joints.

Wrenching pains in the joints of the left hand.

Pains as if from fatigue in both loins, when ascending the stairs.

Drawing and cutting pains from one iliac crest to the other as if a knife had traversed the abdomen; often intermitting and always returning.

LOWER EXTREMITIES.

Painful tension in the muscles of the thigh as if a long walk had been taken.

Wrenching pain on the outside of the right knee extending down the right side of the leg to the malleolus, from thence into the heel, where it ceases.

Trembling of the legs from the knees to the toes so that there is difficulty in walking or raising the feet.

Tearing pains in the calves of the legs, with a feeling of heat, extending down to the toes; the palms of the hands and soles of the feet are very hot.

Tearing pains in the articulations of the feet and in the toes, for several hours.

The back and soles of the feet are swollen, after thirty-four hours, with tearing pains in the ankles and soles of the feet on account of which, though very tired, he was not able to sleep.

A feeling as of electric shocks in all the joints.

GENERALITIES.

General weariness lasting several days.

When sitting down, a feeling as if the whole body were swaying to and fro.

At 4 o'clock in the afternoon great fatigue with profuse cold sweat and somnolence for two hours.

Much of the hair falls out.

Pulse weak and thready and increased in frequency.

Frequent gaping with great somnolence.

Continued yawning, although the joints of the jaw are painful.

She would like to sleep all the time, day and night.

She cannot keep awake and goes to sleep in her chair; her feet go to sleep.

After having passed the night rolling around in bed without waking and passing from one dream to another, she wakes at 5 o'clock, the bed clothing thrown aside and without her night cap, a thing which had never happened to her before.

Sensual lascivious dreams.

PARTHENIUM HYSTEROPHORUS.

NAT. ORD., Synanthereæ.
COMMON NAME, "Bitter broom." Escoba amaya.
PREPARATION.—The dry plant is macerated in five parts by weight of alcohol.

(Dr. Edward Fornias contributed to the *Homœopathic Recorder*, 1886, two papers on this remedy. The first gave the results of physiological experiments; the second is a résumé of those results, including the proving by Dr. B. H. B. Sleght, as follows:)

Résumé of Symptoms.—If we boil down the matter, extracting only the symptoms and changes observed during the above experiments with *Parthenina*, we have the following: *Heaviness and dulness of head, tendency to vertigo, malaise, apathy, lassitude, profuse and very fluid salivation, sensation of heat and weight in the stomach, increased appetite, gastric intolerance, nausea and vomiting. Increased stupor, desire to be quiet, refusal of food, and indifference. Excitation of the heart beats, or slow beating of the heart; depressed circulation, or general functional activity; pulse accelerated, or slow, weak, soft, compressible, without dicrotism; progressive slowing of the pulse, followed by syncope, cardiac paralysis* (and death). *Accelerated, or slow, irregular breathing* (*Cheyne-Stokes*); *rise and fall of temperature, tremors, shivering, diminished perspiration; dilation of the pupils; convulsions* (clonic and tonic); *muscular relaxation, anæsthesia and increased urine and saliva. The kidneys were found enlarged and congested, with evident signs of sanguineous stasis. The process of coagulation of the blood was retarded. The red corpuscles increased in volume. There was a fall of the blood-pressure, and vascular dilatation* (of reflex origin). *The heart was found arrested in diastole, and the brain anæmic. A marked diminution of reflex action in the hips and extinction of the voluntary movements, were noticed. Also a transient excitement of the voluntary movements. And finally the sensibility and the muscular contractility were diminished.*

CASES CURED BY PARTHENINA.—In regard to the therapeutic value of *Parthenina*, little is known as yet, but the plant from which this alkaloid is derived, as said before, has been employed for years in Cuba, both by the people and profession, against fevers of a paludal origin.

Dr. Ramirez Tovar has reported in several numbers of the *Cronica Médico-Quirúrgica*, of Havana, the following cases treated by him with *Parthenina*, with the best results:

CASE I.—"A lady living in the lower part of the city, where the rain always leaves constant channels of infection, was suffering with *daily attacks of intermittent*, which grew more intense every day. She received 1 gram of the salt, divided in six powders, to be taken one every hour after the attack. The next day she had no chill, and the thermometer indicated the absence of fever. She was nursing at the time, and stated that she had noticed a marked increase of milk in her breasts; 50 centigrams more, in doses, were given to her, and the fever did not return again."

CASE II.—"A tailor, 30 years of age, had moved to the lower part of the city and contracted a *tertian intermittent*. He had four paroxysms before the doctor saw him, the last one being *attended by much pain in the left hypochondrium*. He received 1 gram, in 5 doses. There was apyrexia on the day the attack was due, and this did not return again. This man continued to live in the same house, under the same regimen and hygienic conditions."

CASE III,—"A little girl, 6 years of age, lymphatic constitution, living near the beach of the harbor, was brought to Dr. Ramirez Tovar's clinic, suffering for 17 days with *malaise, loss of appetite, sleepiness and fever*. She had taken quinine, both internally and externally, with little benefit, and *was wasting away notably*. At 4 P.M. she commenced to take 50 centigrams of the salt, in 8 doses, and the next day at the same hour the thermometer indicated a fall from 39.5° C. of the previous day to 38.5° C. The mother was ordered to repeat the medicine at longer intervals, but for want of means the child did not take any more. On the 4th or 5th day the temperature went up to 39.5° again, then she was provided with the medicine, and 3 days later the temperature was normal. The action of the alkaloid was aided here by a tonic wine prepared from the extract of the plant."

CASE IV.—"A man 45 years of age, *of delicate constitution, poorly nourished, with a straw yellow face, yellow sclerotics, enlarged liver and spleen, the latter somewhat painful to pressure*, who had contracted *intermittent fever* while in Panama, and had taken quinine, was complaining, when Dr. Ramirez Tovar saw him (middle part of December), *of a pain in the right side* (more severe in some points than in others), which commenced at 1 P.M., with *shiverings*, and which disappeared after two hours to return again the next day at precisely the same time and with the same symptoms. He received 1 gram of *Parthenina*, in 5 doses, one every hour, right after the cessation of the pain. He was seen by the doctor the next day at 4 P.M., and up to that time the pain had not returned. He took then 50 centigrams more, in 5 doses, one every hour, and was free of pain until the latter part of January, when he again consulted the doctor, this time the *pain being located in the stomach*, for which *Parthenina* was repeated (1 gram in 5 doses, one every two hours). The next day the pain had ceased, but returned on the third, and he again received 1 gram, in the same manner as before, and since then he has been free from pain."

CASE V.—"A young lady, 18 years of age, complained of *facial neuralgia with periodical exacerbations,* from which she was suffering four days. She received 1 gram of *Parthenina,* in 5 doses, one every hour, and on the following day she was entirely free from pain. Fifty centigrams more, in 4 doses, were given to this lady to prevent a relapse, and the result was a complete cure."

And to finish this report, I will mention a case which came under my notice: "A little girl, my niece, 5 years old, living in Havana, who, when seen by the late Dr. Govantes, of that city, had been suffering for some time before from *a continued fever, with periodical mid-day exacerbations, which later on, assumed an intermittent type.* She had been saturated with *quinine,* and complained, at the time, of *malaise, lassitude, languor, headache, loss of appetite, gastric intolerance, etc.* The temperature went up as high as 40.6° C. during the hot stage, which was short and was followed by copious sweats, giving relief. *Parthenium hysterophorus* in the form of an extract, prepared and sold at Dr. Villavicenci's Pharmacy, in Havana, was prescribed by Dr. Govantes. Three doses a day, each of the size of a pea, dissolved in water, were given for 4 or 5 days, and at the end of that time she was entirely free of fever and made a quick recovery."

If such results can be ascribed to *Parthenium* and its alkaloid *Parthenina,* I think it would be unjustifiable to set them aside. An early proving of the plant will not only enhance our therapeutic resources, but prevent the non-scrupulous from employing it empirically.

Proving of *Parthenium hysterophorus,* Dr. B. H. B. Sleght.

February 12th.—Until a few days ago had a slight continuous toothache due to a cavity in last molar of lower jaw; cavity recently filled. General health has been excellent for some time.

7:40 A.M. Took 5 drops of tincture. At once have a full feeling in head, especially vertex, pressing from within.

7:45. Ringing in ears, < left.

7:50. Took 10 drops. Ringing and fulness continue and become worse.

7:58. Upper teeth feel "on edge," with slight prickling pains in sockets, which slowly grow more severe.

8:00. Breakfast; above symptoms continue, but grow less severe.

8:10. Loud rumbling in bowels; irrepressible eructations, tasteless.

8:20. 20 drops. A "shivery" feeling runs over limbs and back as this is taken. Singing in ears had ceased but begins again, as does the rumbling.

8:40. "Goneness" in epigastrium, singing ceases; some fulness in head remains.

8:45. Same feeling in teeth as above; singing in ears; head thick, heavy.

8:50. Sharp, aching twinges in upper molars; some sharp pains in ears. Pulse 72.

9:10. 25 drops.

9:15. Stitching pain in left temple, of short duration. Upper incisors tender at sockets when biting.

9:25. Sudden pain in upper teeth with lachrymation, < pressing jaws together.

9:45. 25 drops.

9:55. Aching pain at left supra-orbital foramen. On going into open air no symptoms but taste of drug and fulness of head. A tooth filled yesterday aches slightly, same as before filling.

11:15. 60 drops. Renewed fulness of head. Pulse 76.

11:30. Goneness in epigastrium; vertigo while sitting, with heat of face and blurred vision. Aching at supra-orbital foramen (left), extending to root of nose and becoming more severe there, > eyes closed. Feel dull, stupid. Goneness comes and goes; hunger.

11:45. Aching at lower edge of right ear spreads over side of face; ear feels plugged up. Am drowsy, eyes "heavy;" goneness and unusual craving for food.

11:50. Prickling in skin of back of wrists and hands. A twinge of pain at right infraorbital foramen, gradually increases; cannot fix attention on what I am reading. Hard, painful lump in epigastrium; better after eructations tasting of drug. Slight nausea with some relief.

12 M. 60 drops. Requires much effort to fix attention while counting drops.

12:15 P.M. Head heavy, brain feels loose.

12:30. Stitching pain at lobe of left ear and deep in and above external auditory meatus.

12:45. Dinner.

1:45. 75 drops.

1:50. Hard lump in epigastrium. Head feels as if in a vise. During P.M. only "goneness" and continued taste of drug.

9:00 P.M. 100 drops, followed at once by sudden stitching pains in left frontal eminence, which soon cease.

9:10. Pain in frontal eminence has returned and continues. Teeth "on edge" and tenderness at sockets. Upper incisors ache as after filling. Teeth feel too long.

9:30. Lump in epigastrium. Severe plunging pain in left frontal eminence.

9:45. Stabbing pain runs up rectum after passing flatus.

Mushy stool at 10:30 P.M. (Usually have passage at 10 A.M.; to-day no desire.)

February 13th.—Passed restless night, waking at 3 or 4 o'clock, then dozing and dreaming until 7:30; rose with throbbing deep in brain, as if it would push through top of head; "big" head, > after moving about and washing face. 7:45. 120 drops. 7:55. Breakfast. 8:20. Aching in eyeballs. No further symptoms all day.

9:30 P.M. 5 drops. 9:35. 5 drops.

Same tenderness at sockets of upper incisors when biting.

9:40. 5 drops. Sudden darting pains in right, then in left frontal eminence, with dull heaviness in forehead, gradually increasing.

9:45. 5 drops. Sudden return of pain in frontal eminence. Fulness and aching in ears, coming suddenly. Upper teeth all ache, and feel too long.

9:50. 5 drops. Beating ache in middle of forehead. Bursting pain in right malar bone. Tingling in tip of tongue. Sudden motion increases frontal pain.

9:55. 5 drops. Slight colicky pain at navel. Eructations of drug.

10:00. 5 drops. Same frontal pain, and brief feeling as if blood would burst through face; this returns in a few minutes, especially about nose and root of nose.

10:05. 5 drops. Same frontal pain, and head feels swelled. Pulse, 72.

10:10. 5 drops. Heart-beat all over head, < motion, and over eyes.

10:15. 5 drops. Splitting pain over both ears in spots the size of silver dollar.

10:20. Must look intently to see the words; as I write, letters look pale and eyes ache.

10:25. 5 drops. Eructations tasting of drug. Colicky pains about navel.

10:30. 5 drops. Aching in left lower molars.

10:35. 5 drops. Stabbing pain in left ear. Teeth "on edge."

10:50. All the upper jaw aches, especially at sockets of teeth and on biting. Fulness and pressure in ears. Temples feel as if in a vise. All symptoms < after going up stairs.

February 14th.—Again awoke early, 3 or 4 A.M., and rose at 7:30, after a dreamful sleep, with headache. Felt better after going about. No symptoms during day.

February 15th.—Passed restless night. Fell asleep late, with headache at vertex—a pushing out. Awoke at 4 or 5 A.M. heavy and stupid; then again slept.

February 17th.—5:00 A.M. Took 2-1/2 drachms.

5:02. Eructations taste of drug. Goneness in epigastrium. Pulse, 72. Some rumbling about navel.

5:10. Head heavy; pressure at right frontal eminence, which increases to sharp, penetrating pain, going to root of nose, then to end of nose, where it is most severe. At root of nose, stuffed feeling, as with dry coryza. Pain in nose gets more and more severe; restlessness succeeds; never had such a pain; seems now all in bones of nose and worse on left side. Forehead has ceased to ache. Pain seems to start from supra-orbital foramen now.

5:15. Upper incisors commence to ache. Aching and bursting pain in nose remains; nose feels swollen. Teeth "on edge." Epigastric goneness.

5:25. Sharp pain in left upper and lower molars. Pain in nose has ceased. Bursting pain in left frontal eminence. Upper molars tender at sockets.

February 23d.—12:30. Took 6 No. 40 pills saturated with 6x dil. 2:00 P.M. Same dose. 4:20. Same. 5:00. Sharp, aching pain deep in left ear, gradually grows worse.

5:10. Singing and dull aching in right ear.

5:15. Singing and a pushing out in left ear. Fulness of frontal eminences; thence pains go to root of nose and nose becomes tender to touch. Sharp pain again deep in right ear. Aching of "bridge" of nose and of upper left molars. Hands feel numb, especially dorsal aspects. Rumbling in bowels about navel. Pain again at root of nose. Colic deep in pelvis; pains run down back of thigh to knees.

5:15. Pains again in frontal eminences.

5:25. Aching over eyes; feel like closing them; aching pains run up from above left eye-tooth to eye and over face; occurs by starts and stops. Frontal headache and pains down nose recur at intervals.

5:30. Aching, very severe, at the left side of "bridge" of nose. Sharp stitch deep in left ear. Throbbing in vertex. Sockets of upper teeth tender. Aching at end of nose, which feels full of blood.

5:45. 6 pellets. All pains continue as above. Brain seems loose, < moving head. Front of head feels big.

6:00. P.M. Stabbing deep in left ear, < by pressing teeth together.

6:30. Various pains gradually subside.

PASSIFLORA INCARNATA.

NAT. ORD., Passifloraceæ.
COMMON NAME, Passion flower.
PREPARATION.—The fresh leaves and flowers gathered in May are macerated in two parts by weight of alcohol. A preparation may also be made from the expressed juice of the fresh leaves.

(There has been so much written concerning this unproved remedy that we can only give an abstract of a part of it. Dr. Lindsay, formerly of Bayou Gras, La., was the first to call attention to it a few weeks before his death. He wrote in answer to an inquiry as follows—Hale's New Remedies):

I have much to say. I am satisfied it is no narcotic. It never stupefies or overpowers the senses. A patient under its full influence may be wakened up, and he will talk to you as rationally as ever he did; leave him a moment and he will soon be off to the Elysian Fields again. I have tried it, my friend, in all sorts of neuralgic affections, and have usually astonished my more enlightened patients with it. Many times I have had them to ask me what in the world it was that had such a sweet influence over them.

(Dr. L. Phares, of Newtonia, Miss., states):

I never saw anything act so promptly in erysipelas. I have used it with advantage in ulcers, neuralgias and tetanus. I have seen wonderful effects of it in relieving tetanus, and will mention one case from memory: Some ten years ago I was called to see an old lady, in a distant part of the country, who was reported to be "having fits." I found her to be able to be up most of the time, but, while examining her, convulsions came on, affecting mainly the trunkal muscles, and drawing the head back. I gave her instantly a dose of *Passiflora*. The convulsions subsided, and she has never had one since. I continued the use of the medicine in small doses for a few days. I have used it in treating tetanus in horses—a disease usually considered as inevitably fatal to that noble animal. It has never failed to cure the horse. * * During the late war, my son, Dr. J. H. Phares, had occasion many times to prescribe the *Passiflora* for tetanus in horses, with one invariable result— prompt, perfect, permanent cure. He fortunately saw no case in man. * * * Since the foregoing was written, I have treated with the hydro-alcoholic extract of *Passiflora* several cases of neuralgia, and one of sleeplessness, with incessant motion and suicidal mania. With the same extract during the current week, Dr. J. H. Phares has treated, with the most prompt and satisfactory success, a very virulent and hopeless case of tetanus, with ophisthotonos, trismus and convulsions, in a child two years old. Other most potent remedies, in heroic doses, having failed to produce any effect in this case, he thinks that nothing but the *Passiflora* could possibly have saved the child.

(The editor of the *California Medical Journal* (1889) says):

We have been employing it [*Passiflora*] in some cases of spinal meningitis after the acute symptoms had subsided, when the patients were unable to sleep, either day or night: could not endure the bed, and were unable to maintain the sitting posture, with highly satisfactory results. It is administered in small doses. Add ten drops of the mother tincture (Homœopathic) to half a tumbler of water; teaspoonful every two hours.

(At the meeting of the Homœopathic Medical Society of Delaware and Peninsula, November 14, 1889, Dr. W. D. Troy read a paper on *Passiflora* (see *Homœopathic Recorder*, May, 1890), from which we take the following):

My erysipelatous case was a man of some fifty years. When first seen was a-bed, high fever, facial erysipelas of the flaming, rampant sort, the one eye had disappeared, the other was in rapid retreat. Patient in great anxiety; sharp, stinging pains; could not rest. Was about to give *Apis* when I thought of my *Passion flower*. Gave two-drop doses of the tincture every two hours. Put one-half an ounce of same into one quart of water for local application, to be applied hot by flannels and oiled silk. After six hours patient fell asleep; was awakened for medicine every three hours during the night; went to sleep easily after each dose. Said in morning he had had a night's good rest. Found inflammation markedly reduced. I now changed the remedy—gave *Ham.*, both internally and externally. On next visit found patient every way worse. The disease had sneaked across the scalp and invaded the whole face. The case began to look serious. Returned to the *Passiflora* and kept to it with the most happy results.

My next experience was in a Chorea—a girl budding into womanhood, but in whom the menses had not yet appeared. Child was well developed for her years, fourteen. I learned that for two or three years past the child had "fits," varying at times from moderate to severe. The neurosis was unilateral, the right side alone being affected. The child had had traditional treatment, "off and on," for some time without manifest improvement. I began with the *Passiflora* 1x dil., 10 gtt. doses every three hours. Kept it up for several days, the Choreic symptoms being not quite so violent; still I was growing anxious—wanted more positive results. Added daily a five-drop dose of tincture. After a few more days the mother informed me that there had been a slight "show"—merely enough to stain the diaper, and that for the last two days there had been hardly any "fits." This was encouraging. I judged that the day of deliverance was nigh. Very little more of the drug was given until about the time for next menstrual flux. Then I resumed it with the most satisfactory results. No nervous symptoms save such as are more or lest common to all women at the "periods" subsequently prevailed.

(The following case was reported by Dr. D. C. Buell Dunlevy, of Port Chester, N. Y.—*Homœopathic Recorder*, Nov., 1890):

Mr. D——, æt. 52, sent for me to attend him during the month of May. I found him presenting all the prodromal symptoms of delirium tremens, and at once ordered him to bed, and none too soon, as the event proved. For seven days he tossed about in a wild delirium, which was greatly aggravated by marked gastric irritation. I had him carefully watched, both day and night, until the delirium wore off. The treatment up to this time was *Cannabis Ind.* for the mental trouble and *Nux v.*, which greatly relieved the gastric symptoms. But the moment he began to improve the old cravings for liquor and morphine returned. Right here let me say that for years he has been a great sufferer from piles, and the only rest he could get was to sit propped up in his chair. His sufferings caused him to seek relief during the day in liquor, and at nights in morphine. And this habit had so fastened itself upon him that try as he might he could not give it up. When he came under my treatment I at once put a stop to all stimulants and narcotics, but not without considerable trouble, for he seemed determined to have them. Night after night he would lie there calling for something to make him sleep, and this kept up until he was bordering on a state of insanity. Fully realizing that something must be done, and that quickly, too, I made up my mind to try *Passiflora*. This I did, and from the time I gave him the first dose improvement set in and has continued ever since. I at first gave him a half teaspoonful of the θ at bed time, but this not proving sufficient I increased it to a teaspoonful. He has now been taking it almost constantly for a period of eight weeks and claims he has not had as natural a sleep for years; and lays particular stress on the fact that when he awakes in the morning he feels so refreshed and his mind remains clear. But what seems even more wonderful is that from the day he first took this drug up to the present he has never felt the slightest desire to return to his former habits. The mere mention of liquor or opium seems to sicken him, and I am fully satisfied that he is now cured and will (so far as liquor and opium are concerned) remain so. He now takes special delight in praising the drug to his friends, and really seems never to tire talking about the wonderful help it has been to him. I have also prescribed the drug to others for insomnia and always with success, one case excepted, in which I gave it for hemicrania, and here, although it quieted the patient, it failed to produce the desired sleep.

(The following is extracted from a paper on *Passiflora*, by Dr. C. A. Walters, of Brooklyn. *Homœopathic Recorder*, July, 1890:)

In April, 1888, was called to an infant, 14 months, convulsions, caused by dentition; symptoms called for *Belladonna*, of which the 1x dil., 5 drops in half a glass water, teaspoonful every fifteen minutes until better, then once an hour. The child improved from start, and the convulsions ceased in one hour from commencing the medicine. The next day the child appeared in usual health, and the *Belladonna* was given once in eight hours and discharged from further attendance.

Thirty-six hours after I was recalled, the child was in another spasm. No *Belladonna* symptoms being present I gave 5 drops of *Passiflora* tincture, every fifteen minutes, with the result that it never had another spasm from that day to this. The child slept soundly all through the night and awoke the next morning in its usual good health.

Since then I have prescribed it for the sleeplessness of dentition without a failure, giving it usually in from 5 to 10 drops a dose, to be repeated every fifteen minutes until sleep. I never give it during the day for this purpose, but begin at bedtime.

In the insomnia of adults, from whatsoever cause, I always give 60 drops at bedtime, and if not asleep in half an hour I give the same dose.

Experience has taught me that to give it in smaller doses is a waste of time and disappointing to the patient. Two such doses, *i.e.*, 60 drops a dose, are almost absolutely sure of giving the patient a natural and refreshing sleep. The old school seem to have been forced to resort to *Sulfonal* (whatever that may be) as the only thing capable of producing sleep, and yet, judging from the reports in their journals, it does not seem to "fill the bill." Were they ever to give this a trial we would not hear so much of *Morphine, Chloral, Bromides*, and the like.

I have never used *Passiflora* in erysipelas, having always been able to discharge my patients in from two to four days by giving them *Jaborandi*.

In neuralgia and headache it has acted with wonderful rapidity, even the headache of uterine displacements being brought under its influence. It is almost a daily occurrence to have people whom I never saw before come miles to my office for that "sleeping medicine made from the passion flower."

In conclusion let me say to the brethren, try it. But give it in appreciable doses. Don't be afraid of it. I would not hesitate to give it in four drachm doses, if required. But why give four when one will do?

P. S.—Since writing the foregoing I have used *Passiflora* in two cases of delirium tremens. It acted like a charm in both cases; sent them to sleep in half an hour, and when they awoke, twelve and fourteen hours after, they were themselves again. Sixty drops of tincture a dose, two doses in each.

(The following was reported by Dr. Joseph Adolphus, in *American Medical Journal*.)

A lady who had for several months suffered untold agonies, as she described her sufferings; her pain was described as if a weight of many pounds was lying on her brain; the sense of pressure and tearing inside the skull was fearful; her head felt as if enveloped in ice; the pains ran down the back of her neck, and finally reached the lower end of sacrum, so that a slight touch of the coccyx caused exquisite agony. This was a case in which coccygodinia was associated with the cerebral and spinal disease. I failed to relieve the pain for more than a few hours at a time with all other remedies I had tried; at this juncture, when despair was taking the place of hope, I thought of *Passiflora*, which I then administered in teaspoonful doses every two hours; the result was something to be remembered, for she enjoyed excellent and refreshing night's rest the following night, waking up in the morning much refreshed, nearly free from pain, with a good relish for breakfast. I continued the medicament every four hours for several days, for no further uses for medicine seemed indicated, as there was a rapid and complete recovery.

A lady complained of pain in her rectum continuously; the coccyx was also quite tender to the touch. There were several erosions on the lips of the os uteri; leucorrhœa and severe pain in the small of the back when a certain spot (over last dorsal and first and second lumbar vertebræ) was pressed on. I found she had been treated secundum artem for the uterine trouble, locally and constitutionally, to no certain satisfactory result. Her respirations were often twenty-eight to thirty per minute, much wakefulness, and at times feeling of constriction across her breast and a sense as if her heart would stop beating. Teaspoonful doses of the *Passiflora incar.* was the specific in her case. She continued it every four hours two weeks, but from the outset of treatment she felt the right remedy was administered.

These rectum troubles in women are frequently met with in practice. I find the *Passiflora incar.* the best single remedy I have for them.

Recently a man consulted me for a constant pain in his heart; he described it as sharp and like a pang—often causing a sense of immediate dissolution, and fear of death was on him all the time; pulse irregular in rhythm, now rapid, next slower, occasionally a beat missing; sounds very normal, but accentuated and sharp. *Passiflora incarnata* was a specific in this case; no doubt the center and probably the local ganglia were irritated from some cause, and, whatever it was, the medicament removed both.

By the way, I must not forget to say you will find it a valuable medicament in sleeplessness and tossing restlessness in your fever patients. I use the tincture in teaspoonful doses every four hours. It appears the remedy has a soothing effect on the whole nervous system, without any appreciable narcotic properties.

(From the Transactions of the Twenty-fifth Annual Meeting of the Maine Homœopathic Medical Society we take the following from a paper by Dr. A. I. Harvey on *Passiflora*.)

It does no good where the inability to sleep is due to pain or distress of any kind; but in cases where we find that the nervous erethism is not controlled by the action of *Coffea, Opium, Sulphur,* or other apparently indicated remedy. *Passiflora* is in its place as a succedaneum for *Morphia* or other sedatives. The dose varies from ten drops to one dram of the tincture, according to the age of the patient. I do not hesitate, in the case of an adult, to give dram doses of the tincture every hour until the patient sleeps, and have seen it act in the happiest manner in restoring the rhythm of the heart's action, when that organ has been deranged in its movements by the combined effects of exhaustion and loss of sleep.

Passiflora has also given me much aid in a case of morphine habit of six years' standing, which I cured wholly and entirely by the use of this remedy. It is recommended in the above mentioned doses for delirium tremens, trismus, tetanus and kindred diseases of the nervous system, repeated every hour or half-hour until relief is obtained. The remedy leaves no after effects, is incapable of creating an appetite, and, so far as my observation extends, it is perfectly harmless even in large doses, often repeated.

(Dr. Scudder claimed that the one great indication for *Passiflora* in all cases is *a clean tongue*; when the tongue is foul the remedy will do no good.)

PENTHORUM SEDOIDES.

NAT. ORD., Crassulaceæ.
COMMON NAME, Ditch Stone Crop.
PREPARATION.—The whole fresh plant with the root is macerated in two parts by weight of alcohol.

(The *Medical Advance* for June, 1887, contains a paper by Dr. D. B. Morrow, from which the following is taken.)

The object of this paper is to call attention to the fact that the only proving of *Penthorum* was made on scientific principles, as these verifications demonstrate. If the pathogenesy is carefully studied, it will be seen to meet all the conditions of "common colds," or acute catarrhs, so prevalent in all sections of North America, from the symptoms of chill, malaise, headache, soreness, cough, coryza, dry and flowing, with their secondary consequences of disturbed digestion, constipation, debility, etc. and it will probably cure any or all of these conditions when indicated by correspondence to the pathogenesy.

A medicine having such a catarrhal range is probably a remedy for female troubles equal to *Pulsatilla* or *Calcarea*, and is worthy of a careful proving by women. It cures where antipsoric medicines have failed, and possibly may possess antipsoric qualities.

Authorities.—1, Dr. D. B. Morrow, U. S. Med. Inves., N. S., 3, p. 565 (*Eclectic Med. Jour.*, 1875); effects of tincture, doses of 10 drops, and after one hour 20 drops; on second day, 40 drops; third day, 60 drops at 9 P.M., and 50 drops at 1 P.M.; 1 A.M. same, effects of 100 drops. 2, Dr. Scudder took 20 drops ("a young man took same dose and had similar effects").

MIND.—During both provings the mind was dull and exceedingly depressed and desponding; everything wrong but dinner; reading interfered with because of mental dullness (second day), 1.—Mind became so dull I gave up reading and lay upon the lounge (third day).

HEAD.—On closing my eyes felt like I was floating; vertigo (third day), 1.—Headache continued, could not read; went to hear Boutwell, followed his argument with difficulty, was much annoyed by the little noises made by the audience (second day), 1.—Headache came on again (third day), 1.— When commencing the proving, had a dull, heavy headache, with heat and soreness in the sacrum; this was cured (third day), 1.—An unpleasant heavy pain in the forehead, about the edge of the hair (after four hours), 2.— Catarrhal aching in the forehead, 1a.—[10] The fullness in the sinciput became an ache, as though a weight were pressed down upon it (second day), 1.—Itching of the hairy scalp (second day), 1.

EYE AND EAR.—The inner superior tarsal border of both palpebra itched and burned (third day), 1.—A full sensation in supra-orbital region (a hearty supper), (first day), 1.—Ringing and singing in both ears, 1a.

NOSE.—Discharges from nares thick, pus-like, streaked with blood, and an odor as from an open sore (third day), 1.—A peculiar wet feeling in my nares as though a violent coryza would set in, which did not; the secretion from the nose became thickened and pus-like, but not increased. Wet feeling in trachea and bronchia, passing from above downward, as if a coryza would set in, followed by a slight feeling of constriction, which passed from above downward through the chest (first day), 1.

Catarrhal feeling repeated itself (third day), 1.—Nose felt stuffed, as if swollen (second day), 1.—Sense of fullness of the nose and ears (after four hours), 2.—[20] A secondary symptom, a drawing or contractile feeling of the muscles of the side of the nose affected with catarrh, 1a.—Itching in the nares, 1a.

MOUTH.—Prickling burning sensation on the tongue, as if scalded (first day), 1.—Increased flow of saliva (first day), 1.—The bloody sputa continues, 1a.

THROAT.—The posterior nares feel raw, as if denuded of epithelium, 1a.

STOMACH.—Appetite increased (third day), 1.—Eructations and dejections of little collections of odorless flatus expelled with force (second day), 1.—An unpleasant sensation of disgust and nausea, lasting for three hours, but not interfering with the following meal, which was eaten with greater relish, 2.—Soreness in epigastrium; this symptom appeared at first, not recorded because thought idiopathic, 1a.

ABDOMEN [30].—Borborygmus (second day), 1.—Parietes of abdomen felt thickened (second night), 1.—A clawing, uneasy sensation about the umbilicus, which gradually passed to lower bowel (second day), 1.— Twitching of the muscles in the abdomen (second day), 1.

RECTUM AND ANUS.—A crawling sensation in lower rectum, as though a worm tried to escape (second day), 1.—Burning in rectum at stool, continuing through afternoon, 1a.—Itching of anus; hemorrhoids with aching in sacrum and in sacro-iliac symphysis (some weeks after proving), 1a.

STOOL.—Semi-fluid evacuation of the bowels next morning, having been somewhat constipated, 2.—Some weeks after proving suffered from constipation, an atonic condition of bowels and rectum, 1a.—Was costive when commencing proving; had two natural stools from yesterday's medicine (third day), 1.

URINARY ORGANS [40].—A dull aching in kidneys (third day), 1.—The bladder becomes sore to pressure (third day), 1.—Urine still increased in flow, with burning along the urethra when micturating (third day), 1.— Urine clear, passed more frequently (second day), 1.—Urine actively acid, as shown by litmus; no cloud on boiling; threw down a sediment with *Sulphuric acid, Ammonia,* and *Argentum nitrum* and *Nitric acid,* when boiled; the next day after the dose it was alkaline, as shown by litmus, and only precipitated with *Argentum nitricum;* slightly cloudy, with caloric; unloaded, but increased in quantity, 1a.

SEXUAL ORGANS.—Sexual orgasm (second night), 1.—Erythismus of the sexual system, almost a satyriasis; a slight variocele of long standing was apparently cured (some weeks after proving); this condition was succeeded by a corresponding depression of sexual function, approaching impotency, after months of time returning to the normal condition, 1a.

RESPIRATORY ORGANS.—In the morning a cough seemed to come from deep in the chest, with soreness throughout the chest (third day), 1.

CHEST.—Slight feeling of constriction, which passed from above down through the chest, followed the wet feeling in trachea and bronchia (first day), 1.

PULSE [50].—Pulse regular at 58 (first day), 1.

NECK AND BACK.—Aching through basilar region, from back to front, 1a.—The aching in sacral region reappeared, but subsided as the medicine was eliminated, 1a.—Aching in sacrum and in sacro-iliac symphysis, with the itching of anus, hemorrhoids, 1a.—(When commencing the proving, had heat and soreness in the sacrum, with a dull, heavy headache; this was cured), (third day), 1.

EXTREMITIES.—Arm went to sleep (numb), 1.—Hand felt swollen (second night), 1.—A trembling feeling of legs for several days, with soreness of knees, 1.—While on the lounge the muscles of the leg were suddenly contracted, jerking up the foot as in stepping; in a moment the right one performed the same manœuvre (third day), 1.

SKIN.—A long-cured impetiginous eczema reappeared on both legs, 1a.—[60] A few hot prickings in the skin (second and third days), 1.— Itching of the face and forehead, 1a.—The itchings repeated themselves (third day), 1.

SLEEP AND FEVER.—Fantastic dreams (second night), 1.—Voluptuous dreams and increased sexual desire, sympathetic with urinary excitement, 1a.—A few cold chills rushed up the spinal column (first day), 1.

(In addition to the foregoing we quote the following from same authority):

Prover cured a severe acute flowing coryza, headache, vertigo and cough, with sticking pains throughout the chest, heaviness and trembling of the lower limbs; pulse, 110. *Penthorum* 3x quickly cured.

Miss P——, a blonde of 17, had a severe cough of several weeks duration; worse from talking or singing. Frothy greenish sputa. *Pulsatilla* and afterwards *Phosphorus* were given without benefit. *Penthorum* soon cured.

In the prover it produced a general malaise, headache, weakness of limbs and inability to attend to business, a feeling as though he must give up and be sick. I have promptly relieved several patients having these symptoms with *Penthorum*. It produces a soreness throughout the chest, with a severe dry cough, "as though I would cough my insides out," worse in the morning. Have speedily cured several such coughs with it.

PHASEOLUS NANA.

NAT. ORD., Leguminosæ.
COMMON NAME, Dwarf Bean.
PREPARATION.—The crushed beans are macerated in five parts by weight of alcohol.

(In 1896 and 1897 Dr. A. M. Cushing wrote several articles on this new remedy, and among them the following, which appeared in the *Homœopathic Recorder*, 1897.)

While making a proving of the above remedy I felt a sudden curious sensation in the region of the heart, and immediately felt of my pulse and found it *very weak and fluttering*. I have been asked what that sensation was, but I can't describe it, for, to tell the truth, I believe I was frightened and failed to remember it. Although it is unpleasant to be badly frightened, the nice results I have seen from the use of the remedy and the kind words I have received from the profession in regard to it has more than paid for the little fright. As so little is known of the remedy, I wish to report one case that was not at all indicated by the proving and two cases under the care of an old school doctor. My case was that of a lady aged about forty, who for two years was under the care of a homœopathic doctor for some trouble, I don't know what; then two years under the care of another homœopathic doctor for a fibroid of the uterus. She had twice consulted a specialist in Boston, who said it could not be removed. Then she came under my care with a fibroid as large as a fetus at full term. Suffice it to say, I gave remedies in a higher attenuation than I believed she had taken, and in a few months the tumor had greatly diminished and gave her no trouble. Still she was nervous and had neuralgic pains almost all over her. As remedies did not seem to relieve her for any length of time, I decided to give her *Phaseolus* 9x, as it probably would do as well as what I had given her. The next time I called she met me with "I want a whole bottle like what you gave me last." She does not have to take any medicine now.

I was called in consultation with an old school doctor to a case of confinement. Patient, 26; first child; had been in pain forty-eight hours, but not severe till the last twelve hours. Patient, fleshy; urine heavily loaded with albumen. I knew that trouble was ahead, as she became blind. I found the head jacked firmly in the superior straits, face presentation which I could not change. I decided to wait a little, help what I could and watch the results. In a little while she went to sleep, the first quiet sleep in forty-eight hours; but when she moved it was in a fearful convulsion. I expected the convulsions, but felt that if I applied the forceps, before they appeared some might say if he had let her alone she would not have had them. I immediately turned her upon her left side, well covered up, and adjusted my forceps and soon had the head through the bony parts; and as it is my custom to remove the forceps till the soft parts are dilated to prevent rupture I commenced to do so, when a fearful expulsive convulsion threw forceps and a thirteen-pound child into the bed with a complete rupture of the perineum—my first such case in forty-one years. While she was unconscious I took the necessary stitches, the doctor attending to the medical part. One hour later, when I was in the kitchen helping the nurse and a few damsels dress the baby, the doctor came to me and said her heart was failing in its action fast. I gave him a vial of No. 25 globules medicated with 9x *Phaseolus*, and told him to give her a dose about the size of a bean (being a bean remedy). Ten minutes later he said: "That is wonderful, her heart is all right." Three times during the night he had to repeat it with the same results. Afterwards she had no trouble.

One week later the same doctor came to me saying: "I want a bottle of that remedy." Yesterday I was called to see a lady who was unconscious, pulseless, breathing ten times a minute, beyond hope as I supposed. I gave her three doses of *Phaseolus*, and she is all right.

P. S.—If not too late, I would like to add a little to the paper I sent you not long ago. The same old school doctor to whom I referred in that paper tells me he has used *Phaseolus* in another case of heart disease with a success similar to the others reported.

A few weeks since a lady aged 50, nurse by profession, came to me saying, at times, she had fearful time with her heart palpitating and feeling as if she should die. Being in great haste, I made no examination, but gave her a vial of *Phaseolus* 15x to take a dose three or four times a day, as needed. Yesterday she called, saying she was going out of the city, but did not dare to go without some more of the medicine, for she *never took anything in her life that did so much good as that.*

(Dr. Cushing also read the following paper before the Massachusetts Homœopathic Medical Society, which we take from the *New England Medical Gazette*. January, 1897:)

By request I appear before you to-day, and I presume you will be disappointed if my paper is not on some new remedy; and such it is,—a remedy, I think, worthy the careful investigation of every homœopathic physician,—phaseolus nana, or the common white bean. It is unnecessary for me to say to you that Boston is called a bean-eating city, or refer to the many sudden deaths there or in its vicinity from brain or heart trouble, nor how in a certain way young men grow old. Can you tell me the cause? I shall not take the time to report the proving I made, nor why I began it, nor how I prepared it, nor its wonderful effects upon the nervous system, the genital organs, stomach, bowels, or kidneys, in the provings, referring only to three symptoms. A medical student has made a short but interesting proving of the remedy, confirming some of my symptoms. While my proving was going on nicely, I suddenly felt a curious sensation in the region of the heart. It was so sudden and strange I immediately felt of my pulse and found it very irregular and feeble, so much so I think I was frightened, at least I did not take any more of the medicine. Never before had I had any irregular action of the heart. Soon after, I read that foreign physicians were using a decoction of the growing bean and pod for dropsy.

About that time I was called to see a hopeless case of uterine cancer with severe general dropsy. I prescribed the best I knew and decided to try the bean remedy. Several days elapsed before I could get any, and then only the dry pods, as it was in December. I steeped them and gave it with apparent relief. I report this case more especially to speak of the final result. I called one day expecting to find her quite comfortable, but found her dead. She suddenly screamed, "Oh, my head!" grasped it with both hands and was dead.

Months later, after an experience with another patient which I will report later, it suddenly dawned upon me that possibly the bean decoction might have hastened her death.

I was called to see a man about forty-five, suffering from general dropsy with heart and other complications, who had been under the care of a homœopathic physician some time. Although he had taken *Digitalis*, *Strophanthus*, *Strychnia*, *Nitroglycerine*, salts, etc., he had been unable to lie down for two weeks. I prescribed for him, but as soon as I could I prepared and gave him the bean-pod decoction. In about one week he was able to lie down in bed, and his legs, which at my first visit measured over twenty-one inches in circumference, measured fifteen inches. Then hay fever appeared, and by the advice of nineteen or twenty-five women an old-school expert from New York was called and I was left out.

The following cases, having symptoms similar to those developed in the proving, were given the same preparations as those used in the proving.

A man aged sixty-nine, a retired clergyman on account of a heart disease that had troubled him many years, yet no physician had been able to satisfactorily diagnose, came home from a trip where he had unwisely preached twice, greatly exhausted. The heart's action was weak and irregular, growing weaker each day for a few days, when he was entirely pulseless at both wrists, which continued four days in spite of my best efforts. I then gave him *Phaseolus* 9x, and in a few hours there was an improvement, and in thirty-six hours his pulse was regular and strong, about seventy per minute; and it remained so till my last visit, one-half hour before his death, two weeks after beginning the medicine. I was called to New York and returned too late to make a *post-mortem* examination. Among his children were a public school teacher and a college professor. I told them what I was giving, and they watched the case very closely and were surprised at its effects. Later they asked me if I would send some of the same medicine to a friend in Connecticut who had no money but a bad heart, said by the doctor there and an expert in Boston to be a weak heart. I sent the medicine and two weeks later they wrote: "His breath is not as short, his limbs were not as badly swollen, could walk and sleep better, but they did not know as he was any better." I sent more medicine and have not heard from that.

A lady living in the West, aged about fifty, had been ailing several years. Her greatest complaint was a weak, bad-aching heart. I treated her a few months with general improvement, but she complained of a weak, tired, bad-acting and bad-feeling heart. I sent her *Phaseolus* 9x, and later she wrote me that forty-eight hours after commencing the last medicine sent her heart wheeled into line all right and remains so.

A lady, aged eighty-seven, had diarrhœa, which was soon relieved; then I found her heart acted badly, about every third beat omitted, and she said it had been so for a year or more. I gave her *Phaseolus*, and two days later her pulse was all right.

Dr. Brown, of Springfield, reported a case of a young man that only once in two weeks did he get his pulse up to sixty, ranging from fifty to fifty-five the two weeks. He gave *Phaseolus* 6, which I furnished him, and the next forenoon his pulse was seventy-two and remained so.

I will report only one more case, treated with this remedy, one which I think very interesting.

A lady physician, aged thirty, married, no children, never has been sick except with childhood diseases. Two years ago had considerable mental trouble and rode a bicycle a good deal. Since that time, two years ago, five times each minute, or about that, her heart would give one hard unpleasant throb, then omit one beat, this in the day time, but much worse at night, preventing sleep. Being in somewhat of a hurry, I did not examine the heart, thinking there would be a plenty of time later, but gave her *Phaseolus*, the 10th I think. Thirty-six hours later the heart would beat one hundred consecutive times without the slightest variation, and it continued to improve, although after taking the medicine thirty-six hours she was obliged to desist on account of a severe headache. She is never subject to headaches, but it was so bad she dared not take any more of the medicine. It was as if something was pressing hard against each temple, much worse soon after taking each dose of the medicine. This headache led me to fear that the death I mentioned might have been hastened by the medicine.

A medical conundrum. A lady, aged about thirty, decided she would investigate the next world to see if she could enjoy it better than this, and called in the aid of morphine to help her along. Not being in the habit of taking morphine, to disguise the bitter of it, placed a tablet of morphine in the middle of a baked bean and swallowed it whole. She took her little dose in the evening, having eaten nothing since noon, and went to sleep. At seven in the morning she awoke and was surprised to find herself in this world. When asked if she would get up, replied, no, she would sleep a little longer. At eleven A.M. she awoke and tried to get up, but could not walk, so crawled to the door and opened it to let in fresh air. A servant found her there, and at her request handed her the camphor bottle, and she took a little. Dr. Rowe was called and said she vomited a little mucus, some dark specks that looked like blood, and a small piece of lettuce she ate the noon before. She had taken twelve and one-half grains of morphine. Did the lettuce antidote it? Did the bean destroy its power? Why did it not kill her?

POTHOS.

NAT. ORD., Araceæ.
COMMON NAME, Skunk Cabbage.
PREPARATION.—The fresh root gathered in spring is macerated in twice its weight of alcohol.

(Contributed by Dr. S. A. Jones to the *Homœopathic Recorder*, 1889.)

This perennial, odorous member of the natural order *Araceæ* is one of our most common meadow and bog plants. From its very realistic, skunk-like odor when cut or bruised, and its resemblance in shape of leaf and mode of growth to the cabbage, it has been commonly well known as the skunk cabbage.

Belonging to the same family as the Calla lily and Indian turnip, the shape of its flower becomes at once familiar to anyone who observes it. Among the first plants to flower in spring is this species, and by closely observing the surface of any boggy meadow in the latter part of March or early April one will find irrupting the earth like mushroom the points of many beautiful spathes gaping open to extend invitations to the earliest slugs and carrion beetles of the season. These are the flowers of Pothos appearing some time before the leaves, and when divested of the mud that clings to them, and polished with a damp cloth, as the apple-woman serves her pippins, they shine out in beautiful mottled purple, orange, and deep red, and, being very fleshy, will keep up appearances many days if cut deep and placed in hyacinth jars.

The root is large, thick, and cylindrical, giving off its lower end numerous long, cylindrical branches; the leaves which appear on the fertilization of the ovary are large, smooth, entire, and deeply plaited into rounded folds. On opening the pointed spathe or floral envelope, a club-like mass will be noted arising from its base. This is the spadix bearing the naked flowers, which are perfect, consisting of a four-angled style and four awl-shaped stamens. The fruit, when mature, is a globular, ill-smelling, glutinous mass, consisting of the enlarged, fleshy spadix and changed perianths, and enclosing several large bullet-like seeds.

The roots are easily gathered, one alone being sufficient to make a year's stock of tincture for the most lavish practitioner.

THE TINCTURE.

Take the fresh root stalks and rootlets, gathered in spring on the first appearance of the flowers, and chop and pound them to a pulp, and weigh. Then taking two parts, by weight, of alcohol, mix the pulp with one-sixth part of it, add the balance, and, after stirring the whole well, pour it into a well-stoppered bottle and let it stand for eight days in a dark, cool place. After straining and filtering, the resulting tincture should be of a light brown color and have a slightly acrid taste and a neutral reaction.

CHEMISTRY.

The active principle of this plant is doubtless volatile, as the dried root presents none of the acridity of the fresh, and is odorless as well. Dr. J. M. Turner determined in the root a volatile fatty body, a volatile oil, a fixed oil, and a specific resin.

On the 16th of December, 1887, there came into my hands a case that the family physician (a homœopath) had pronounced epilepsy and declared incurable. Upon being consulted, his diagnosis had been confirmed and his prognosis corroborated by the late Prof. E. S. Dunster, of the University of Michigan.

Up to date that identical patient has had neither a "fit" nor any approximation thereto, and that fact is an occasion of this paper. One who already discerns the first gray shadows of that night which comes to all, does not now write at the urging, or the *itching*, of the Ego. He disclaims any merit, having evinced only a monkey-like imitativeness. He had from the Infinite, the gift of a good memory, and an old book, picked up one happy day at a street stall, flashed into recollection some twelve years later, and enabled him then to imitate the much earlier doing of its worthy author—

"Only the actions of the just Smell sweet and blossom in the dust."

This dead worthy—he that was James Thacher, M. D.—more than any other, made known the virtues of *Pothos fœtida*, and gratitude for what his book had taught me to do made me feel that to write up this forgotten remedy were the fittest return that I could make for his well doing.

A second incentive, ample enough, is found in the fact that the first homœopathic paper on *Pothos fœt.* has never had a faithful translation into our language, and has not been critically reproduced in any other. A study of the *Homœopathic Bibliography*, as given in this paper, will teach an impressive lesson not only to the *real* student of Materia Medica, but also to those who assume the responsibilities of editorship.

A third inducement, and perhaps a pardonable, is the singular fact that much search in our literature has not enabled me to find any assistance of the clinical application of *Pothos fœt.* by a homœopathic practitioner. If any reader knows of any such, he will greatly gratify the writer by making it known.

AN EMPIRICAL BIBLIOGRAPHY.[K]

1785. Rev. Dr. M. Cutler.—*Memoirs of the American Academy of Arts and Sciences.* Boston.

1787. D. J. D. Schoepf, M. D.—*Materia Medica Americana potissimum Regni Vegetabilis.* Erlangen. (Not in my possession. Quoted from Barton.)

1813. James Thacher, M. D.—*The American New Dispensatory.* Boston. (This is the second edition wherein Pothos is mentioned for the first time. Our citations are from the fourth edition. Boston, 1821.)

1817. James Thacher, M. D.—*American Modern Practice, etc.* Boston.

1818. Jacob Bigelow, M. D.—*American Medical Botany, etc.* Vol. 2. Boston.

1820. Wm. M. Hand.—*The House-Surgeon and Physician.* Second edition. New Haven.

1822. Jacob Bigelow, M. D.—*A Sequel to the Pharmacopœia of the U. S.* Boston.

1822. John Eberle, M. D.—*Materia Medica and Therapeutics.* Philadelphia. (The citations are from the fourth edition. Philadelphia, 1836.)

1825. Ansel W. Ives, M. D.—*Paris' Pharmacologia.* Third American edition. New York.

1830. Elisha Smith.—*The Botanic Physician, etc.* New York. (The title page proclaims him "president of the New York Association of Botanic Physicians.")

1838. C. S. Rafinesque.—*Medical Flora, etc.* Philadelphia.

It was admitted into the *catalogus secundarius* of the second edition of *The Pharmacopœia of the United States of America,* and dropped into the dust-heap when the men who knew how to use it had passed away.

FOOTNOTES:

[K] As my researches are confined to my own library, I do not profess to be exhaustive. I have not given all the references at my command, but have aimed to include such writers as have made positive contributions to our knowledge of this drug. Of my list, only Rafinesque is a mere (but a useful) compiler.

EMPIRICAL APPLICATIONS.

In dealing with authors who have gone to their reward, it has always seemed to me a duty to give their own words as far as possible. It brings them face to face with the reader, and is as if one brushed the moss from their gravestones, or perhaps, like Old Mortality, carved afresh a half-obliterated name.

It is not the briefest way, but it has the merit of showing from whence the bricks came of which the edifice is built. I shall, then, cite the authorities in chronological order, and copiously enough to include essentials.

Cutler.—The roots dried and powdered are an excellent medicine in asthmatic cases, and often give relief when other means are ineffectual. It may be given with safety to children as well as to adults; to the former, in doses of four, five or six grains, and to the latter in doses of twenty grains and upwards. It is given in the fit, and repeated as the case may require. This knowledge is said to have been obtained from the Indians, who, it is likewise said, repeat the dose, after the paroxysm (*sic*) is gone off, several mornings, then miss as many, and repeat it again; thus continuing the medicine until the patient is perfectly recovered. It appears to be anti-spasmodic, and bids fair to be useful in many other disorders.—*Op. cit.*, 1,409.

Schoepf.—I am obliged to cite at second hand, as I have never been able to find a copy of his *opus*. One may judge of its rarity, when a foreign advertisement by a German bookseller some years since failed to obtain it for me.

Prof. W. P. C. Barton, *op. cit.*, gives the gist of the Hessian surgeon's contribution in a style and manner as prim and orderly as that of Surgeon Schoepf himself on a dress parade.

"Phar
m.   *Dracontii Radix.*

Qual.   *Acris, alliacea, nauseosa.*

Vis.   *Incidens, califaciens, expectorans.*

Usus: *fol. contrita ad vulnera recentia et ulcera. Tussis consumptiva Scorbutus et elii morbi radix. Ari officin. utilis."*

"Incidens": Young reader, you must go back more than a century to understand the "pathology" that is wrapped up in that word like a mummy in its cerements. Don't laugh at *that* "pathology," for some graceless graduate will laugh at yours in 1989. Note, however, in passing, that Schoepf says nothing, save *tussis*, that suggests the *vis anti-spasmodica* of Cutler.

Thacher.—The roots and seeds, when fresh, impart to the mouth a sensation of pungency and acrimony similar to Arum.

It may be ranked high as an anti-spasmodic, experience having evinced that it is not inferior to the most esteemed remedies of that class. In cases of asthmatic affections, it alleviates the most distressing symptoms, and shortens the duration of the paroxysms. * * * Rev. Dr. Cutler experienced in his own particular case very considerable relief from this medicine, after others had disappointed his expectations. * * * The seeds of this plant are said by some to afford more relief in asthmatic cases than the root.

In obstinate hysteric affections this medicine has surpassed in efficacy all those anti-spasmodics which have generally been employed, and in several instances it has displayed its powers like a charm. In one of the most violent hysteric cases I ever met with, says a correspondent, where the usual anti-spasmodics, and even musk had failed, two teaspoonfuls of the powdered root procured immediate relief; and on repeating the trials with the same patient, it afforded more lasting benefit than any other medicine. In those spasmodic affections of the abdominal muscles during parturition, or after delivery, this root has proved an effectual remedy. In chronic rheumatism, and erratic pains of a spasmodic nature, it often performs a cure, or affords essential relief.

It has in some cases of epilepsy suspended the fits, and greatly alleviated the symptoms.

In whooping cough, and other pulmonic affections, it proves beneficial in the form of syrup.

During every stage of nervous and hysteric complaints, and in cramps and spasms, this medicine is strongly recommended as a valuable substitute for the various anti-spasmodic remedies commonly employed. It is free from the heating and constipating qualities of Opium. [Yet Schoepf endowed it with the *vis colifaciers*.]

Having in a few instances tested its virtues in subsultus tendinum, attending typhus fever, its pleasing effects will encourage the future employment of it in similar cases.

Two instances have been related in which this medicine has been supposed to be remarkably efficacious in the cure of dropsy.

The roots should be taken up in the autumn or spring, before the leaves appear, and carefully dried for use. Its strength is impaired by long keeping, especially in a powdered state.—*Mat. Med.*, 4th ed., p. 249.

A young woman, about eighteen years of age, was harassed by severe convulsive and hysteric paroxysms, almost incessantly, insomuch that her friends estimated the number at seven hundred in the course of a few weeks; her abdomen was remarkably tumefied and tense, and there was a singular bloatedness of the whole surface of her body, and the slightest touch would occasion intolerable pain. At length her extremities became rigid and immovable (*sic*), and her jaw was so completely locked that she was unable to articulate, and liquids could only be introduced through the vacuity of a lost tooth. She had been treated with a variety of anti-spasmodic and other medicines, by an experienced physician, without relief. Having prepared a strong infusion of the dried root of skunk cabbage, I directed half a teacupful to be given every few hours, without any other medicine; the favorable effects of which were soon observable, and by persisting in the use of it about ten days the muscular contractions were removed, the jaw was relaxed, and her faculty of speech and swallowing, with the use of all her limbs, were completely effected.

Another young woman had been exercised with the most distressing paroxysms of hysteria for several days, without obtaining relief by the medicines prescribed, when the skunk cabbage infusion was so successfully directed that her fits were immediately arrested, and in a few days a cure was completely effected.

The brother of this patient was seized with violent convulsions of the whole body, in consequence of a cut on his foot; the skunk cabbage was administered, and he was speedily restored to perfect health.

A woman was affected with violent spasmodic pains, twenty-four hours after parturition; six doses of skunk cabbage entirely removed her complaints.—*American Modern Practice*, p. 530.

Barton.—The smell from spathe and flowers is pungent and very subtle. Experience leads me to believe they possess a great share of acridity; *having been seized with a very violent inflammation of my eyes* (for the first time in my life), which deprived me of the use of them for a month, by making the original drawings of these plates. The pungency of the plant was probably concentrated by the closeness of the room, in which many specimens were at the time shut up.—*Veg. Mat. Med.*, 1, 128. [The italics are not in the original text.]

The seeds are said to afford more relief in asthmatic cases than the root; and this I believe very probable, for they are remarkably active, pungent, and, as has before been mentioned, exhale the odor of Asafœtida.—*Op. cit.*, p. 131.

The bruised leaves are frequently applied to ulcers and recent wounds, and, it is said, with good effect. They are also used as an external application in cutaneous affections; and I have heard of the expressed juice being successfully applied to different species of herpes. The leaves are also used in the country to dress blisters, with the view of promoting their discharge. * * * For this purpose I can recommend them where it is desirable to promote a large and speedy discharge, and no stimulating ointment is at hand.

Colden recommends the skunk cabbage in scurvy.—*Op. cit.*, p. 132.

Bigelow.—The odor of the Ictodes resides in a principle which is extremely volatile. I have not been able to separate it by distillation from any part of the plant, the decoction and the distilled water being in my experiments but slightly impregnated with its sensible character. Alcohol, digested on the plant, retains its odors for a time, but this is soon dissipated by exposure to the air.

An acrid principle resides in the root, even when perfectly dry, producing an effect like that of the Arum and the Ranunculi. When chewed in the mouth, the root is slow in manifesting its peculiar taste; but after some moments a pricking sensation is felt, which soon amounts to a disagreeable smarting, and continues for some time. This acrimony is readily dissipated by heat. The decoction retains none of it. The distilled water is impregnated with it, if the process be carefully conducted, but loses it on standing a short time.—*Amer. Med. Bot.*, 2, 45.

To insure a tolerably uniform activity of this medicine, the root should be kept in dried slices, and not reduced to powder until it is wanted for use.—*Op. cit.*, p. 49.

A number of cases have fallen under my own observation of the catarrhal affections of old people, in which a syrup prepared from the root in substance has alleviated and removed the complaint.—*Op. cit.*, p. 48.

In delicate stomachs I have found it frequently to occasion vomiting even in a small quantity. In several cases of gastrodynia, where it was given with a view to its anti-spasmodic effect, it was ejected from the stomach more speedily than common cathartic medicines. I have known it in a dose of thirty grains to bring on not only vomiting, but headache (*sic*), vertigo and temporary blindness.—*Op. cit.*, pp. 48-49.

Hand.—The root is a pungent anti-spasmodic in colics and griping of the bowels.

Leaves bruised relieve painful swellings, whitlows, etc.—*House Surg. and Phys.*, p. 250.

Eberle.—In chronic cough attended with a cold, phlegmatic habit of body, I have employed the powdered root of this plant with the most decided benefit. In an old man who had been for many years afflicted with a very troublesome cough and difficulty of breathing, I found nothing to give so much relief as this substance.

In cases of chronic catarrhal and asthmatic affections, and very generally with evident advantage.—*Mat. Med. and Thur.*, 2, 154.

Ives.—The root loses its pungent taste, and appears to be nearly inert in a few weeks after it is gathered. I prepared, however, an alcoholic extract some years ago, by digesting the fresh roots and evaporating the tincture in the sun, which possessed and retained all the acrimony of the recent root. The fresh leaves are actively rubefacient.—*Pharmacologia*, p. 147.

Smith.—Skunk cabbage is not only a good anti-spasmodic in all cases where such are indicated, but it is also a powerful emmenagogue, anthelmintic, and a valuable remedy in dropsy, in spasms, rheumatism, palpitations, etc. It is frequently used in childbed to promote the birth. * * * * For expelling worms, the pulverized root should be administered in molasses for a sufficient length of time, following it up with a purge.—*Op. cit.*, p. 511.

Rafinesque.—Powerful anti-spasmodic, expectorant, incisive, vermifuge, menagogue, sudorific, etc. Used with success in spasmodic asthmas and coughs, hysterics, pertussis, epilepsy, dropsy, scurvy, chronic rheumatism, erradic and spasmodic pains, parturition, amenorrhœa, worms, etc.—*Op. cit.*, 2, 230.

III.

THE HOMŒOPATHIC BIBLIOGRAPHY.[L]

1837. *Correspondenzblatt der Hom. Aerzte*, January 18th, 2d part, No. 1, p. 6. Allentown, Pa. Hering, Humphreys, and Lingen.

1843. *Symptomus Kodex*, vol. 2, p. 392. Jahr. (Taken from the *Correspondenzblatt*, and not correctly.) *Handbuch der Hom. Arzneimittellehre*, vol. 3, p. 613. Noack and Trinks. (Taken from the *Correspondenzblatt*, and incompletely.)

1847. *Manual of Hom. Mat. Met.—Jahr.* Translated by Curie, 2d ed., vol. 1, p. 462. London. (This is the first appearance of the Allentown "abstract of symptoms" in English. *Curie* credits his *data* to some "United States' Journal," probably meaning the *Correspondenzblatt*. His translation is erroneous, and yet, up to date, it is the fullest source of information for him who reads English only.)

1848. *New Manual or Symptomen Codex.—Jahr.* Translated by Hempel, vol. 2, p. 573. (This is a singularly incomplete translation from the German *Kodex*, with no reference to any source. A literal copy of this translation is all there is of *Pothos fœt.* in the *Encyclopædia*. It omits the only symptom in the *Correspondenzblatt* abstract that made my application of this remedy not purely empirical.)

1851. *Jahr's New Manual.* Edited by Hull, 3d ed., vol. 1, p. 797.

1851. *Characteristik der Hom. Arzneien.* Possart, part 2, p. 506.

1860. *"Hull's Jahr."* *A New Manual of Hom. Practice.* Edited by Snelling, 4th ed., vol. 1, p. 977.

1866. *Text-Book of Mat. Med.* Lippe, p. 545.

1878. *Encyclopædia of Pure Materia Medica.* Allen, vol. 9, p. 155.

1884. *American Medicinal Plants.* Millspaugh, vol. 1, p. 169.

FOOTNOTES:

[L] The definite article is used because it is believed to be complete, thanks to the scholarship and courtesy of Dr. Henry M. Smith, of New York. To him, also, am I indebted for the original text of *Pothos fœt.* from the *Correspondenzblatt.*

POTHOS FŒTIDA SYMPTOMATOLOGY.

Translated from the *Correspondenzblatt* by T. C. Fanning, M. D., Tarrytown, N. Y.[M]

Because the odor is quite like Mephitis it is considered a so-called anti-spasmodic.

Abstract of symptoms from Hering, Humphreys, and Lingen.

So absent-minded and thoughtless that he enters the sick rooms without knocking; pays no attention to those speaking to him. Irritable, inclined to contradict; violent.

Headache of brief duration, in single spots, now here, now there, with confusion. Pressure in both temples, harder on one side than on the other alternately, with violent pulsation of the temporal arteries.

Drawing in the forehead in two lines from the frontal eminences to the glabella, where there is a strong outward drawing as if by a magnet.

Red swelling, like a saddle, across the bridge of the nose, painful to the touch, especially on the left side near the forehead, while the cartilaginous portion is cold and bloodless; with red spots on the cheek, on the left little pimples; swelling of the cervical and sub-maxillary glands.

Unpleasant numb sensation in the tongue; cannot project it against the teeth; papillæ elevated; tongue redder, with sore pain at point and edge.

Burning sensation from the fauces down through the chest. With the desire to smoke, tobacco tastes badly.

Pain in the scrobiculus cordis as if something broke loose, on stepping hard.

Inflation and tension in the abdomen; bellyache here and there in single spots; on walking, feeling as if the bowels shook, without pain.

Stool earlier (in the morning), frequent, softer.

Urging to urinate; very dark urine.

Painful, voluptuous tickling in the whole of the glans penis.

Violent sneezing, causing pain in the roof of the mouth, the fauces and œsophagus all the way to the stomach, followed by long-continued pains at the cardiac orifice.

Pain in chest and *mediastinum posticum*, less in the *anticum*, with pain under the shoulders, which seems to be in connection with burning in the œsophagus. Pressing pain on the sternum.

Sudden feeling of anxiety, with difficult (or oppressed) respiration and sweat, followed by stool and the subsidence of these and other pains.

Inclination to take deep inspirations with hollow feeling in the chest, later with contraction in the fauces and chest.

The difficulty of breathing is better in the open air.

Pain in the crest of the right tibia.

Rheumatic troubles increased.

Sleepy early in the evening.

All troubles disappear in the open air.

In attempting to analyze this "abstract of symptoms," to see if the internal evidence tends to show that the recorded effects are genuine results of the drug, it is well to remember that these provings—for we infer that three observers participated therein—were made in the light of the empirical history of *Pothos fœt.* The said history was on record before the date of these provings, and it cannot have escaped Hering's eye; he was too wide a reader for that. He was, beyond doubt, aware of the pathogenetic effects observed by Bigelow—*headache, vertigo, temporary blindness, vomiting, even from small quantities.* Having, then, this clue to its physiological action, these symptoms should reappear in his proving *if his imagination furnished his symptoms.* As only a mild headache is noted in the *Correspondenzblatt*, it is evident that these provers did not *work from a pattern.* It is also evident that the *usus in morbis* did not suggest the Allentown symptomatology, for the anti-asthmatic virtue of *Pothos fœt.* is one feature on which the greatest stress had been laid, and yet the only *pathogenetic* suggestion of its applicability in asthma is: "*Sudden feeling of anxiety with difficult* (or oppressed) respiration and sweat, followed by stool and the *subsidence of these and other pains.*" Who ever heard of an asthma relieved by stool? Who could have *invented* such an odd modality? As it stands it is an *unicum*, and by every rule of criticism this single symptom-group gives the stamp of verity to the Allentown "abstract of symptoms." But there is other and singularly convincing evidence of the genuineness of this abstract. As the reader is aware, Thacher had emphasized the efficiency of *Pothos fœt.* as an anti-spasmodic in hysteria, although the "key-note" that indicates it in hysteria had wholly escaped his discernment.

Now this very "key-note" appears in the Allentown pathogenesis, but so unobtrusively as to show most conclusively that the prover who furnished it did not recognize its singular import and value. Such testimony is absolutely unimpugnable by honest and intelligent criticism.

It is also apparent that some of the less pronounced of its empirical virtues are reflected in the proving. For instance, Thacher found it efficacious in "erratick pains of a spasmodick nature." Is not this "erratic" feature reproduced in such conditions as:

"Headache, of brief duration, in single spots, now here, now there?"

"Pressure in both temples alternately, harder on one side than on the other?"

"Bellyache, here and there, in single spots?"

Brevity of duration and recurrence "in single spots, now here, now there," are phenomena at once *spasmodic* and *erratic*. It must be admitted that the trend of its pathogenetic action and the lines of its therapeutical application are parallel, and, therefore, that the latter are confirmatory of the former.

With such an anti-hysterical reputation as the empirical use had given to *Pothos fœt.*, it might fairly be anticipated that its pathogenesis would be distinguished by a paucity of objective *data*, for only a tyro in pharmacodynamics, or a "Regular," would expect to find a full-lined picture of hysteria in any "proving." And so we have in the "abstract" a flux of subjective symptoms, "erratic" enough for hysterical elements, and still further characterized by an apparent evanescence, as if its phenomena of sensory disturbance were as fleeting and unsubstantial as those of an hysterical storm.

The *will-o'-the-wisp-like* character of its subjective symptoms, and its physometric property (hinted at in the pathogenesis and emphasized in Thacher's case) are the features that will chiefly impress one in studying this distinctively American remedy.

That the "abstract of symptomes" evinces a cautious trial of this drug, and that more heroic experiments will add to our knowledge of its pathogenetic properties, are plain deductions from the absence in the "abstract" of such pronounced effects as Bigelow observed and also from the evidence of the *usus in morbis*. The remedy needs an efficient proving, especially in the female organism.

FOOTNOTES:

[M] Literalness rather than elegance has been sought in the translating.

AN APPLICATION OF POTHOS FŒTIDA.

Miss B——, æt. 20; a tall, spare brunette, and a good specimen of Fothergill's *Arab type*, brainy and vivacious. General health has been good, but she was never robust; could not go to school regularly. Between her thirteenth and fifteenth years grew rapidly in stature, and then she was easily wearied on walking; knees tired and limbs ached. Had good digestion through the growing period, but subsequently became subject to "bloat of wind" in abdomen. These meteoristic attacks came when lying down. A "weight rises from the abdomen up to the heart." She must at once spring up. This condition is relieved by eructating, by liquor, and by drinking hot water. The night attacks of meteorism are by far the worst. *She is now subject to them.*

[Her grand-mother had such "spells of bloating;" would spring out of bed at night, lose consciousness, and "bloat up suddenly." If she had such an attack when dressed, they had often been obliged to cut open her clothes.]

Patient has found that apples, tomatoes, cabbage and onions disagree with her; no other food. She is constipated—"wants to and can't."

Her hair is unusually dry; scalp full of dandruff; skin, generally, soft and flexible.

She has frequent epistaxis; has had four and five attacks a day. Blood bright red, "runs a perfect stream," does not clot at the nostrils. Has previously a "heavy feeling" in the head, which the bleeding relieves.

In appearance she is "the picture of health;" good complexion, fairly ruddy cheeks, sparkling eyes—in a word, she is an incarnated protest against "single blessedness."

In the latter part of July, 1886, had her first "fit." She had arisen with a headache, which kept on increasing in severity. Just after a light meal had the attack; "Oh, dear! Oh, dear!" and fell insensible. Stiffened at first, then had clonic spasms. Neither bit the tongue nor frothed at the mouth. No micturition or defecation. On coming to, did not remember that she had fallen, but recollected being borne up stairs. Had a "dreadful nosebleed" after the attack. Left her very weak; could hardly lift her feet from the floor. Before the "fit" the headache had become unbearably severe.

Had her second "fit" on August 7th, 1887. Headache came on and kept growing worse; was in temples, beating and throbbing, and in eyes, "light hurt"—also on vertex, "pressing-down" pain. At 4 P.M. suddenly fell down insensible. No cry. Tongue bitten. Slight frothing at the mouth. First "stiff all over," then clonic spasms. After the "fit" knew that something had happened to her. Was prostrated for nearly a month, but not so much as after first attack.

December 10th, 1887, third "fit." On the night of the 9th her mother had been very ill, and she herself was very uneasy and alarmed. Had the attack before breakfast. Blurred vision, headache, fall; no biting of tongue, nor frothing. First rigid, then clonic spasms; after attack, nose bled profusely, head ached all day, face flushed and dark. Prostrated as usual.

In none of the attacks was there any involuntary micturition or defecation, nor was it ever necessary to use any force to hold her on the bed.

One other fact I gathered from her brother, namely: during her "fits" her abdomen bloated so rapidly and to such a degree that the family had learned to remove her clothing as soon as possible after she fell.

Of course, Thacher's case, wherein the "abdomen was remarkably tumefied and tense," came into memory at once. The old volume was taken down, and that case re-read. Then followed the *Encyclopædia*, and then the English *Symptomen Codex*. No pathogenetic light or corroboration *there*. Then Curie's "Jahr." Ah! "*Inflation and tension in the abdomen.*" Only a straw, but a pathogenetic, and I grasped it thankfully. I found also, "*aching in the temples with violent arterial pulsation.*"

It was an open winter; my son dug some skunk cabbage roots in a swamp; a tincture was made; ten-drop doses, four times daily, were taken until six ounces had been consumed.

No "fit" up to date; no epistaxis; only once a slight headache.

I never made a diagnosis in this case; have not reached one yet, nor am I grieving over that omission. I did rashly declare that it was not epilepsy, because Sauvages *tympanites intestinalis* is a feature of hysteria, but not of epilepsy. But not a word of this was said to the patient. It was not a "mind cure," for I have no "mind" to spare; nor was it "Christian science," for I am not up to that. I had an *amnesis* in which grand-mother and grand-daughter participated. Nature had put the "key-note" in italics, not only in the patient but also in the drug. Thacher stumbled upon it empirically; Hering found it pathogenetically, and that led to its application under the guidance of the only approximation to *a law* in therapeutics that has yet been discovered by any of woman born: *similia similibus curantur!*

(Anent the foregoing paper Dr. W. C. Campbell sent the following to the same journal:)

POTHOS FŒTIDA, HYSTERIA.

November 6, 1889, was called in haste to see Miss N——, aged 19 years. Found her lying upon the floor, exhibiting all the phenomena of epilepsy, clenched hands, frothing at the mouth, clonic spasm, etc.

On questioning the family, I learned that she had been subject to such seizures for about two years, and that they were increasing in frequency. She had been dismissed from the various cotton mills in which she had been employed because of them. The father had been informed that she had epilepsy, and she had been treated accordingly by three old school physicians.

The sister informed me that although she had frequently fallen near the stove she had never struck it. Further questioning elicited the fact of her never having injured herself more seriously than to bite her tongue. It was then I became suspicious, and later felt convinced that it was hysteria and not epilepsy with which I had to deal.

I remembered having read in *The Recorder* an article by Dr. S. A. Jones, of Ann Arbor, on *Pothos fœtida*, with the record of a case in some respects similar to mine. After again reading it up, I made a tincture of the roots and tendrils gathered at the time, of which I gave her a two drachm phial, directing her to take ten drops three times per day.

On the second day she had a slight seizure while at dinner. After two months she again resumed her place in the mill, where she has since been steadily employed, and is strong and well in every way.

Have used *Pothos* in epilepsy, also in dropsy, with negative results.

PRIMULA OBCONICA.

NAT. ORD., Primulaceæ.
COMMON NAME, Primrose var. obconica.
PREPARATION.—The entire fresh plant in flower with root is macerated in twice its weight of alcohol.

(Dr. E. V. Ross, of Rochester, N. Y., thus summarizes the various papers that have appeared on this remedy—sources of papers named in his article:)

The following summary of the pathogenetic effects of *Primula* were produced from handling and in otherwise coming in contact with the plant, and so far as known the poisonous properties are wholly confined to the leaves.

The effects bear a close resemblance to *Anacardium, Euphorbium, Ranunculus, Rhus*, etc. It is evidently deserving of a thorough proving, and it is our intention to attempt one as soon as a reliable preparation can be had.

References: (1) *Syme, British Medical Journal;* (2) *London Lancet;* (3) *Homœopathic World*, March, 1892; (4) *American Homœopathist*, 1897, p. 429; (5) *New York Medical Journal*, January, 1898, p. 68.

(1) 1. Eczema on face.

2. Eczema on face and arms.

3. Moist eczema on face and forearms, papular and excoriated.

4. Severe cracking over joints and fingers as from frost.

5. Great itching of the skin.

6. Eruption appears at night.

7. Eruption and itching worse at night.

8. The itching was intolerable at night.

(2) 9. Irritable papular eruption on both hands, followed by desquamation.

10. Papular eruption on chin.

11. Eruption of small papules on a raised base with intolerable itching.

(3) 12. Papular eruption (eczematous) on hands, wrists and fingers.

13. Skin red and swollen and itching violently.

14. At night she became feverish, hands and face would burn, then intolerable itching followed by erythema with small papules becoming pustular.

15. Papular eruption itching violently.

(4) 16. Confluent blotches on face resembling urticaria.

17. Eruption between fingers which resembles scabies.

18. Desquamation.

19. Purple blotches on dorsal surface of hands.

20. Palmar surface of hands and fingers are stiff and unusable.

21. Deep-seated blisters form on tip of each finger and above and below each phalangeal flexure.

22. Blisters on fingers from which a clear fluid escapes on being pricked.

23. Intense itching and burning accompanies the eruption.

(5) 24. Eruption preceded by pricking sensation which gradually changes to a smarting.

25. Skin tumefied and diffuse infiltration with a red serosity, with here and there small fullæ filled with a limpid liquid.

26. Eyelids greatly swollen and covered with large fullæ, eyes half closed.

27. Great tension and redness of skin resembling erysipeias.

28. Desquamation sometimes furfuraceous, sometimes lamellar, involving all of the epidermic layer in such a manner that in some places the papillary layer was exposed.

29. Eyelids stiff and immovable, resembling ptosis.

30. Dryness and heat in palms of hands.

31. Deep infiltration of tissues rendering the parts stiff and immovable.

32. Skin symptoms accompanied by pronounced febrile symptoms.

From symptoms Nos. 5, 6, 7, 8, 14, 15, 23 it would appear the time of aggravation is at night, and the most prominent sensation is *itching* and less prominent is burning. This is characteristic of the *Arsenicum* eruption, also of *Anacardium*, *Rhus tox.*, and some others. The eruption also bears a strong resemblance to these remedies, and if one may judge from the symptoms enumerated ought to prove a potent rival in erysipelas and eczematous complaints. *Rhus* poisoning will no doubt find a new and efficient remedy in *Primula*.

PYRUS AMERICANA.

NAT. ORD., Rosacæ.
COMMON NAME, Mountain ash.
PREPARATION.—The fresh bark is macerated in twice its weight of alcohol.

(We find the following in the *American Observer*, 1878, credited to *Northwestern Analist* and written by Dr. H. P. Gatchell. Allen, in the *Encyclopædia* has not mentioned the drug, and we can find no mention in any of the dispensatories consulted. Dr. Fernie, in his excellent book, *Herbal simples* devotes some space to it. We quote: "'There is,' says an old writer, 'in every berry the exhilaration of wine, and the satisfying of old mead; and whosoever shall eat three berries of them, if he has completed a hundred years, he will return to the age of thirty.' At the same time it must be noted that the *leaves* of the Mountain ash are of a poisonous quality, and contain prussic acid like those of the laurel." The following is Dr. Gatchell's paper, the proving, be it noted, is made from a tincture of the bark:)

My memory of details, never remarkable, except as the details belonged to some system, is not as good as in earlier life, and in the matter of disconnected or partially connected incidents, the widow Bedott could, at any time, have given me five points in ten, and then have beaten me easily.

No. 1 of the provers was a married lady; No. 2 and No. 3 were lads. The tincture of the bark was used, several drops being put in a cup of water, of which teaspoonful doses were given and repeated at, I do not remember what, intervals. Myself experienced some irritation of the eyes; no other symptoms.

No. 1. Feels like crying. Feels as if the knees are immensely swollen, as if the toes the same. Knees and toes ache. Feels constricted around the waist, obliged to loosen the clothes at once. Headache begins over the eyes, left side of head aches terribly, like a tooth ache. Aches everywhere, in every joint. Left great toe feels as if torn from the socket. Sense of prolapsus of womb, bearing down and pressing out, as if swollen, and burning all over. Pains in the head knife-like. All the pains intense, acute. Thinks the conditions that of inflammatory rheumatism as if the lungs were congested, especially at the base. Can hardly breathe, as if cold water in the stomach. Thinks mucus accumulated in the cold stomach. Craves hot teas. Headache extends to the right side. Head feels as if it would burst. Great weight on top of head. Toes burn. Aching at heart. Twinging pains in arms, legs and toes. As if rectum were shrunken, dried up. Bearing down pains and pressing out, like labor pains. Feels gloomy and discouraged, but can't cry. Very cold, shivers internally; thinks she must look blue. Cold creeping all over. Pain in knees subsides, and is succeeded by pain as in the tendons and along the calves. "Oh, such a drawing pain, cutting and darting also, like that in the head." Feels resolute, as full of a gloomy determination. Stomach cold again. Thinks meat bad for her, would not digest; needs soft, mild food. Irritation of bladder and urethra; feels as if prolapsus of bladder. Dreads to move, especially on account of the joints. Sensitive to cold. Stomach still feels as if full of cold water. Sick feeling under right scapula. Thinks bile deficient. Shooting pains in forehead. Feeling as if coldness in stomach extends up under the sternum. Same feeling in the gullet. Excessive aching of bones of toes; seems unendurable. Thinks the stomach very weak, as if it would digest nothing; thinks it is dry and wrinkled. Hypochondriac, not nervous. Feels lazy, as if she would like to lie in bed and be waited on. Selfish. Headache penetrating in temples. Thinks she is clairvoyant, can read character and understand motions; can see into herself; thinks the blood dark blue. Feels pains drawing, rending along posterior aspect of thighs and down to toes. Left side most affected. Feels as if the left leg were drawn up, and would never straighten again. Pains seem to move in meandering lines. Seems to be able to go out of herself for a short distance, to walk around and return into the body. Thinks she is looking down upon her own body. Seems to her that the fundus of the stomach is depressed in the abdomen, as if on fire at the pyloric end of stomach. Thinks there is a red spot there, looking like raw beef, as if the stomach burnt up with raw whisky. Exclaims in a plaintive tone, "Don't get out of patience with me" (of which I had given no indications). Cries, feels babyish. Apprehension; fears something terrible is about to occur. Very chilly. Can't talk loud; voice gone. She feels so weak, as if about to die. Moans and groans, calls for help. Oppression about the heart, as if it had stopped beating, as going into convulsions. Feels as if a spasm of the heart, tetanic. As if the blood too thick to circulate. Thinks she would have died but for the *Camphor* I gave her. Felt as she did when near dying of hemorrhage. Brain is active, intellect clear, thoughts vivid, the whole being intensified. Next morning, sense of constriction at base of lungs. Some cough. Clammy feeling of skin. Very sensitive to air.

No. 2. Causes a glow all over, hands sweat. Some pain in finger joints. Throat feels obstructed. Some hoarseness. Dry cough, as if pharynx stuffed with cotton. It is an effort to talk. Tongue feels partially paralyzed, cannot direct it. Throws the paper down, has lost inclination to read. Feels indolent, indifferent. Feels chills when air strikes. Spasmodic breathing, like a nervous woman—silly, mystical. Pain in finger joints continues. Feels like crying. Sad, weeping mood. Tears will come. Eyes smart. Heart aches, as from some great sorrow. Eyes feel as if had been crying a long time, as if swollen, burning. Very sensitive to cold, easily chilled. Chills down the back and both legs. Ends with a very tranquil feeling, particularly of consciousness. Next morning, tight feeling of patella. Joints all feel constricted and sore.

No. 3. Very chilly. Can't endure cold at all. Other symptoms not recorded.

In all three, pains and chilliness much increased by moving about.

No. 1. Subsequently her muscular condition was much improved. Her muscles did not ache from work as formerly.

A cut bled less freely than usual, bled scarcely any, and healed very quickly.

SALIX NIGRA AMENTS.

NAT. ORD., Salicaceæ.
COMMON NAME, White Willow.
PREPARATION.—The fresh aments are macerated in twice their weight of alcohol.

(Dr. John Fearns writes of this remedy in *Chicago Medical Times*, 1896:)

At this writing I wish to speak not of the tonic and antiseptic properties of this species of *Salix*, but of its usefulness as a sedative to the generative system. As a sedative on these lines I have had very good results from its use.

In cases of acute gonorrhœa with much errotic trouble. Also in cases of chordee with great irritation; for these purposes I have given it in doses of thirty to sixty drops on retiring, and repeat at midnight or towards morning, if needed; in these cases nothing has given me more satisfaction than this remedy. It answers the purpose, it robs night of its terrors, and it leaves no unpleasant consequences in its train.

In cases of excessive venereal desire, amounting to satyriasis, from experience I would use this remedy first. I have seen it control the venereal appetite in a very satisfactory manner. It can be given in cases where the bromides have always been considered appropriate, and it can be given where the bromides would be very inappropriate and there is no reflex effect on the brain or nervous system.

SALVIA OFFICINALIS.

NAT. ORD., Labiatæ.
COMMON NAME, Common sage.
PREPARATION.—The fresh leaves are macerated in twice their weight of alcohol.

(Although scarcely used in the present day sage runs back in medical history to the Greeks, and, according to Fernie, is still held in the highest esteem by country people in many parts of Europe. Quoting Gerard: "Sage is singularly good for the head and brain; it quickeneth the senses and memory; strengtheneth the sinews; restoreth health to those that have palsy; and takes away shaky trembling of the members." The following appeared in *Echo Med. du Nord*, 1897, concerning this remedy:)

This remedy (in English, *Sage*) has been almost forgotten in modern medical art, but still remains in high repute as a domestic medicine. Lately, French physicians have called attention to it, and not only for gargling in cases of inflammation of the throat and for washing the mouth in affections of the gums, but more especially as an unfailing remedy for night-sweats in persons suffering from affections of the respiratory organs. In the numerous experiments made with it, there were never any disagreeable concomitant effects. On the contrary, it was found that *Salvia* acts even more favorably on the tickling coughs with consumptives than *Belladonna, Rumex crispus*, etc., so that preparations of *Morphine* and *Codeine* could be dispensed with.

Salvia should be used in the form of the tincture, and, indeed, the tincture prepared from the fresh leaves and the blossom tips, as we find it in homœopathic pharmacies. It should be given in doses of 20, 30, or 40 drops, in a tablespoonful of water. The effects manifest themselves very quickly, two hours after taking a dose, and these effects persist for two to six days.

SAURURUS CERNUUS.

NAT. ORD., Piperaceæ.
COMMON NAME, Lizard's Tail.
PREPARATION.—The entire plant including the root is macerated in twice its weight of alcohol.

(The following short notice of this almost unknown remedy appeared in the *Homœopathic Recorder*, 1895:)

Readers who are interested in the remedies of nature rather than those produced in the laboratory and sold under trademarks will remember that it was Dr. D. L. Phares, of Mississippi, who, over half a century ago, pointed out the wonderful virtues of *Passiflora incarnata*, so much used to-day. What Dr. Phares said of the remedy laid dormant until Hale, in his ever perennial *New Remedies*, rescued it from the dusty pages of old medical journals, in which so much of value is buried awaiting resurrection. Among such buried remedies is *Saururus cernuus* or, as it is more commonly known, "lizard's tail." Dr. Phares, who seems to have been an unusually keen observer, used *Saururus cer.* in his practice, as he did *Passiflora*, for many years before he communicated his observations to the medical journals, and the *Saururus* seems to be quite as important and useful a remedy in its sphere as is *Passiflora,* and one quite as worthy of a thorough proving. In absence of proving it may be said that Dr. Phares used it for years with marked success in all irritation and inflammation of the kidneys, bladder, prostate and urinary passages. He considered it peculiarly adapted to all such cases if they were attended by strangury, or painful and difficult urination. Dr. Phares used the remedy both externally and internally and he found that the stomach was very tolerant of the rather heroic doses he prescribed.

The plant is an indigenous perennial found in swampy localities, in some parts of the United States, and has been, and is still, used in domestic practice for those conditions for which Dr. Phares commends it.

SCOLOPENDRA MORSITANS.

PREPARATION.—The insect is triturated with sugar of milk in the usual way.

(In the case of a man bitten in the arm by a centipede, reported in *Nashville Journal of Medicine*, 1870, among the striking symptoms was no perspiration in the arm for three months. Dr. Sherman, of California (*Med. Advance*), reports the following symptoms as prominent in a woman bitten by a centipede:)

Head.—Vertigo, with blindness, worse in the morning.

Stomach.—Nausea and vomiting; unable to retain either food or liquid.

Back.—Terrible pains in back and loins, spasmodic and irregular, at times extending down the limbs. Pains returned every few days for three weeks, commencing in the head and going out at the toes. "Resembled labor pains as nearly as anything I ever saw."

SCUTELLARIA LATERIFOLIA.

NAT. ORD., Labiatæ.

COMMON NAME, Mad-dog skullcap.

PREPARATION.—The whole fresh plant is macerated in twice its weight of alcohol.

(The following proving of *Scutellaria lat.*, from *University Bulletin*, 1897, was made, under the auspices of Dr. Geo. Royal, by nine provers:)

No symptom has been recorded unless experienced by two provers. When experienced by two provers, and not often repeated, the symptom is recorded in common type. When often repeated in two provings is found in italics. When often repeated in three provings, or found in four or more, the symptoms appear in black type.

MIND.—**Inability to study or fix the attention on one's work.** *Confusion of mind. Apathy.* Irritability.

HEAD.—**A full or throbbing sensation in head. A dull heavy headache mostly in the forehead and temples.** Sharp shooting pain in the head. Pain in the occiput. Headache relieved in the open air. Headache relieved by eating. Headache aggravated by motion.

EYES.—*Aching in the eyeballs.* Eyeballs painful to touch. Eyeballs feel too large.

FACE.—Flushed.

MOUTH.—*Bad taste; sour; bitter.*

THROAT.—Sensation of lump in throat which could not be swallowed.

STOMACH.—**Nausea. Sour eructions.** *Poor appetite.* Vomiting of sour ingesta, hiccoughs, pain and distress in stomach.

ABDOMEN.—**Gas in bowels.** *Colicky pain in abdomen. Fullness or distension of abdomen. Uneasiness in abdomen.* Pain in the abdomen.

STOOLS.—**Diarrhœa.** *Light colored.* Stools preceded by colicky pain in abdomen.

URINARY ORGANS.—**Quantity of urine diminished. Biliary salts increased.** Frequent micturition but quantity small.

CHEST.—Pain in chest.

HEART AND PULSE.—Pulse rate irregular.

BACK.—Pain in back.

UPPER EXTREMITIES.—*Sharp stinging pains.* Aching.

LOWER EXTREMITIES.—**Weakness. Aching.** *Uneasiness.*

SLEEP.—**Restless. Unrefreshing.** *Disturbed.*

GENERAL SYMPTOMS.—**Restlessness. Tired weak feeling.** *Uneasiness. Languor.*

The remedy seems most suitable to persons of a nervo-bilious temperament. All the symptoms seem to be aggravated by work or excitement and ameliorated by sleep.

SISYRINCHIUM.

NAT. ORD., Iridaceæ.
COMMON NAME, Blue-eyed grass.
PREPARATION.—The fresh root is macerated in twice its weight of alcohol.

(Dr. W. U. Reed, of Northmanchester, Ind., contributed the following in 1892 to the *Hom. Recorder*, concerning this little known remedy. *Sisyrinchium* was one of the old "Thompsonians." From what Dr. Reed says of it the remedy must be a very powerful one and worthy of full investigation.)

Numerous articles have appeared in our medical journals during the past few months relative to the treatment of persons bitten by venomous reptiles, especially the rattlesnake. Whether the rattlesnakes found in the marshes of Indiana are in any respect different from those found in Oregon, or in the mountains of Pennsylvania, I do not know. The bite of the Indiana rattler has been known to prove fatal to both man and beast. Notwithstanding we have growing in our woods and fields a small plant, which I believe to be a specific for the treatment of persons or animals bitten by the rattlesnake. From my own experience and observation in the use of this remedy, I believe it to be a positive cure in all cases if exhibited in any reasonable time. I have never known it to fail in a single instance, even where the alcoholic treatment and many other kinds had failed.

The plant referred to, the roots of which are used in the treatment of snake bites; or a tincture made from the roots, is the *Sisyrinchium* of the *Iris* family, I think, and is said to have been used by the Indians in treating snake bites, by bruising and moistening the roots and applying to the wound. I am not aware of its ever having been used as a medicine by the profession, and, so far as I know, I am the first to prepare and use it in the form of a tincture. By your kind permission I will report, through the columns of your valuable journal, a few cases treated by this remedy, which for convenience I will call *Sisyrinchium*.

Case 1. Bessie A., aged six years, while playing in the yard on a farm, some twelve miles in the country, was bitten in the hand by a rattlesnake which was killed a moment after by the mother of the little girl who was attracted by the screams of the child. Sixteen hours after I arrived, everything having been done in the meantime that had ever been heard of by the parents, even to poulticing the wound with entrails of a black chicken. The little sufferer was, indeed, an object of pity. The hand and arm were swollen almost to bursting, the swelling extending to the shoulder and spine, being of a bluish black color as if dreadfully bruised. This discoloration extended over the back to the hips. Skin hot and dry, face flushed, pulse quick and hard. Child unconscious. I felt that the case was hopeless. But through the earnest entreaties of the mother, I proceeded to do what I could. Saturating a piece of cotton with the tincture I had prepared, I bound it on the wound; then dropping twelve drops in a glass of water I directed that a teaspoonful be given every hour, the compress to be renewed every hour also, until my return. I confess I had little hope of seeing my little patient alive again, but on my return the following day I was much rejoiced to find a decided change for the better in the condition of the little sufferer. The swelling was not nearly so tense, the fever had subsided, the delirium gone, and the danger seemed past. The treatment was continued, and a speedy and permanent recovery followed.

Case 2. Burt Whitten, aged ten, while out in a marsh with a number of older boys gathering huckleberries, was bitten in the right ankle by a rattler. He was so frightened when he saw the snake, as it bit him, that he ran all the way home, a distance of nearly a mile; although the day was very hot. This patient came to my hands after the usual alcoholic treatment for twenty-four hours by an Allopathic physician, with the patient growing worse all the time. I found this patient in about the same condition as the first. The leg and foot were enormously swollen and of the same general appearance; the foot, calf of the leg and thigh were black; the whole body was very red, hot and dry; face dark red; pulse quick and hard; patient delirious but would cry out if touched. Fifteen drops in a glass of water. Teaspoonful every hour, with cotton saturated with the tincture applied to the wound. In this case the change, I was informed by the father, was quite noticeable in two hours. The boy had been in a wild delirium all night and up to the time he received the first dose of *Sisyrinchium*. After the second dose he became quiet, and in two hours the delirium had passed away. Under this treatment the patient was able to be out on the streets again in four days, though the discoloration did not disappear for some time after.

Many more cases might be given where this remedy has been given to both man and beast with the same results.

SKOOKUM CHUCK.

(Some readers may be startled at this name, applied to a remedy, but under that name it came before the profession and the name has stuck. It is the Western Indian's designation of the waters of what is now known as "Medical Lake." The following by Dr. W. D. Gentry appeared in the *U. S. Med. Investigator*, 1889:)

The water is of a deep amber and almost red in the sunlight. The following is an analysis of the salts, obtained by evaporation of the water; the proportion being in grains per U. S. gallon 231 cubic inches:

Sodic chloride,	16.370
Potassic chloride,	9.241
Sodic carbonate,	63.543
Magnesic carbonate,	.233
Ferrous carbonate,	.526
Calcic carbonate,	.186
Aluminic oxide,	.175
Sodic silicate,	10.638
Organic matter,	.551
	————
	101.463

Lithic carbonate,

Potassic sulphate,   } Each a trace.

Sodic bi-borate,

The lake has no outlet, but is fed by two enormous springs. It contains no living things with the exception of axolotl, a kind of salamander, such as are found in the lakes of the Mexican Cordilleras.

The medical and curative properties of this remarkable lake was known to the Indians of the northwest as far back as they have any legends or tribal history, and it was held in such reverence by them that the country around this lake was called 'Sahala Lyee Illihe,' or 'Sacred Grounds,' and no matter how hostile the tribes were to each other no Indians journeying to or from the 'Skookum Limechen Chuck,' or 'strong medicine water,' were ever molested.

When the Indians were considering the transfer of their lands to the government, many years ago, it is recorded as a matter of history, that old Quetahlguin, father of the present Chief Moses, and 'Old Joseph,' father of Chief Joseph, lately a prisoner of war, with the broken remnants of his band, after weeks of deliberation and consideration, with the 'Sahala Lyee,' or Great Spirit, through their medicine-men, or prophets, firmly said: 'We have talked with the Great Spirit and we have slept with his words in our ears. The Great Spirit is our father and the earth is our mother. We have a good home and it was made for us by the Great Spirit; it is a part of us; it is our mother. In Wallowa Lake are an abundance of fish created especially for our tribe. None other of his red children have such fish. In the 'Skookum Chuck' we have a remedy for all our ailments. We only have to bathe in and drink its water and we are made well. If we sign the treaty we will forever offend the Great Spirit; we will sign away our mother and she will cry. Her tears will dry up these lakes and we will be hungry and sick. We will go to the Skookum Chuck only to find that its waters have disappeared.'

The story is told of a Frenchman passing the lake many years ago, before the properties of the water became known to the whites, with a drove of sheep afflicted with a skin disease called 'the scab.' As soon as the sheep saw the water they ran to it, but would not drink. They stood in the water for some time, and in a few days they were well of the 'scab.' The Frenchman was suffering with rheumatism. He concluded to try the water of the lake for his disease. He was speedily cured. The whites were soon attracted to this lake by the stories of marvellous cures reported by the Indians, and by seeing Indians return in health and vigor from the lake, who had been taken there on litters, appearing at the point of death. It is estimated that over 20,000 people have visited this lake since 'Joseph's Band' were driven from that section of the country, and it is fast becoming as popular as any other of our great health resorts.

My attention was called to *Skookum chuck* some time since, and I procured some of the salts and triturated a quantity, making the first, second, third and sixth potencies. I partially proved the first potency by taking two grains every two hours. The first effect produced was a profuse coryza with constant sneezing, as in hay fever. This continued until the medicine was antidoted by tobacco. My appetite was greatly increased. Some rheumatic pains in limbs, and heaviness about the sacrum. The catarrhal effects were so severe I could not continue the remedy. I have used the third and sixth potency in my practice and have cured a number of cases of catarrh, and am confident that the remedy will be curative in hay fever.

(Later investigation, however, demonstrated that the chief curative action of the salts was in skin diseases. Dr. D. De Forest Cole, of Albion, N. Y., wrote the following to the firm from whom he procured the remedy:)

Some time since I received from you one bottle *Skookum chuck* 3x trit. I had a very bad case of urticaria which resisted the usual remedies as *Apis*, *Urtica ur.*, etc., and I gave her (a girl twelve years old) four powders of about four grains each of the *Skookum chuck*, instructing her to take one powder in one-half glass water, one teaspoonful every two hours, and she returned in a week free from any urticaria. I gave her four powders more, and no appearance of urticaria since. Besides curing the urticaria the patient's health is in every way improving. I write this thinking you might desire to know of its value in urticaria, as well as eczema.

(The following cases were contributed by Dr. D. W. Ingalls, Bridgeport, to *N. Y. Med. Times*, 1894:)

CASE 1. Mrs. D., aged forty-eight years, suffered four years with eczema plantaris, fissured, red and painful, which gave forth a viscid secretion, drying into scales half an inch in thickness. For the past two years the patient had not been able to wear shoes nor walk any distance, owing to the excessive soreness of the feet.

Patient consulted me March 1st, and the following treatment was given: Two-grain powders of the 2x trituration of *Skookum chuck* every two hours, and an ointment applied nightly consisting of *Skookum salt*, one drachm to the ounce of *Vaseline*. In the morning the feet were washed with *Skookum chuck* soap. April 1st the patient walked to the dispensary in felt shoes. The fissures and greenish tinge of the crusts had nearly disappeared. The two-grain powders were then given every four hours and the former treatment continued. On May 1st, patient walked to the dispensary wearing leather shoes for the first time, the ointment was stopped, the fissures and crevices being hardly perceptible. The patient was advised to wash the feet night and morning with the *Skookum chuck* soap.

June 1st patient presented herself, stating that she had very little trouble with her feet, except some tenderness upon a misstep. Appearance good.

A powder of the 3x was given every night, together with the continued washing of the feet night and morning. July 1st the patient was discharged cured.

CASE 2. Mrs. B., aged twenty-eight, eczema of the nose of one year's standing. The usual ointments were given, but without result. March 15th the following treatment was given: Five-grain powder of the 2x trituration *Skookum chuck* four times a day, together with the *Skookum* ointment applied nightly. This case was entirely cured in six weeks.

CASE 3. Mrs. H., aged twenty-three, benign growth in left breast about the size of a walnut; first noticed about eight months previously. Upon strict inquiry, no history of cancer or tuberculosis was given. One-grain powders of the 1x were given, the first week every four hours. Two-grain powders of the 2x were given every four hours the second week. Five-grain powders of the 3x were given the third week and continued seven weeks, when the patient was discharged cured.

CASE 4. Mr. S. was afflicted with eczema of the scalp, which spread from back of the ears to the eyebrows, covering the entire scalp with a squamous or scabby eczema, accompanied with a constant itching and shedding of scales. On March 18th the following treatment was given: Head to be washed four times a day with *Skookum chuck* soap. A five-grain powder 2x trituration was given every hour during the first week, when *Sulphur*, third decimal, was given for three days, and *Skookum chuck*, second decimal, was continued for one week. One-grain powder of the 1x was given in water four times a day for two weeks; then the third decimal trituration was used until June 1st, when patient was discharged cured.

CASE 5. Mr. J., nasal catarrh, of years' standing. A greenish-yellow discharge having the odor of a slight ozœna. The patient had been so much relieved that he is at present writing very comfortable, and believes that he will be permanently cured.

CASE 6. Mrs. D., aged thirty-six, prolonged suppuration due to abscess of the axilla; nine months' standing. June 20th the following treatment was given: The abscess was washed four times a day with the solution of *Skookum* salts, five grains to one quart of water, and the 2x given internally every two hours until July 10th, when the abscess was healed. A two-grain powder was then continued, night and morning for one month, with no return of the abscess. To sum up, I have simply verified what Dr. Gentry and others have given us about the remedy. I have used it with gratifying success in all suppurating wounds. It evidently has a great sphere of action, and I hope some day to see a good proving.

(The following was contributed by Dr. B. F. Bailey, Lincoln, Neb.:)

We have many remedies brought to our notice in an empirical way, which soon lose their prominence, first because we have no provings, and second, having no provings, clinical study is not close enough. When *Skookum chuck* was first written up, I began to use it and watch its effects, that it might be possible to find its proper niche in practice. The following two cases will, I think, give an idea of the cases in which it may always be depended upon:

Case No. 1.—A married woman of 40 years of age. History and present condition show a lithæmic diathesis. For years has never been free from eczematous troubles. At times suffers much from rheumatism, not infrequently, rheumatism disappears to be immediately followed by hordeoli upon eyelids. Has been treated long and faithfully by Allopaths, and now for some years by our own school. Prescribed *Skookum* 3x—one powder every 4 hours. Improvement was soon evident. Persisted in this treatment for three months, and now for two years patient has been perfectly well.

Case No. 2.—Patient, married woman of about 26 years, comes to me with urine, sp. grav. 1.030, marked uric acid deposits, flushed face upon a yellowish background—so often seen in lithæmic cases. Much difficulty of digestion. Great dryness of skin, especially of scalp, with great trouble from falling out of hair—in short a thoroughly lithæmic case. *Skookum chuck* 3x every four hours. Satisfactory improvement. Has feared head will become entirely bald. Now no loss of hair, and a loss of the heated, congested feeling of face and head. In fact, a satisfactory recovery now of some weeks standing. These cases briefly stated ought to be of interest, in that they show it to be probable that we will find the sphere of action of *Skookum* to be in lithæmic cases, and for the treatment of these cases we have but a few clearly defined reliable remedies.

SOLANUM CAROLINENSE.

NAT. ORD., Solanaceæ.
COMMON NAME, Horse-nettle.
PREPARATION.—The fresh, ripe berries are macerated in twice their weight of alcohol.

(In 1889 Dr. Napier called attention to *Solanum Carolinense* as a remedy in the treatment of epilepsy, stating that it was used as a domestic remedy in the South for convulsions and "that he had successfully prescribed it in his practice." Dr. Charles S. Potts, of the University of Pennsylvania, contributes a paper *Therap. Gazette*, Dec., 1895, on the remedy, giving some new points, from which the following is condensed:)

At the clinic for nervous diseases of the University Hospital, *Solanum Carolinense* was tried in a series of twenty-five cases, twenty-one of which were idiopathic, three organic, and one probably so. Of these, eight of the idiopathic cases either did not return after the first visit or else were not under observation sufficiently long to offer a fair test. In the remaining seventeen cases the following results were obtained—viz., five, two of them organic, were not improved. In the remaining twelve the results showed more or less benefit from the use of the drug. The five cases in which no improvement was noted were afterwards placed upon other treatment, either antipyrin and bromide of ammonium or the mixed bromides with amelioration of the symptoms in four; in the remaining one no drug seemed to be of service. The dose used at first was 10 drops. This dose was found to be useless, and after the first few cases they varied from 30 drops to teaspoonful three or four times daily. No unpleasant effects were observed, excepting a mild diarrhœa in some cases. This was also noticed by Dr. Herdman. He also noticed that in large doses the temperature was lowered and the pulse slowed.

In many epileptics diarrhœa is more of a benefit than otherwise.

The conclusions derived from the results obtained in seventeen cases are:—

1. That the drug has a decided influence for good upon the epileptic paroxysm.

2. That this influence is probably not so great or so sure as that obtained by the use of antipyrin and the bromide salts or even of the mixed bromides.

3. That in those cases in which it is of service it relieves the paroxysms, without causing any other unpleasant symptoms, such as are sometimes caused by the use of large doses of the bromides.

4. That the dose ordinarily recommended is too small, and that as much as a teaspoonful or more four times daily is often needed to secure results.

The following are some of the cases in which the remedy seemed to act beneficially:

H. T., male, aged thirteen years. Idiopathic epilepsy; had his first spell when five years of age; averages one paroxysm daily. The *Solanum* was first given in 10 drop doses *t. i. d.* without effect. When increased to 25 drops the spells were lighter in severity, but occurred about as often. The dose was finally increased to a teaspoonful four times daily. After being put upon this dose he was under observation six weeks, during which time he had six seizures much lighter in severity.

T. H., male, aged twenty-eight years. He had epileptic seizures for the past three years. They followed an injury to the head which rendered him unconscious, but produced no other visible injury. Since this, however, has had almost constant headache. First spell six month after the injury, and have been very frequent since, averaging three to four weekly; they are of ordinary type. *Solanum* in 40 drop doses three times daily was ordered. Spells at once decreased in frequency and severity. During the last six weeks he was under observation he only had three spells, very mild in type.

C. R., male, aged twenty-one years. Epileptic seizures for past three years following an injury. Had been trephined in right parietal region before coming under our observation. After trephining the symptom improved, but got worse again; when seen by us was having one daily. 40-drop doses of *Solanum* caused diarrhœa, and dose was reduced to 30 drops *t. i. d.*, when diarrhœa ceased. Under this treatment he had no spell for two weeks. In the following month he had three spells; was then lost to observation.

A. N., male, aged thirty years. First spell one year ago; have since occurred every two weeks; good deal of headache. Ordered *Solanum* 30 drops *t. i. d.* No spells for one month and headache ceased. He then stopped attendance.

J. D., female, aged eighteen years. First spell when thirteen years old; has one spell a month at the time of her menstrual period. About a week before this period was given 40 drops *t. i. d.*, and escaped the usual spell. The following month, however, she had one.

I. K., female, aged twenty-five years. Nocturnal epilepsy for past three years; about one spell a month. While using 40 drops *t. i. d.* went three weeks longer than usual without a spell. The dose was then increased to 1 fluid drachm *t. i. d.*; she then ceased her visits.

F. S., female, aged twelve years. First spell five weeks ago; has been having them daily since. *Solanum* 30 drops *t. i. d.*, ordered; this dose was gradually increased to 1 fluid drachm *t. i. d.* During the three months that she was under observation her spells averaged in number about one a week.

H. B., male, aged eighteen years. First convulsion at age of ten years; then had none until three months ago; has had general convulsions about once daily since. *Solanum*, 40 drops *t. i. d.*, ordered. He was only under observation nine days, having during that time four spells, much milder in character.

A. C., female, aged fifteen years. First convulsion one year ago; they have been increasing in frequency; now has one about every three days. During the three weeks she was taking 30 drops of *Solanum* three times a day she had one spell, that occurring during the third week.

H. K., male, aged eighteen years. First spell when fourteen years old. Every three or four days has several attacks in succession, an average of about one daily. While taking *Solanum* in 40-drop—afterwards increased to teaspoonful—doses he had twelve in thirty-eight days, an average of a little less than one in three days, going six without having any.

SPIRITUS GLANDIUM QUERCUS.

NAT. ORD.—Cupuliferæ.
COMMON NAME—European or English oak.
PREPARATION.—The spirit is destilled from the tincture prepared by macerating the acorn kernals from the Quercus robur, in five times their weight of dilute alcohol.

(The following, from Rademacher, is quoted and translated by Dr. J. C. Burnett in his *Diseases of the Spleen*).

I became acquainted with this remedy in a wonderful way. Many years ago (I do not remember the exact time) a working carpenter, who had previously lived at Crefeld, came to seek my advice for his bellyache, which was of long standing. According to his own statement, he had long been under Sanitary Councillor Schneider in Crefeld, who was not able to help him, and so sent him to Professor Günther in Duisberg. Ten journeys thither were likewise in vain.

I tried my usual remedies for seemingly such cases, but to no good; and as I noticed he was a good cabinetmaker, and dabbled a bit in upholstery, I told him it would be a good plan if he were to hire himself out to a country squire as joiner, thinking that the food of the servants' hall would suit his sick stomach better than the beans, black bread, and potatoes of the master carpenter. The good fellow followed my advice, and lived with a squire for many years; and I heard nothing more about him. Finally, he married the parlormaid, and settled here in this town as a joiner. One day when visiting his sick wife I remembered the old story of his bellyache, and wanted to know how it then was. "All right," said he, "I have not had it for years." It seems that a local surgeon, being one day at the squire's, told him to get some acorns, and scrape them with a knife, and then put the scrapings into brandy and leave them to draw for a day, and then to drink a small glass of this spirit several times a day. He did as he was advised, and was forthwith relieved, and very soon entirely freed from his old trouble.

From what I knew of the surgeon, I was very sure he could not give me any intelligent reason for his prescription. I should only have heard that acorn scrapings in brandy were good for the bellyache, or, at the most, I may have ascertained from what doctor, or peasant, or old wife he had got the tip.

But this would have done me but poor service; and as I had in the meantime become much more cunning, I questioned the joiner himself afresh as to the kind of his old pain, particularly as to the part of the belly where the pain was *last felt* when he had had a bad attack. He was in no doubt about it, but at once pointed to the part of the belly nearest the left hypochondrium. So I very shrewdly suspected that the abdominal pains were really owing to a primary affection of the spleen, in which notion I was strengthened by remembering that the best pain-killing hepatic and enteric remedies had done him no good.

To get as soon as possible to the bottom of the thing, I set about preparing a tincture of acorns, and gave a teaspoonful five times a day in water to an old brandy drunkard, who was sick unto death, and of whom I knew that he had suffered from the spleen for a very long time, the spleen being from time to time painful. He had likewise ascites, and his legs were dropsical as far as the knees. It occurred to me that if the acorn tincture were to act curatively on the spleen the consensual kidney affection and its dependent dropsy would mend. I soon saw that I had reckoned rightly. The urinary secretion was at once augmented, but the patient complained that each time after taking the medicine he felt a constriction of the chest. I ascribed this to the astringent matter of the acorns, and thinking the really curative principle thereof would most likely be volatile I caused the tincture to be distilled. This acorn spirit caused no further constriction, and the urinary secretion was still more markedly increased, the tension in the præcordia became less and less, and this hopelessly incurable drunkard got quite well, much to the surprise of all who knew him, and, honestly speaking, much to my own surprise also.

Having thus put the spirit of acorns to such a severe test, and that in a case that I already knew so well, in which it was impossible to make a mistake as to the primary affection, I went further, and used it by degrees in all sorts of spleen affections, and that not only in painful ones, but in painless ones, in the evident ones, and in those of a more problematical kind. Gradually I became convinced that it is a remedy, the place of which no other can take. More particularly is it of great, nay, of inestimable value in spleen-dropsy. Later on, I found that the volatile curative principle of acorns may be still better extracted with water with the addition of alcohol. [The *aqua glandium* is thus prepared:—One pound of peeled and crushed acorns to the pound of distillate.] Perhaps water alone might extract the healing principle, but it would not keep thus, and so the cures would be uncertain, not to mention the fact that such-like decaying medicines are a great trouble to the chemists. The dose of the spirituous acorn-water (the only preparation I have used of late years) is half a tablespoonful in water four times a day. It has not much taste; some would even say it has none, but the doubter may make a solution of alcohol and water in the same proportions, and he will soon find that it has quite a taste of its own.

I must make mention of two of its peculiar effects. Certain people feel, as soon as they have taken it, a peculiar sensation in the head, lasting hardly a minute or two, which they say is like being drunk.

With a few people, particularly with those who have suffered from old spleen engorgements, diarrhœa sets in after using it for two or three weeks that makes them feel better. It seldom lasts more than a day, and is not weakening, but moderate. Hence it is not needful either to stop the acorn water or to lessen the dose.

I could add many instructive cases of spleen-dropsies and other spleen affections in which the volatile principle of acorns proved curative, but as I have so much more to say on other subjects I dare not be too discursive on this one point; besides, what I have already said will suffice for common-sense physicians. Still I cannot forbear noticing a few bagatelles. For instance, I have found that the acute spleen fevers that occur intercurrently with epidemic liver fevers are best cured with *aqua glandium*—at least that is my experience.

Furthermore, I am of opinion that the three *splenics* of which I have made mention are curative of three different morbid states of the spleen, and I know well from my own experience that acorns are indicated in the most common spleen affections; and, finally, I am not acquainted with any positive signs whereby those three separate morbid states of spleen can with certainty be differentiated from one another.

(In a later work, *Gout and its Cure*, by Burnett, the remedy is again brought up as follows:)

For some years past I have been acquainted with a remedy that antidotes the effect of alcohol very prettily, as I will show. I enter upon the subject in this place, because it deserves to be widely known, and also because in the treatment of gout, the alcoholism not infrequently bars the way. The remedy I refer to is the distilled spirit of acorns—*Spiritus glandium quercus*. My first account will be found in my "Diseases of the Spleen," where *Spiritus glandium quercus* is dealt with as a spleen medicine. I speak of set purpose of the homœopathic antidote, because alcoholism is a disease, and as such must be met by specific medication.

Some of Rademacher's patients complained to him that while taking his acorn medicine they felt in their heads somewhat as if they were drunk; but as Rademacher did not believe in the law of similars—indeed, knew but little about it—their complaint had no ulterior significance to him, but still it struck him as worthy of record. "A few, but not many, of those who take it immediately feel a peculiar sensation in the head, which they say is like they feel when they are drunk, the sensation lasting only a minute or two."

Now, in the light of the homœopathic law, this symptom is eminently suggestive, but whether any one beside myself has ever noticed this symptom I am not aware. Rademacher had previously related the following brilliant cure. * * * He says that in order to get a clear idea of the action of the remedy he caused to be prepared a tincture of acorns, of which he gave a teaspoonful in water five times a day to an almost moribund brandy toper, who had long been suffering from a spleen affection that at times caused him a good deal of pain, and who, at the time in question, had severe ascites and whose lower extremities were dropsical up as far as the knees. Our author was of opinion that the affection was a primary disease of the spleen, and reasoned that if the tincture of acorns cured the spleen the kidneys would duly resume work and the ascitic and anasarcous state would disappear. He soon found he was right; patient at once began to pass more urine, but he complained that every time he took a dose of the medicine he got a constriction about the chest, and this Rademacher ascribed to the astringent quality of the acorns, and to avoid this he had the tincture of acorns distilled. The administration of this distilled preparation was not followed by any unpleasant symptom, and the quantity of urine passed increased still more, the tension on the præcordia slowly lessened and this inveterate drunkard got quite well, much to the amazement of everybody, Rademacher included, for he did not at all expect him to recover.

Now, it must be admitted that a remedy that can cure an old drunkard of general dropsy and restore him to health deserves closer acquaintance, and when we first regard it from the pathogenetic side as producing, of course, contingently, a cephalic state, resembling alcoholic intoxication, and then from the clinical side as having cured an abandoned drunkard, it looks very much as if we had a remedy homœopathic to alcoholism. I may add that Rademacher nowhere hints that the *Spiritus glandium quercus* stands in any relation to alcoholism; he regards it merely as a spleen medicine, specially indicated in dropsy due to a primary spleen affection. At first I regarded it merely in the same light, but when I really gripped the significance of the pathogenetic symptoms just quoted I thought we might find in our common acorns a notable homœopathic anti-alcoholic.

(It is not fair to quote further from Burnett, but we may add that in his book, *Gout and Its Cure*, there are given a number of clinical cases in which the remedy acted brilliantly in those addicted to tippling, or drinking hard. It is not so much that the remedy extirpates the habit, but it enables those afflicted to easily control their appetite and drink "like other people," without that insatiable craving. The dose is about ten drops in water three to four times a day.)

SOLIDAGO VIRGA-AUREA.

NAT. ORD., Compositæ.
COMMON NAME, Golden Rod
PREPARATION.—The fresh blossoms are macerated in twice their weight of alcohol.

(The following is to be found on p. 131 of Dr. Gallavardin's "Homœopathic Treatment of Alcoholism:")

"A lady, by administering, morning and evening, an infusion of the dry leaves and flowers of Golden Rod (*Solidago virga-aurea*) tells me that she cured her husband of an affection of the bladder which had compelled him to use a catheter for a year or more. A friend of Homœopathy, not a physician, desired to test the efficaciousness of this plant. He caused the first dilution of its tincture to be taken three times a day by seven patients of from forty-two to seventy-four years of age, who had been obliged to catheterize themselves for weeks, months and years, and cured them so thoroughly that they had no relapses. Surgeons who spend much time in catheterizing such patients for months and years could often cure them much more rapidly by prescribing for them the remedy just mentioned."

(Dr. A. E. White, *Homœopathic Recorder*, July, 1891, relates the following case:)

Mrs.——, age 37, married, has had seven children. Came to me December 10, 1890, with the following history: "Had not had her menses for four months. Thought she was in a family way. Abdomen bloated up every P.M.; sick at her stomach all of the time; frontal headache, P.M.; felt better when first getting up in the morning, at which time her abdomen was almost normal in size.

"Her water she complained of more than anything else. Had to pass it every half hour during day and several times during night.

"Backache all of the time, which was not decreased by passing water. Urine had a white, slimy deposit on standing a short time.

"Requested an examination, but could not discover that she was in a family way. Found her back very sensitive in region of kidneys, trace of albumin in urine.

"I gave her a vial of *Solidago* 1x, told her to take two disks every four hours and report in three or four days. She came back December 13th, 'the medicine went right to the spot.' From the second dose her water became natural and she did not bloat so much in P.M. Her stomach did not bother

her any more. I gave her a bottle of *Puls.* 3x to take with the *Solidago*, and she reported December 17th, that her menses had come on.

"I have used it in several other cases where it seemed indicated by the tenderness in kidney region and the inability to control the water from whatever cause, always with perfect satisfaction to patient and myself."

(The following paper on the use of *Solidago virga-aurea* is by Dr. M. Gucken, of Eupen, Germany:)

The Golden Rod is in Homœopathy, according to my opinion, not as much made use of as it deserves. Foh. Gottfr. Rademacher, who has many admirers among us, says, in his *Justification of Experience in Medicine*, about *Virga-aurea*: "This herb is a very old and good kidney medicine. It is a specific for kidneys, and brings the patients back to the normal condition." I have used the Golden Rod for a long time, and have to make favorable reports. The results of extensive homœopathic proving of this remedy on healthy persons cannot be found in our literature, but a Würtemburg physician, Dr. Buck, has given us a list of cures with the Golden Rod in the popular homœopathic paper edited by Dr. Bolle, which wholly confirms the statements of Rademacher, besides the cases reported by Dr. Buck.

According to this last, *Virga-aurea* is especially adapted for scrofulous subjects; at the same time other constitutions do not exclude the use of this remedy. In the first place, *the condition and the action of the kidneys and the quality of their secretions* are to be considered in the selection of this remedy. The symptoms on the part of the kidneys and the urinary organs, which point to *Virga-aurea*, are as follows:

Pains in the kidneys; region of kidneys painful upon pressure; feeling of enlargement and tension in the kidneys, also pains in the kidneys which extend forward to the abdomen and to the bladder. Dysuria, difficult and scanty urination; urine dark, red-brown, with thick sediment; stone and gravel, albumen, blood or slime in the urine; urine dark, with sediments of phosphates; slightly sour, neutral or alkaline; urine with numerous epithelial cells or small mucous particles. Epithelial cells with gravel of triple phosphates, or phosphate of lime. Bright's disease.

Side symptoms which point to this remedy:

Skin.—Scrofulous rash; little blotches on hands and feet, itching very much; very obstinate, itching exanthemas; exanthema of the lower extremities without swelling of the inguinal glands, but with disturbance in urinating (catarrh of the kidneys).

Sleep.—Insomnia.

Fever.—Rheumatic fever; very frequent pulse; high fever.

Head.—Headache.

Eyes.—Scrofulous, herpetic inflammation.

Ears.—Sudden deafness, with ringing in the ears and albuminous urine.

Nose.—Dry; the inner surface of the nose covered with blood crust; scalding and very scanty brown urine.

Mouth.—Flat ulcers in the mouth and throat.

Gastric: Stomach, Abdomen and Stool.—Continuous bitter taste, disturbing the rest, especially nights; heavily covered tongue, which does not become clean in spite of the use of anti-gastric remedies, and only cleanses itself at the return of abundant urinating; chronic catarrh of the bowels; diarrhœa, with scanty, dark urine; dysentery; costiveness; sensation of pain in the abdomen on both sides of the navel, upon deep pressure; physconia of the abdomen by gases; severe pricking in both hypochondria to the region of the kidneys, reaching to the lower extremities, with continued bitter taste in the mouth, especially at night, with very scanty brown and sour urine.

Female Parts.—Hæmorrhage, chronic leucorrhœa, in connection with copious, watery urine and sediments of mucous particles and uriniferous tubules; epithelium.

Respiratory Organs.—Heavy expectoration in coughing; croup, with little blotches on the hands and diminished urine; chronic catarrh of the lungs; continuous dyspnœa; periodical asthma, with nightly dysuria.

Trunk and Lower Limbs.—Rheumatism of the intercostal muscles; chronic pains in the loins; limping, dragging gait; rheumatic pains in the legs; pains in the thighs; the legs can be moved horizontally, but when moved perpendicularly they feel lame.

In connection with these symptoms the description of a few cases of sickness, in which *Virga-aurea* proved itself, might be of some interest.

CLINICAL.

During the spring of 1886 scarlet-diphtheria appeared in this place. On March 28th I was called to attend the 8-year old son Matthias, of Wernerus, a weaver, in the hamlet of Niepert, that showed symptoms of the above disease. Cynanche was at high degree, and the throat was filled with diphtheritic coating, so much so that I had reason to fear the worst, on account of the accompanying fever and of the choked-up condition and weakly (scrofulous) habit of the patient. But the well-known remedy of Viller, given alternately with *Belladonna*, proved itself also in this case, and the symptoms in the throat assumed, after a few days, a less dangerous character. Not so with the fever, which gradually assumed the form of typhoid, and ran very high, while the scarlet-rash grew quite pale. On the morning of April 5th, his temperature was 42.5°, the patient unconscious, the pulse weak and intermittent, the feet swollen. Upon inquiry the parents told me that the boy urinated very little. His urine, of which I had taken a quantity the day previous for examination, contained a considerable amount of albuminous sediments. I prescribed *Kali arsenicosum* in the fourth centesimal potency, which had been recommended in similar cases by Dr. Hock in the international homœopathic press; but, although the temperature decreased after using this remedy, the dropsical swelling of the feet increased more and more, and after a few days the entire body of the patient was swollen very much. The discharge of urine grew continually less. Under these circumstances I examined the patient again thoroughly, and found great sensitiveness of the kidneys against pressure, in spite of his otherwise apathetic condition. These symptoms reminded me of *Virga-aurea*. This remedy was immediately applied, and I had no reason to regret it. Within one day the urinal discharge became profuse, the general condition improving at the same time; the peeling off took place without further trouble, and after the patient had taken *Virga-aurea* for two weeks, and, on account of anæmia, for one week three times a day, a dose of *Ferrum peroxydatum* in the 2d trituration, he had so far recovered that I did not consider it necessary to give further medicine.

In 1885 a 45-year-old Belgian mine official (his work was office-work) consulted me on account of sleeplessness and pain in the back. The patient had no other complaints, only he carelessly added it sometimes took him a long time to urinate, because of want of the necessary pressure. He considered this weakness as the result of gonorrhœa, from which he had suffered years ago. The sleeplessness, for which he had tried all remedies possible, would make itself known from the time he went to bed until 3 o'clock in the morning, at which time he could get sleep, but not a refreshing one, and on arising he would feel very tired, especially in the upper part of the thighs, and then would commence the pain in the back, which extended to the loins, and lasted until he went to bed in the evening, without being prompted by external influences (warmth, cold, rest, motion). Also sleeplessness nights, pain in the back daytimes. At first I considered *Nux vom.* proper, and I prescribed the same for the patient, in the 3d decimal potency, four drops twice a day. At the same time I requested the patient to bring a sample of his urine at his next visit. After some time he came back with the sample, and declared that the prescribed remedy had not shown the least effect.

The urine was dark and slimy, reddish, slightly acid, and had at the bottom of the bottle brick-dust settlings. Heat did not show albumen, but by heating it the dark urine became clearer, and contained also salts of uric acid. I examined the kidneys of the patient, found them sensitive against pressure, and the diagnosis pointed to chronic catarrh of the kidneys. Sleeplessness, pain in the back and the tired feeling in the upper parts of the thigh were additional symptoms of this malady, and I determined to use *Virga-aurea*. The patient took this for three months three times a day, after which he wrote me that he was entirely well. About a year afterwards he had a relapse, but not in the form of former symptoms, but in the form of ischias, against which disease Golden Rod proved itself beneficial.

In conclusion, may be mentioned a double case of the curative power of *Virga-aurea*, which also contributes to the heredity of disease. Some time ago, the wife of a farmer, 53 years old, asked me for a prescription for a trouble which she had had for twenty-six years, since her first confinement. The patient, a stout and fresh-looking person, made the following statement: After the confinement, which was very laborious, and which was followed by prolapsus uteri, the latter still existing, her legs began to swell, and an itching rash broke out by degrees. Menstruation had always come at the proper time, but suddenly stopped six months ago.

Since that time the itching had become almost intolerable, the legs more swollen and always cold, but she did not feel a continuous heat in her head. The appetite was very poor; she had always a bitter taste in the mouth, and the tongue was thickly coated. At the same time she had rising from the stomach, as if she should suffocate, and at the least exertion she lost her breath. She urinated very little, and this mostly at night. My question, if there were pains in the back, was answered in the negative, but the kidneys of this patient were also sensitive against pressure. The appearance of the lower limbs of the patient frightened me. From knee to heel they formed a bluish-red mass in the shape of a stove-pipe, which were covered with little blotches and crusts. This kind of an eruption, together with the other symptoms, led me to the use of *Virga-aurea*, the prolonged use of which, although it did not affect a cure, produced a mitigation of the whole body, so that the lady induced her eldest son to come to me for help. This man had also trouble in his lower limbs not unlike his mother. He had a year ago passed through a severe throat difficulty, after which his lower limbs began to swell and to itch; they were also tainted bluish-red and covered with vesicles; he also complained of scanty urine, and his kidneys were sensitive against pressure. What better could I, under the circumstances, prescribe than *Virga-aurea*?

The result was good. After a few months the patient had no more difficulty.

In the cases above mentioned, I prescribed the 3d decimal dilution of the tincture of the whole plant of Golden Rod. The water of Golden Rod, recommended by Rademacher and others, I have never tried.

STELLARIA MEDIA.

NAT. ORD.—Caryophyllaceæ.
COMMON NAME.—Common Chickweed.
PREPARATION.—The whole fresh plant in bloom is macerated in twice its weight of alcohol.

(Frederick Kopp proved this remedy and the results were published in the *Homœopathic World*, 1896, as follows:)

"It has proved to me a matter of impossibility to answer all the letters that have been sent to me by readers of the *Homœopathic World* on the subject of the use of *Stellaria media* in the treatment of rheumatism, but I trust that the information given below will satisfy all the correspondents. It will be remembered by my readers that the new drug was first proved by me in 1893, consequent on my attention being drawn to the weed by our esteemed friend, the Rev. F. H. Brett. I made a thorough proving of the drug, not only once, but several times, so as to satisfy myself beyond a doubt as to the symptoms peculiar to it, and the excruciating rheumatic-like pains developed at the time are still vividly remembered by me; in fact, they were so severe and intense as not to be easily forgotten when once experienced. There is no mistaking the *rheumatic* symptoms of the drug. They come on very rapidly, and the sharp, darting pains so peculiar to rheumatism are experienced, not only in almost every part of the body, but the symptoms of soreness of the parts to the touch, stiffness of the joints, and aggravation of the pains by motion are also present. These pains may be described as follows:

"Rheumatic-like pains over the right side of the head; especially towards the back, with the parts sore to the touch; rheumatic-like pains darting through the whole head, worse on right side; rheumatic-like pains left half of forehead, over the eye, with the parts sore to the touch; rheumatic-like pains in the left foot; rheumatic-like pains in the ankles; sharp, darting, rheumatic-like pains in the left knee, gradually extending above along the thigh; rheumatic-like pains below the right knee-cap; rheumatic-like, darting pains through various parts of the body, especially down the right arm and the middle and index fingers of the left hand; stiffness of the joints in general; rheumatic-like pains in the calves of the legs, which are sensitive to the touch; rheumatic-like pains in the right hip; rheumatic-like pains across the small of the back, aggravated by bending or stooping; stiffness in lumbar region with soreness; darting, rheumatic-like pains through right thigh; rheumatic-like pains in right groin.

"It will be seen by the above symptoms that almost every part of the body in which it is possible for rheumatic pains to occur is affected, the rheumatic-like pains darting from one part to another. My correspondents all being readers of *The Homœopathic World* will remember a case reported in the January number of the journal (1896), by Mr. R. H. Bellairs, in which the pains were 'now in ankle, now in knee, now in arm, wrist, or fingers.' This case fully illustrates the symptoms borne out in my proving of the drug, and it but naturally followed, according to the law of similars, that the disease should yield to the month's treatment with *Stellaria media.* Mr. Bellairs says he thinks that possibly 'shifting pain' is a key-note, and I am glad that I am able to inform him that he is correct in his supposition. I am pleased to hear that he has often given *Stellaria media* in chronic rheumatism, and now looks upon it as a specific. It is these things that gladden the heart of the prover of new drugs—the news of the practical triumph of a new drug over symptoms of disease similar to those it is itself capable of developing in a healthy body—and one feels amply repaid for the hours and days of pain and suffering that one has inevitably to put up with in the vocation of 'proving.' I heartily congratulate Mr. Bellairs on his success in curing the above case.

"I have been asked by one correspondent whether a changeable climate—one with sudden changes of temperature occurring every day, for instance—would prevent the drug from taking effect in the treatment of rheumatism. To this question I can promptly return an answer in the negative. I have proof upon proof lying before me to testify that *Stellaria media* is just as efficacious in a changeable climate as in any other. Reports of cases cured have come to me from various parts of the world, under varying changes of climate, and the result has always been the same, namely, 'the cure of the case.'

"For *internal* administration I have always found the 2x tincture the most efficacious, given in from one to two drop doses every two, three, or four hours, according to the severity of the symptoms. For *external* purposes I strongly advise the θ tincture. It may be employed either in the form of a lotion (20 to 60 minims of θ tincture to a tumblerful of water), the ointment or the liniment (30 to 40 minims of the θ tincture to ʒj of pure olive oil). Cloths steeped in the lotion and renewed when dry may be applied to the painful parts, or the ointment or liniment may be rubbed well in. Experience has taught me that external treatment combined with internal greatly assists in hastening the cure. In the treatment of rheumatism *Stellaria media* is a very active drug, acting very promptly; a low dilution of the mother tincture of the drug taken internally is very apt, therefore, to intensify the pains, and these should therefore be avoided and the 2x dilution used."

STIGMATA MAIDIS.

A Tincture of the Fresh Corn Silk.

NAT. ORD.—Gramineæ.

COMMON NAME.—Corn Silk.

PREPARATION.—One part of fresh corn silk is macerated in two parts by weight of alcohol.

(A great deal has been published lately concerning this remedy. The following by Dr. Dufan, *London Medical Record*, seems to give the best outline of its uses:)

1. The stigmata of maize have a very marked, though not always a favorable, action in all affections of the bladder, whether acute or chronic.

2. In acute traumatic cystitis, and also in gonorrhœal cystitis, they have a very marked diuretic action, but, at the same time, increase the pain; hence they should not be employed in these cases.

3. The best results have been obtained in cases of uric or phosphatic gravel, of chronic cystitis, whether simple or consecutive to gravel, and of mucous or muco-purulent catarrh. All the symptoms of the disease, the vesical pains, the dysuria, the excretion of sand, the ammoniacal odor, etc., rapidly disappear under the influence of the medicine.

4. The retention of urine dependent on these various affections often disappears as improvement progresses, but the use of the sound must sometimes be continued, in order to empty the bladder completely.

5. The stigmata maize have very often produced a cure after all the usual internal remedies had been tried in vain, or with only partial success. In other cases, the ordinary methods of treatment, which had at first proved more or less entirely useless, became efficacious after stigmata had been administered for a time, and had, as it were, broken the ground for them. Most frequently the stigmata alone sufficed for the cure, but still in some cases the effect was incomplete, and it was found that the treatment could be varied with benefit. Injections and irrigations of the bladder also proved useful adjuncts to the maize.

6. As the stigmata of maize are a very powerful, though at the same time entirely inoffensive diuretic, they have also been employed with the best results in cases of heart disease, albuminuria, and other affections requiring diuretics. Cases have been reported in which the urinary secretion was tripled and even quintupled in the first twenty-four hours, and others where

the exhibition of the drug was continued for two or three months without the slightest untoward effect.

(Though Dr. Dufan condemns the use of the remedy in gonorrhœa, other practitioners have commended it for that very purpose. Dr. Leo Bennett, *Therapeutic Gazette*, 1893, having had "unusual success" in the treatment of that disease with the *Stigmata maidis*.)

SUCCINIC ACID.

PREPARATION.—The pure chemical is triturated in the usual way.

(The following is by Dr. Morris Weiner, of Baltimore, 1892:)

About twelve years ago I decided to prove *Succinic acid* (*Acidum succinicum*). *Agricola* mentions this acid, 1546, as *Salt of amber. Boyle*, towards the close of the 17th century, was the first who pronounced it to be acid, and *Stecker de Neuform* confirmed this statement, after repeated investigations, calling it a *true* acid. *Berzelius* published its elemental composition, $C_4H_2O_3$.

This acid was long ago laid aside as obsolete, and not without good reason, because since the Puritans in chemistry commenced to rule over every laboratory of pharmacy, by trying to redistill this crude acid and changing its yellowish color to snowy whiteness, they drove out every trace of the *oily matter* which alone constitutes its medical action. The whiter this acid becomes the larger doses can be taken without any action on the human system. Knowing that this *oil of amber* is driven out totally by redistillation I was compelled to prepare the crude acid myself.

The expense is considerable. One pound of amber yields about half an ounce of crude acid, and the glass retort, after dry distillation, must be broken to collect the acid.

The fumes of *Acidum succinicum crudum* are inflammable, producing asthma, cough, sneezing, weeping, dropping of watery mucus from the nostrils, pain in chest and headache.

None of our remedies gives a truer picture of hay fever, and since the *oil of amber* must be securely inclosed in the amber itself, it was but natural to conclude that by trituration I may receive all the virtue of the remedy.

At the same time I remembered that necklaces and earrings of amber are considered a popular protection agent against neuralgia, colds, and even hay fever.

Since that time I prescribed in cases of hay fever the third decimal trituration, one or two grains dissolved in twelve teaspoonfuls of distilled water, one teaspoonful every two hours, with the best results, and have cured more than thirty persons, who were formerly obliged to go to the mountains to get temporary relief. Already after the first week most of them experienced decided relief.

SYMPHYTUM OFFICINALIS.

NAT. ORD.—Borraginaceæ.
COMMON NAME.—Comfrey, Healing Herb.
PREPARATION.—One part of the fresh root gathered just before blooming is macerated in two parts by weight of alcohol.

(The following concerning this remedy, which dates back to Dioscorides, we find in *American Journal of Homœopathy*, 1846:)

The Homœopathic Examiner for August contains a paper entitled "*Connection of Homœopathy with Surgery*," by *Croserio*, translated by P. P. Wells, M. D. It is there stated that "injuries of the bones are healed most promptly by *Symphytum officinale* 30 internally once a day. This remedy accelerates the consolidation of fractures surprisingly." The translator adds a note as follows: "I have had repeated opportunities of verifying this declaration of Croserio. A boy, fourteen years old, broke the bones of the forearm, at the junction of the lower and middle thirds, two years ago. He had twice repeated the fracture by slight falls. The ends of the fragments are now slightly movable on each other, and the arm is weak and admits of little use. Three doses of *Symphytum* effected a perfect cure. The lad became more robust, and has since had better general health than ever before."

A boy, eight years old, fractured the humerus, near the junction of the condyles and shaft. *Arnica* 30 immediately arrested the spasmodic jerks of the muscles of the injured arm. This remedy was continued the first three days, when the traumatic fever had entirely subsided. He then had *Symphyt.* 3, gtt. i., in half a tumbler of water, a teaspoonful every morning and evening. The splints were removed the *ninth day*, and the bone was found consolidated. The cure was entirely without pain. How much earlier than this the fragments ceased to be movable is not known. Well may the author say it heals broken bones surprisingly. Let it be remembered that the discovery of this specific is but one of the many rich fruits of *Hahnemannism*.

(The following appeared in the *Homœopathic World*, 1890, under the signature F. H. B.:)

In none of the Homœopathic treatises that I possess do I find any mention of the above remedy. I am surprised at this, for I believe it to be a very valuable one in certain cases. Its common name of *knitbone* seems to point to popular experience of one of its uses; but I believe its knitting, or uniting, power extends to muscular and other tissues of the body, as well as to the bones. Let me give two instances of my own personal experience.

Many years ago I had an inguinal rupture on each side, not extensive ones, but causing a protrusion about the size of half a small walnut. After wearing a truss for some time, I bethought me of what I had heard of the uniting power of Comfrey, and made some tincture from the root, and rubbed it in. After doing so two or three times, the signs of rupture quite disappeared, and the parts remained sound for about three years; when, from some cause or other, the right side broke out again, but as it did not give much trouble I neglected it for some time, and then tried the Comfrey tincture again, but this time without success. I suppose the ruptured edges had got too far asunder. The left side, however, which originally was the worse of the two, has kept sound ever since. I think this shows that a rupture, if not too extensive, and if taken in time, may often be cured by this remedy. The other case I have to relate was of a different kind. Five weeks ago I had a fall on my back, the whole force of which was concentrated on a small portion of the lower spine, through the intervention of the back pad of my truss. I thought for the moment my back must have been broken, the pain was so excessive; and not only the back, but diaphragm and all the organs below it suffered acutely for three or four weeks after the fall. But a fortnight after the fall I was for the first time conscious of a pain and tenderness higher up the spine, at a point, I think, where ribs commence, and on feeling I found a protuberance there, as if a partial dislocation had taken place there. I again thought of Comfrey, and had some of the tincture applied. The tenderness at the point subsided after two or three applications, and in a few days the protuberance disappeared. * * * On more careful examination I find that the point of secondary disturbance was higher up than I have described—two or three inches higher than the first insertion of the ribs in the spinal column.

(Dr. Gottweis, in *Hom. Zeitung*, vol. vii., says:)

An old and very valuable remedy. This plant is found all over Europe (and in some parts of North America), in wet fields and ditches. We make a tincture out of it which has marvelous healing and cicatrizing properties. *Symphytum* must be a very old popular remedy; its reputation is well established, and it is mentioned in all the old medical "tomes." The decoction acts as an effective demulcent and pain-killer in severe bruises. It diminishes the irritation in wounds and ulcers, ameliorates and lessens too copious suppuration and promotes the healing processes. In homœopathic practice the tincture diluted with water is used with great success in fractures and bruises or other injuries of bones. Its effect is really extraordinary in injuries to sinews, tendons and the periosteum.

A few days ago a colleague consulted me about a horse with a stab wound in the fetlock which would not heal, do what he would, and which rendered locomotion impossible. (The doctor is by no means a young or inexperienced veterinarian.) I examined the wound, and at once recommended *Symphytum* θ. Within two weeks the animal was cured. This remedy really cannot be overestimated.

(Dr. W. H. Thompson, President of Royal College of Surgeons in Ireland, in an address reported in London *Lancet*, 1896, reports a case of which the following is the gist:)

Early in 1895 he saw a man who was suffering from a malignant growth in the nose—"a malignant tumor of the antrum, which had extended to the nose." An exploratory operation confirmed this diagnosis. "He refused the larger operation. The exploration was made by Dr. Woods. We found that the tumor did extend from the antrum, into which I could bore my finger easily. Dr. O'Sullivan, Professor of Pathology in Trinity College, declared the growth to be a round-celled sarcoma. Of that there is no doubt. The tumor returned in a couple of months, and the patient then saw Dr. Semon, in London, who advised immediate removal. He returned home, and after a further delay he asked to have the operation performed. I did this in May last by the usual method. I found the tumor occupying the whole of the antrum. The base of the skull was everywhere infiltrated. The tumor had passed into the right nose and perforated the septum so as to extend into the left. It adhered to the septum around the site of perforation. This was all removed, leaving a hole in the septum about the size of a florin. He went home within a fortnight. In a month the growth showed signs of return. It bulged through the incision and protruded upon the face. Dr. Woods saw him soon afterwards, as I had declared by letter that a further operation would be of no avail. The tumor had now almost closed the right eye. It was blue, tense, firm, and lobulated, but it did not break. Dr. Woods reported the result of his visit to me, and we agreed as to the prognosis. Early in October the patient walked into my study after a visit to Dr. Woods. He looked in better health than I had ever seen him. The tumor had completely disappeared from the face, and I could not identify any trace of it in the mouth. He said he had no pain of any kind. He could speak well when the opening remaining after the removal of the hard palate was plugged, and he was in town to have an obturator made. He has since gone home apparently well."

The patient told Dr. Thompson that he had applied poultices of *Comfrey* (or *Symphytum*) and that was all.

"Now this was a case of which none of us had any doubt at all, and our first view was confirmed by the distinguished pathologist whom I have mentioned and by our own observation at the time of the major operation. Here, then, was another 'surprise.' I am satisfied as I can be of anything that the growth was malignant and of a bad type. Of course, we know in the history of some tumors that growth is delayed and that in the sarcomata recurrence is often late. But this is a case in which the recurrence occurred twice—the second time to an extreme degree; and yet this recurrent tumor has vanished. What has produced this atrophy and disappearance? I do not know. I know nothing of the effects of comfrey root, but I do not believe that it can remove a sarcomatous tumor. Of course, the time that has so far elapsed is very short; but the fact that this big recurrent growth no longer exists—that it has not ulcerated or sloughed away, but simply, with unbroken covering, disappeared—is to me one of the greatest 'surprises' and puzzles that I have met with."

SYMPHORICARPUS RACEMOSUS.

NAT. ORD., Caprifoliaceæ.
COMMON NAME, Snow Berry.
PREPARATION.—One part of the fresh ripe berries is macerated in two parts by weight of alcohol.

(In 1882 Dr. Edward V. Moffat read the following paper on this remedy before the Homœopathic Medical Society of New York:)

Let us go back about fifteen years and sketch a history of this drug. At that time Prof. S. P. Burdick investigated the medicinal of many plants hitherto unused by the profession, among others chanced to be the snow berry, or *Symphoricarpus racemosus*. He gave some of the drug to the first prover, an intelligent lady, who on feeling the marked nausea, which it soon produced, exclaimed: "Doctor, this is precisely like the morning sickness I always experienced during pregnancy." Dr. Burdick became more interested, repeated the experiment with other provers, obtained almost uniform results, viz., a feeling varying from qualmishness to intense vomiting. It was given to female provers only and merely tested far enough to verify that symptom.

Upon this clue Dr. Burdick gave it in the higher potencies to patients suffering from the vomiting of pregnancy with most satisfactory results. Indeed, after a trial of many years, he has found it so far superior to other remedies that he now relies on it altogether with rarely any but entirely satisfactory results.

He mentioned the drug in his course of lectures, so I bore it in mind waiting for a test case. Soon that came in the person of a young lady three months advanced in her first pregnancy who was suffering from a deathly nausea, with vomiting and retching so prolonged and violent as to produce hæmatemesis. The smell or thought of food was repugnant in the extreme. An examination disclosed no malposition or apparent cause for the trouble, so I procured some *Symphoricarpus* (200) from Dr. Burdick and gave her one dose in the midst of a violent paroxysm. In a few minutes she stopped vomiting and said she felt soothed and quieted all over. In half an hour the nausea began again, but a few pellets checked it promptly and she fell asleep. Once during the night she awoke distressed and took a dose, but slept again quite soon. For a month or so she felt very well until after over-exerting herself she became nauseated once more; but it was promptly checked, nor did it return during her pregnancy.

After this I had the opportunity of prescribing it in a number of cases with such gratifying results that I gave some of the drug to a number of physicians, requesting a faithful trial. Among them were my father, brother, Dr. Danforth, Dr. McClelland, of Pittsburg, and several others. All reported favorably and some enthusiastically, and so I have been led to bring this subject before this society. The indications as far as I have observed them in cases of pregnancy are a feeling of qualmishness with indifference to food. In more severe cases, like the above, there is a deathly nausea; the vomiting is continuous violent retching, but it covers every graduation between these extremes; it does not seem to be confined to any particular *morning* aggravation; a prominent symptom is the disgust at the sight, smell or thought of food. One case I remember where the patient was comparatively comfortable while lying on the back, but would be nauseated by the slightest motion of the arms, particularly raising them. The case was completely relieved by a few doses. And so the cases might be multiplied.

Thinking that if the irritation of pregnancy were thus subdued, that of menstruation might be as well, I have given it repeatedly in such cases of nausea or vomiting just before, during or after catamenia, with admirable results.

TELA ARANEARUM.

COMMON NAMES, Spider's Web, Cobweb.
PREPARATION.—Triturate in the usual way.

(The following paper is by Dr. S. A. Jones, it was published in the *American Observer*, 1876):

Dr. Gillespie, of Edinburgh, "cured an obstinate intermittent with cobweb after other means had failed." Dr. Robert Jackson was led from this to try it himself. He told his success to Dr. Chapman, of Philadelphia, who requested one of his pupils, Dr. Broughton, to investigate the subject, which he did, and wrote his Inaugural Thesis thereon in 1818. From these and other authorities we can gather enough testimony to show that it is well worth while to make a systematic proving of this animal product, thereby predicating its sphere and precisioning its employment.

In a work on fevers—which particular edition I have not been able to consult—Dr. Jackson writes: "I think I may venture to say that it prevents the recurrence of febrile paroxysms more abruptly, and more effectually, than bark or arsenic, or any other remedy employed for that purpose with which I am acquainted: that, like all other remedies of the kind, it is only effectual as applied under a certain condition of habit; *but that the condition of susceptibility for cobweb is at the same time of more latitude than for any other of the known remedies.*"

If we bear in mind Grauvogl's constitution-classification of *Diadema aranea* as an hydrogenoid remedy, and recall how generally the hydrogenoid constitution is induced by intermittent fever, we shall be ready to acknowledge the truth of the passage which I have placed in italics, and with this evidence of a truthful beginning we shall be more ready to accept the subsequent testimony.

"If the cobweb," continues Dr. Jackson, "was given in the time of perfect intermission, the return of paroxysm was prevented; if given under the first symptoms of a commencing paroxysm, the symptoms were suppressed, and the course of the paroxysm was so much interrupted that the disease, for the most part, lost its characteristic symptoms. If it was not given until the paroxysm was advanced in progress the symptoms of irritation, viz.: tremors, startings, spasms, and delirium, if such existed as forms of febrile action, were usually reduced in violence, sometimes entirely removed. In this case sleep, calm and refreshing, usually followed the sudden and perfect removal of pain and irritation. Vomiting, spasms, and twisting in the bowels, appearing as modes of febrile irritation, were also usually allayed by it; there was no effect from it where the vomiting or pain was connected with real inflammation or progress to disorganization."

"In cases of febrile depression, deficient animation, or indifference to surrounding objects, the exhibition of eight or ten grains of cobweb was often followed by exhilaration: the eyes sparkled; the countenance assumed a temporary animation, and, though the course of the disease might not be changed, or the danger averted, more respite was obtained than is gotten from wine, opium, or anything else within my knowledge."

"In spasmodic affections of various kinds, in asthma, in periodic headaches, in general restlessness and muscular irritabilities its good effects are often signal. The cobweb gives sleep, but not by narcotic power;— tranquillity and sleep here appear to be the simple consequence of release from pain and irritation."

"The changes induced on the existing state of the system, as the effect of its operation, characterize it as powerfully stimulant: 1. Where the pulses of the arteries are quick, irregular, and irritated, they become calm, regular, and slow, almost instantaneously after the cobweb has passed into the stomach: the effect is moreover accompanied, for the most part, with perspiration and perfect relaxation of the surface. 2. When the pulses are slow, regular, and nearly natural they usually become frequent, small, irregular, sometimes intermitting. 3. When languor and depression characterize the disease, sensations of warmth and comfort are diffused about the stomach, and increased animation is conspicuous in the appearance of the eye and countenance."

Dr. J. likewise "effected perfect cures with it in some troublesome spasmodic affections, and gave it with the most marked benefit in dry, irritating coughs, usually termed nervous. In the advanced stage of phthisis it procured a respite beyond his expectation. He also found it useful in restraining a troublesome hiccough."

Remembering the fame of *Mygale avicularia* in chorea we may well expect this other spider to be of use "in some troublesome *spasmodic* affections."

Dr. Chapman writes of it: "I have cured some obstinate intermittents, suspended the paroxysms of hectic, overcome morbid vigilance from excessive nervous mobility, and quieted irritation of the system from other causes, and particularly as connected with protracted coughs and other chronic pectoral affections. * * * * Some consider it as highly stimulant, invigorating the force of the pulse, increasing the temperature of the surface, and heightening excitement generally—others, witnessing no such effects, are disposed to assort it with those remedies which seem to do good *chiefly by soothing the agitations of the system.* I confess that I concur in the latter view of its properties."

How unconsciously the Philistines of Old Physic bear testimony to the truth of our therapeutic law. Given where "heightened excitement" obtained, Chapman saw it "do good chiefly by soothing the agitations of the system," and to him, of course, cobweb was a sedative.

Dr. Broughton, in his Thesis, says: "In all the cases of disease in which I have seen or heard of the exhibition of the web, no sensible, or at least no uniform, operation could be observed. Some patients were sensible of none, others of a slight sudorific, and some a nauseatic effect; and one or two thought it proved cathartic after remaining in the system for the space of twelve or fifteen hours. These accounts being so incorrect and various, I determined to ascertain (if possible) the correct operation by giving the web to healthy persons."

"I found from these experiments that the operation of the web appeared principally to be upon the arterial system; and perhaps in less time than any article already known: the force and frequency of the pulse being uniformly reduced in some cases ten, in others fifteen strokes in a minute; and in one case, the pulse, from being strong and full, became soft, small, and very compressible; all which operation took place within the space of two hours, after which time the artery gradually regained its former force and frequency. This has been the only invariable effect I could observe, all others appearing but anomalous."

Dr. Thacher cites the following case from a paper of Dr. Jackson's: "W. Sands has been afflicted for many years with a distressing asthma, which has proved fatal to his father and two sisters. The complaint being hereditary, and aggravated by malformation of the thorax, no remedy gave any permanent relief, nor did change of climate procure any alleviation of symptoms. For a considerable time back he has never been able to lie down in bed on account of a sense of suffocation, but is obliged to be supported half sitting by pillows, and is seldom able to sleep. He swallowed nearly a scruple of the spider's web, he swallowed it at bed time, and to his utter astonishment enjoyed sound and uninterrupted sleep all night; a blessing to which he had been an entire stranger above six years. Since he began with the cobweb thinks his health is improved; the cough has certainly abated, but whenever the remedy is omitted the complaint returns."

Dr. Oliver found that "by the use of this remedy a patient laboring under organic disease of the heart and hydrothorax obtained great relief and refreshing sleep, who had not before slept for three nights. Another, under similar affection, experienced uncommon relief from the same prescription. To one suffering much pain from cancer it afforded ease and comfortable sleep. A patient in phthisis pulmonalis being affected with distressing agitation of mind and nervous irritation, it answered like a charm, and soon induced great sleep like a moderate dose of opium."

THALLIUM.

PREPARATION.—Triturate the pure metal in the usual way.

(The following is from the *Homœopathic World*, 1893):

In the "French News" column of the *Chemist and Druggist* we came across a note on the effect of *Thallium*, which we have no doubt homœopaths will soon turn to good account. Here is the paragraph:—

CURIOUS EFFECT OF A REMEDY.

"Dr. Huchard read a paper at the last meeting of the Paris Academy of Medicine on *Acetate of Thallium*, which was formerly advocated by Dr. Combemale, of Lille, as a medicament against profuse perspiration in certain cases of serious illness. It appears, however, that its useful influence is counterbalanced by the fact that it causes the hair to fall off with great rapidity. Dr. Huchard exhibited at the meeting several photographs of patients who had become quite bald in several days. He was consequently very emphatic against the use of the remedy."

There is all the difference between the two schools in this note. To the allopath this is a "curious effect" merely, and serves to condemn the drug. To the homœopathic it brings to light a new remedy for a troublesome affection which is by no means too well provided for.

Thallium is a rare metal, whose atomic weight is 204.2, its symbol being Tl. It receives its name (θαλλός, a green shoot) from the green line it gives on the spectrum, through which it was discovered by Crookes in the residuum left from the distillation of selenium. *Thallium* has a bluish white tint and the lustre of lead; is so soft that it can be scratched by the finger nail. Specific gravity, 11.8. It belongs to the lead group of metals, but has peculiar reactions of its own. It is used in the manufacture of glass of high refractive power.

THLASPI BURSA PASTORIS.

NAT. ORD., Cruciferæ.
COMMON NAME, Shepherd's Purse.
PREPARATION.—Three parts of the fresh plant in flower are macerated in two parts by weight of alcohol.

(The following paper on this remedy is by Dr. E. R. Dudgeon and appeared in the *Monthly Homœopathic Review*, 1888):

The *Art Médical*, for July, 1888, contains a paper on this plant by Dr. Imbert Gourbeyre, displaying all his well-known ability and erudition. Although an unproved remedy, its sphere of specific action is pretty accurately known, and in former days it was frequently employed by many eminent medical authorities. In our own days, though almost unknown to "scientific" medicine, it enjoys a considerable reputation in popular medicine, chiefly for hæmorrhages, and profuse menstruation, and metrorrhagia.

According to Dioscorides, it is emmenagogue and abortive, anti-hæmorrhagic, and a remedy for sciatica. In Salmon's *Doren Medicum* (1683) it is said: "The seed provokes urine and the courses, kills the *fœtus*, resists poyson, breaks inward apostems, and, being taken in ʒij, it purges cholera." In Vogel's *Historia Materiæ Medicæ* we read of the seed: "Ischiaticis infusum prodesse, et menses ciere (Dioscorides). Sudorem pellere, et ad scorbutum posse, si eb vius teratur, adiecto saccharo (Bœrhaav)." It was called by the old herbalists *sanguinaria*—"quia sanguinem sistet." Murray, at the end of last century, pronounced it useless; but De Maza, arguing against this opinion, relates a case of metrorrhagia cured by it, applied as a cataplasm to the loins, on the recommendation of an old woman, after the doctor had tried several medicines without effect. Lejeune (1822) says he has seen good results from its employment in hæmoptysis.

Rademacher has a great opinion of it. He says: "This plant was held to be an anti-hæmorrhagic medicine by the ancients. The superior wisdom of later physicians has pronounced it to have no such power, *because it contains no astringent principle*! (Carheuser's *Mat. Med.*) A second property attributed to it was that of stopping diarrhœa; a third, that of cutting short agues. I have lately used it repeatedly in chronic diarrhœa, when this is purely a primary affection of the bowels, with surprising benefit; but it is useless in consensual diarrhœa. I have not yet used it in ague, but would not dissuade others from trying it. But the most important remedial power of this common innocuous plant I learned from no medical author; the knowledge of it was actually forced upon me by the following case: I was called to see a poor woman from whom, eight or ten years before, I had brought away a large quantity of urinary sand by means of magnesia and cochineal, and thereby cured her. Now, the tiresome sand had again accumulated in the kidneys, and the patient was in a pitiable state. The abdominal cavity was full of water, the lower extremities swollen by œdema, and the urine of a bright red color, which formed, on standing, a sediment unmistakably of blood. I prescribed tincture of *Brusa pastoris*, 30 drops, 5 times a day, solely with the intention of stopping the hæmaturia as a preliminary; but imagine my astonishment when I found that the tincture caused a more copious discharge of renal sand than I had ever witnessed. Paracelsus's words occurred to me: 'A physician should overlook nothing; he should look down before him like a maiden, and he will find at his feet a more valuable treasure for all diseases than India, Egypt, Greece or Barbary can furnish.' I should certainly have been a careless fool had I, with this striking effect before me, changed to another medicine. I continued to give the tincture; I saw the urinary secretion increase with the copious discharge of sand; the water disappeared from the abdomen and extremities, and health was restored. I went on with the tincture until no more sand appeared in the urine, and I had every reason to suppose that the deposit of sand was completely removed. Since then I have used this remedy in so many cases with success that I can conscientiously recommend it to my colleagues as a most reliable remedy. Among these cases was one which appeared to me very striking. It was that of a woman, aged 30, who came to me for a complication of diseases. I examined the urine for sand, but found none. I gave her the tincture of *Brusa pastoris*, and a quantity of sand came away. On continuing the tincture much more sand came away, and her other morbid symptoms disappeared."

It was stated some time ago that Mattei's *anti-angioitico* was a tincture of *Thlaspi bursa pastoris*, but, if we are to credit the statement of a periodical lately published, entitled *General Review of Electro-Homœopathic Medicine*, this is not so, for *anti-angioitico* is there stated to be a medicine compounded of *Aconite, Belladonna, Nux vomica, Veratrum album*, and *Ferrum metallicum*. I mention this inadvertently, but I do not suppose it is of much consequence, and my first experience of the remedial action of *Thlaspi* was anterior to the information that it was one of Mattei's remedies.

In the 3d volume of the *British Journal of Homœopathy*, page 63, there is an observation taken from the Berlin *Med. Zeit.*, to the effect that Dr. Lange found the greatest benefit from "a decoction of the whole plant in cases of passive hæmorrhage generally, and especially in too frequent and too copious menstruation." In the *Zeitsch. f. Erfahrungsheild.*, the periodical published by the followers of Rademacher, Dr. Kinil relates the case of a woman who, three weeks after accouchement, was affected with strangury.

She could not retain her urine, which dribbled away, drop by drop, with constant pain in the urethra. The urine was turbid and had a deep red sediment. She got 30 drops of the *tincture of Thlaspi* five times a day. The strangury disappeared at once, the urine could be retained after a few days, and after eight days it became clear and without sediment.

Dr. Hannon (*Presse Med. Belge*, 1853) mentions that he had found *Thlaspi* very useful in hæmorrhage when the blood was poor in fibrine. Dr. Heer (Berlin *Med. Zeit.*, 1857) found *Thlaspi* efficacious in the dysuria of old persons, when the passage of the urine is painful and there is at the same time spasmodic retention of it. On giving the medicine, a large quantity of white or red sand is discharged, and the troublesome symptoms disappear. Dr. Joussett (*Bull. de la Soc. Hom. de France*, 1866) had a case of hæmorrhage, after miscarriage, at three months. He tried *Sabina*, *Secale*, *Crocus*, tampons soaked in chloride of iron, but all in vain. He consulted Dr. Tessier, who recommended him to try *Thlaspi*, 20 drops of the mother tincture in a draught; at the second spoonful the hæmorrhage ceased. He found it useful in hæmorrhage with severe uterine colic, with clots of blood, in that following miscarriage, in the metrorrhagias at the menopause, and in those associated with cancer of the neck of the uterus. He found good effects from the dilutions in some of these cases. Dr. Jousset, in his *Elements de Med. Prat.*, repeats his recommendation of *Thlaspi* in hæmorrhages.

My own experience of *Thlaspi* is very small. In one case Dr. Rafinesque, of Paris, cleverly "wiped my eye," to use a sporting term, with this medicine. A young French widow was treated by me for a severe attack of jaundice, from which she made a good recovery. But after this she suffered for a couple of months from a very peculiar discharge after the catamenial flux. It had the appearance of brownish, grumous blood, and was attended with obscure abdominal pains. The cervix uteri was swollen and soft, but not ulcerated. I tried and tried to stop this discharge, but without success. She went back to Paris and put herself under the care of Dr. Rafinesque, who was her ordinary medical attendant. He tried several different medicines without any effect on the discharge. At last he gave *Thlaspi*, 6th dilution, and this had an immediate good effect. Afterwards he gave the mother tincture, 10 drops in 200 grms. of water, by spoonfuls, and again in the 6th dilution, and after keeping her on this medicine for some weeks the discharge was completely cured. The full details of the case will be found in the *Brit. Journ. of Hom.*, vol. 32, p. 370.

One other case I have had illustrative of its action in the presence of excessive quantities of uric acid in the urine: A lady, æt 76, was under my care for a very curious affection. She had considerable rheumatic muscular pains in various parts, and constant profuse perspirations day and night. Along with this she had the most abundant secretion of uric acid, which passed away with every discharge of urine. Sometimes the uric acid formed small calculi, which gave much pain in their passage down the ureter, but it generally appeared in the form of coarse sand, which formed a thick layer at the bottom of the utensil. This sand continued to pass after the cessation of the sweats and rheumatic pains, which lasted six or seven weeks. I tried various remedies—*Pulsatilla, Picric acid, Lycopodium,* etc., but without effect. At last I bethought me of Rademacher's recommendation of *Thlaspi,* and after a few doses of the 1st dilution the sand diminished very much, and, indeed, sometimes disappeared altogether, and when it did return, it was in insignificant quantity.

On the whole, I think this medicine deserves a thorough and complete proving. It is evidently a powerful anti-hæmorrhagic, and its influence on the urinary organs, more particularly in bringing away and in curing excess of uric acid in the urine, is very remarkable.

I have elsewhere mentioned the power of this substance to affect the secretion of uric acid, and then I have seen several cases corroborative of its medicinal virtues in this direction. One, a gentleman, æt. 57, who, in addition to other dyspeptic symptoms, had occasionally large discharges of coarse uric acid, coming away in masses the size of a good big pin's head, but curiously enough without pain. I prescribed *Thlaspi,* which he said soon stopped the uric acid. Nearly a year after this he called on me for a different affection, and informed me that the uric acid had reappeared several times in his urine, but that a few doses of *Thlaspi* 1 stopped it, and it never came to the height it attained when I first gave it to him. A lady, nearly eighty years of age, was suffering from the pressure of a calculus in the left ureter, which I knew to be of uric acid, as she had previously passed much 'sand.' The urine showed no sand, and was very scanty. I tried several remedies, among the rest the Borocitrate of magnesia, but it was not till I gave *Thlaspi* 1 that a great discharge of coarse brick-colored sand took place, with speedy relief to her pain. At the same time, indeed, I made her drink copiously of distilled water, which has a powerfully disintegrating effect on uric acid sometimes, but, as she had already been taking this for several days without effect, I am inclined to give the whole credit of the cure to *Thlaspi.*

It is not alone in such cases that *Thlaspi* is useful. Its ancient use as a hæmostatic has been confirmed in modern times and in my own experience, and my friend, Dr. Harper, related to me lately a most interesting cure he had effected by its means of a very prolonged and serious affection. The case was that of an elderly lady who for years had suffered from a large discharge of muco-pus, sometimes mixed with blood, sometimes apparently nearly all blood, which poured from the bowels after each evacuation. She had been many months under the medical treatment of the late Dr. D. Wilson, who at last told her he considered her disease incurable. She then put herself under the treatment of a practitioner who relies chiefly on oxygen gas for his cures; but she was no better—rather worse—after his treatment. She then came to Dr. Harper, who worked away at her with all the ordinary remedies without doing a bit of good. At last he bethought him of *Thlaspi*, led thereto by my remarks on its anti-hæmorrhagic properties in my "therapeutic notes" in *The Monthly Homœopathic Review* of October, 1888, and he found that, from the time she commenced using this remedy, the discharge from the bowels gradually declined and ultimately ceased, and there has been no return of it.

No doubt *Thlaspi* is a great remedy, and until it is satisfactorily proved, we may employ it with advantage in cases similar to those I have mentioned. But it is to be hoped that some of our colleagues endowed with youth, health and zeal, will ere long favor us with a good proving of it, whereby its curative powers may be precisionized. At present we only partially know these from the less satisfactory results of clinical experience.

(The following is from a paper by Dr. Millie J. Chapman in Transactions of American Institute of Homœopathy, 1897:)

The provings are brief and do not furnish very full indications for its use. However, from them we learn of its effectiveness in expelling accumulations of sand and uric-acid crystals from the kidneys and bladder, also in controlling hemorrhage from the nose, kidneys, or uterus.

My attention was first called to this remedy in cases of sub-involution following either abortion or labor at full term, where it many a time induced recovery.

I have since witnessed equal success in hemorrhage from uterine fibroid where the flow was controlled, and the growth was greatly reduced in size before the age of the individual would naturally produce these changes. Also uterine hemorrhage, attended with cramps and expulsion of clots, has been relieved by it after curetting had failed.

A member of the Women's Provers' Association took five drops of the tincture three times a day for ten days. This was followed by a great increase of urine and a menstrual flow lasting fifteen days. She became alarmed and could not be persuaded to continue the proving.

Another took ten drops, three times a day, for five days, when the quantity of urine and brick dust deposit were so unusual that her interest in scientific investigation suddenly ceased.

About a year since, there came for treatment a patient who had suffered long from both disease and treatment of the bladder. *Thlaspi* 2x and later five drop doses of the tincture expelled great quantities of sand, and was followed by complete relief of the bladder symptoms and the disappearance of rheumatic pains that had been supposed incurable.

Another case of similar bladder irritation and marked evidences of gout was promptly relieved.

Thlaspi also has a reputation in the cure of urethritis.

THYROID.

PREPARATION.—The dried thyroid gland of the sheep is triturated in the usual way or an extract may be prepared from the fresh gland.

(The following paper on the effects of *Thyroid* was written by Dr. F. G. Œhme, Roseburg, Oregon:)

The *Thyroid*, especially if used continually or in large doses, *causes* the following *symptoms*:

1. Elevation of the temperature.

2. Increase of the heart's action and of the frequency and volume of the pulse, which, however, is more compressible. Walking, even standing, after taking a dose is apt to cause a feeling of faintness and even complete syncope. The heart may become so weak that it cannot endure any overexertion without danger, even death may result.

3. Shortness of breath.

4. Increase or decrease of appetite, sometimes nausea, less frequently vomiting, still less diarrhœa.

5. Improvement in body nutrition generally, more complete absorption of nitrogenous food. But later on nitrogen is excreted in excess of that taken in the food.

6. Loss of weight.

7. Increase of sexual desire.

8. Menses profuse, prolonged or more frequent, rarely amenorrhœa.

9. Increased activity of the mucous membrane, kidneys and skin, which becomes moist and oily, sometimes exfoliation of the epidermis.

10. Rapid growth of the skeleton in the young with softening and bending of those bones which have to bear weight.

11. A disease closely resembling exophthalmic goitre. A cataleptic improved under large doses of *Thyroid*, but when the dose of 75 grs. a day was reached symptoms like those of exophthalmic goitre developed with a pulse of 160, but no glandular swelling. When the *Thyroid* was discontinued the catalepsy grew worse, the exophthalmic goitre better; when resumed the catalepsy better, the exophthalmic goitre worse.

A patient, while under *Thyroid* treatment for myxœdema, took, through a misunderstanding, in eleven days nearly 3 ounces of the dessicated *Thyroid*, whereupon tachycardia, pyrexia, insomnia, tremor of the limbs, polyuria, albuminuria, and glucosuria, in short, a disease similar to exophthalmic goitre developed.

Thyroid has been *used* with benefit in the following *diseases*:

1. Arrested development in children, cretinism, idiotism.

2. Myxœdema. [The extirpation of the entire *Thyroid* produces a disease resembling myxœdema.]

3. Simple goitre.

4. Excessive obesity with tendency to weakness and anæmia.

5. Melancholia functional insanity, where improvement has taken place up to a certain point and then remains so.

6. Defective secretion of milk during lactation when connected with reappearance of menses. *Thyroid* will suppress the latter and increase and enrich the milk.

7. In fractures of the bones in which consolidation does not promptly occur.

8. Hypertrophy of cicatricial tissue resembling keloid, possibly true keloid.

Doses: Either the fresh gland of the sheep prepared like food or the extract, or in the dessicated state, of the latter may be given from 2-3 grs., or more or less, once a day (at night) or oftener.

The *Thyroid* is *contra-indicated* in tuberculous persons, as they are apt to lose quickly in weight, over two pounds in twenty-four hours.

Rheumatic and anæmic symptoms are more frequently aggravated than improved.

As the *Thyroid* is a powerful remedy, the following should be always remembered:

There is a decided difference with regard to individual toleration, some are very susceptible.

The pulse should be watched regarding frequency and quality. The least effort or exertion will increase it even to 160, hence some cases should be kept in bed or at least very quiet and tranquil even for a time after the remedy has been discontinued. Deaths have taken place after a few days' treatment.

If *Thyroid* is not taken for myxœdema the patient should be weighed at least every two weeks, and if pathogenetic symptoms, called thyroidism, appear the remedy should be discontinued or reduced.

If softening of the bones has been caused it may be necessary to restrict the use of the legs or to use splints.

Thyroid seems to have a cumulative effect.

In many cases a liberal diet should be prescribed to avoid injurious consequences.

TRYCHOSANTHES DIOICA.

NAT. ORD., Cucurbitaceæ.
COMMON NAME, Patal.
PREPARATION.—One part of the entire fresh plant is macerated in two parts by weight of alcohol.

(In 1893 H. L. Saha, homœopathic practitioner, Pabna, Bengal, sent the following to *Hom. Recorder.*)

Trychosanthes dioica (Bengali name, Patal). It belongs to the order of *Cucurbitaeæ*, is a creeper, flowering in all seasons, but chiefly in spring. It is a native of Bengal. Its fruit is called Patal, and is used by the natives as one of their chief curry.

The plant and its root are used by the native physicians in various maladies. Its action is mainly upon the liver and intestines. The decoction of the root is generally used by the mother physicians for removing costiveness, especially where there is a derangement of the functions of the liver.

A boy of fourteen years of age, who had habitual constipation, took, at the advice of a quack native physician, about three or four ounces of the decoction of its root, which produced profuse diarrhœa. After four or five stools I was called. I saw him weak and dejected, using abusive language to his native physician. His face was very pale. Stools were profuse, frequent, gushing, yellowish, watery. Much pain and cutting about the umbilicus during and before stool. After every stool he felt dizziness of the brain. This case struck me that *Trychosanthes dioica* will prove a grand remedy for diarrhœa. I prepared its tincture from the root and used it in 3x potency, in some cases with great satisfaction. The following cases will show its curative power:

1. A girl, aged 6 years, was attacked with diarrhœa; stools were profuse, thin, yellowish, watery, mixed with little white mucous; very offensive smell; cutting pain about umbilicus during and after stool. Pain in liver and eyes; jaundice; face yellowish; very weak; did not wish to answer questions: sad and peevish. On the fifth day I was called. I prescribed *Trychosanthes dioica* 3x every three hours. I saw the patient much better next day. Within a day or two the patient was all right.

2. A boy, aged 16 years, suffering from chronic diarrhœa; passed from four to five stools in a day. The character of the stool was yellowish, watery, mixed with a little white and greenish mucus. Smell offensive; dull, aching pain in the region of the liver. Face very pale; eyes jaundiced. He was very

sad and dejected. His appetite little; taste bitter. He had been at first treated by an allopath, then, afterwards, by a homœopath. The latter showed some improvement. I was called on the thirteenth day, when I noticed the above symptoms. I prescribed *Trychosanthes* 3x every four hours. The patient was completely cured within four days.

I cured some cases of choleric diarrhœa by this medicine, but those cases were vaguely reported to me.

I hope that, when proven, *Trychosanthes dioica* will show its large sphere of action and give our Materia Medica a new remedy for looseness of bowels.

USNEA BARBATA.

NAT. ORD., Lichens.
PREPARATION.—The fresh lichen is macerated in five times its weight of alcohol.

(This appeared in No. 284 of the *U. S. Med. Investigator* signed "—— M. D."):

In March, 1878, I was cutting wood. I cut down a soft maple; the top was well loaded with moss. It attracted my attention; I viewed it closely. I ate a little, about the size of a hickory nut, as I trimmed up my tree. My head began to ache. I cut off one log, and had to go to the house. I could feel the blood press to the brain. My wife worked over me, and I got to sleep. Next morning felt well; never felt better. I did not think of the moss I had eaten. I went on a visit and was gone five days. On my return I went to my tree. The first sight of it reminded me of my headache.

I gathered some of the moss and made a tincture. I soon had a case of headache to try my remedy on; it stopped at once.

In the fall, about September, a load of young folks came to pick cranberries. Two of the young ladies had headache from riding in the hot sun. Both took to the lounge. Now for my remedy. I put one drop of tincture in a goblet of water, gave a teaspoonful; ordered another in fifteen minutes. The second dose stopped the pain.

A young married lady came on a visit to a relative—was having pains in her head. I was sent for; found her wild with pain. She said she had been subject to headache for five years; had got tired of doctoring. Gave her one drop in a cup of water, teaspoonful in twenty minutes; no more pain. I put ten drops in a two-drachm vial of alcohol, directed her to take one drop when she felt her headache coming on. One year after she wrote her friend it had cured headache; sent thanks to me.

I could give many more cases where the pain is over the entire head, or front head, with a feeling as if the temples would burst or the eyes would burst out of their sockets. I have always used the tincture. I have not noticed any other effect from it; would like to see a proving.

VERBENA HASTATA.

NAT. ORD., Verbenaceæ.
COMMON NAMES, Blue Vervain, Purvain, Wild Hyssop.
PREPARATION.—One part of the fresh plant, in flower, is macerated in two parts by weight of alcohol.

(An extract from a paper by Dr. J. N. White, Queen City, Texas, detailing at length the case of a five-year-old boy, who, after six weeks of whooping cough, developed epileptic symptoms, having as high as twelve spasms in twenty-four hours. After two months of treatment with such remedies as *Solanum Car.*, *Sulphonal*, *Hyoscyamus*, *Cannabis Ind.*, *Calomel*, *Zinc*, etc., with no results, the case was given *Verbena hastata*. Another doctor was in consultation and we quote:)

I told my friend (the Doctor) that when he became satisfied with the zinc treatment I wanted to try another eclectic remedy. (The Doctor was an allopath.) He was perfectly willing and I put him on *Verbena hastata*, 12 minims every four hours, skipping the dose at midnight. After we both took the case we decided, as there were no curative properties in the sulfonal, we would drop it, and not use anything to control the paroxysms, and consequently the boy seemed to get worse to the parents, as he would have several falling spells a day. From the first dose of the *Verbena hastata* the boy began to improve. He would have contractions of the muscles of the arms and legs and look wild for a minute or more for the first week, but after that he never had another symptom. We kept him on the medicine, as above, for six weeks, and now he takes twelve drops three times a day.

He has not had any symptom in over two months, and all that wild vacant look is gone, and he plays, eats, sleeps, etc., as if he had never been troubled with epilepsy.

VISCUM ALBUM.

NAT. ORD., Loranthaceæ.
COMMON NAME, Mistletoe.
PREPARATION.—One part of the fresh leaves and berries is macerated in twice its weight of alcohol.

(The following account of this ancient remedy was published in the *Allgemeine Hom. Zeitung*, 1886:)

The Grand Universal Panacea of the old Gauls and Germans.—By *Dr. v. Gerstel*, of Regensburg.—This parasite shrub belongs to the 22d class, Linné, is found on various trees, and was prized above all others as a healing remedy in the Gallic and German antiquity. The Druids—their priests—were at the same time naturalists, metaphysicians, doctors and sorcerers, and to the mistletoe growing on oaks were ascribed, above all other plants, marvelous healing powers. That the oak mistletoe was prized above all those growing on fruit or other trees, as a remedy, may be due to the fact that in ancient times all oaks and oak groves were regarded with a holy veneration, being considered the favorite abodes of the old German deities. The mistletoe growing on oaks was therefore venerated by the ancient Gauls and Germans as the holiest of heaven-sent gifts to mankind. It was applied in all diseases, and without it no religious service could be conducted. From the Germanic mythology we know that as a priest—a Druid—discovered a mistletoe growing on an oak, he at once called up all the brethren of his order of the neighborhood. They doffed the many-colored garments in daily use, and donned flowing white robes as a sign of humility in the presence of the divine plant. The highest in rank approached the tree provided with a golden sickle, bent his knees, and was then lifted by his companions on high until he could reach the plant. This was then cut with the golden sickle and prepared and preserved for sacred and for healing purposes.

If it could be secured six days after the new moon, the most exhalted healing properties were attributed to it, and it was at once made into a potion which, mixed with the blood of steers that had never done any work and which had been immolated beneath the oaks, formed a draught which brought blessings, fruitfulness, health and prosperity to all who could partake of it.

As at that time, and for a long time after, the origin and propagation of the parasitic plant was unknown, it was surrounded with a magic halo, and by virtue of its undoubted healing qualities, especially in gout, rheumatism, nerve pains of various kinds, neuralgias, especially of the rheumatic and gouty variety, as well as of its close affinity with and influence upon the female sexual system, it was accorded the highest rank among all remedies by the Priestesses, the female Druids.

About the year 1857-58, I passed one year in the town of Steger, in upper Austria, as physician to Prince Lamberg; there I became well acquainted with Dr. W. Huber, at the time physician to the Homœopathic Hospital of the "Sisters of Mercy," and found in him also an antiquary of considerable learning. His researches brought to his notice in what high veneration the mistletoe was held by the ancient Germans and Gauls and its employment as a universal healing remedy. Dr. Huber, who was a man of unusual intelligence and of high scientific acquirements, desired to learn the true sphere of action of this important remedy, and preparing a mother-tincture from the mistletoe—*lege artis*—he proved the several dilutions on himself and others, men and women, thus truly following the example of Hahnemann and his disciples. I still possess some of this identical tincture as prepared by Dr. Huber, who, I am grieved to say, died suddenly of apoplexy during my sojourn, in the year 1858.

Dr. Huber carefully collated all the symptoms experienced by his provers; he had a great predilection for the mistletoe, which he prescribed in many different ailments. He frequently conversed with me about its healing properties, and often gave it in his hospital and in his private practice. He used it chiefly in the 3d and 6th decimal dilution. According to Dr. Huber, the symptoms of *Viscum album* are similar to those of *Aconite, Bryonia, Pulsatilla, Rhododendron, Rhus* and *Spigelia, i.e.,* are in accord with our foremost anti-arthritic and anti-rheumatic remedies. *Viscum* has symptoms in common with each of these remedies, and is thus particularly useful in gouty and rheumatic complaints, in acute as well as in chronic cases; more particularly in those having *tearing pains* in no matter what part of the body. It follows well after *Aconite* in acute rheumatism. It is also very effective in different neuralgias of a gouty or rheumatic origin, as in ischias, prosopalgia, periostitis, and especially in earache, tearing pains in the ears, and otitis. It is a sovereign remedy in rheumatic deafness. As *causa excitans* of diseases amenable to it may be regarded high winds, *i.e.,* all gouty, rheumatic or other ailments which, similarly to *Rhus* and *Rhododendron,* are aggravated by sharp north or northwest winds, such as we have in winter. For this reason *Viscum* is more often applicable in the colder season than in summer, or at time when gouty or rheumatic affections or pains are usually aggravated. It has also been found beneficial in asthmatic complaints if connected with gout or rheumatism.

The mistletoe moreover stands in a peculiarly close relation to the female sexual system (uterus), and especially to the climacteric period, when women cease to menstruate and chronic or periodical hæmorrhages are often met with. *Viscum* also promotes labor pains similarly to *Pulsatilla* and *Secale*, and is especially efficient in effecting the expulsion of the placenta, also in incarcerated placenta.

When the great army of gouty and rheumatic ailments which may befall all parts of the body are taken into consideration, as well as the manifold sufferings originating in the female sexual system, which manifest themselves as menorrhagias as well as amenorrhœa, but more often are caused by congestive states,—when we consider the powerful influence of the mistletoe on these forms of diseases as brought out by the careful homœopathic provings on the healthy, is it to be marvelled at that the old Gauls and Germans venerated it, by whose mysterious origin they were overawed, as a sovereign remedy for their ailments and sufferings, as a sacred gift presented by the gods of mankind?

(The following clinical case is from *Hom. World*, 1876, by Dr. Ivatts:)

October 24, 1875.—T. H———, æt. about fifty. Rheumatism for the last six years of ankle, wrists, and knuckle joints, also pains across the lumbar muscles. Extreme distress on motion, with weariness and pain. Great pain in walking. Worse on commencing to move, but after continuing the movement for a time the pain diminishes. No pain when at rest except when warm in bed, when the ankle and wrist joints are occasionally very bad. Patient holds a degree L.R.C.S.I., but has relinquished practice for fifteen years and travelled abroad. Never could get relief from the rheumatism.—*Viscum album* No. 1, five drops twice a day. November 14.— After taking medicine for ten days the weary feeling gradually diminished, and the muscular motion became free from distress. Has now continued medicine for three weeks, and he says, "I am quite free from rheumatic pains." February 18, 1876.—Saw patient to-day, and he tells me he has continued quite free from the rheumatic pains since November.

(Dr. E. M. Holland wrote as follows concerning the remedy, *Medical Summary*, 1898:)

My first case of child birth in which I used *Mistletoe* (*Viscum album*) was May 30, 1897. Was called to see Mrs. C.; second confinement; there was but little advancement; I sent the husband to my office, three blocks away, for some *Mistletoe*, and I gave the lady half a teaspoonful with a swallow of water every twenty minutes, and before one hour had passed labor was on in good shape, and in half an hour longer all was over.

I returned to my office, and in less than half an hour I was called to see a colored woman, much of a lady, mother of two children; on examination I found only a slight advancement of the child, mouth of the womb but little dilated. I learned that she had been just about the same for twelve hours. I prepared a mixture and ordered a teaspoonful every twenty minutes; this dose contained 30 drops of the *Mistletoe*. I was not well, and returned to my office, leaving instructions to notify me when labor was well on; my office was four blocks from her residence. I reclined on a lounge, intending to return in about an hour, but dropped into a doze, and in about one and a half hours the husband came on the run, notwithstanding they had sent a little girl for me. He reached my office panting, and exclaimed: 'For God's sake, hurry, for her insides have all come out.' On my arrival, I found the child and afterbirth all in a pile. The confusion was soon calmed down by the assurance that all was well.

Soon after this I was called to see Mrs. M., the mother of seven children. I had been with her in six of the seven confinements, and knowing that she had always been tedious I gave the messenger a small vial of the same mixture and same dose, labelled it teaspoonful every twenty minutes, stating that I would be there in an hour or two, and I was; but the child was born about fifteen minutes before.

On the 14th day of July of the present year I was called to attend Mrs. B. in her third labor, some two miles in the country. I left home at 3:30 A.M. When I arrived at the house I found nothing to indicate that I would be permitted to return home sooner than—I will say a number of hours. I found presentation all right, some dilatation, but there was but little advancement. The pains seemed to be of excruciating character, but not the kind to do more than wear the patient out. She told me that the same kind of pains had been on for a day and night, so I continued with the *Mistletoe* in half-teaspoonful doses every twenty minutes. Pains came on; in just one hour her extreme agony ceased. Labor came on, and in half an hour more the child was born.

In all these cases the placenta came readily and everything progressed well after birth. I said I left my office at 3:30 A.M., and I was at home again by 7 A.M. It may be that four cases are not sufficient to decide on the merits of a remedy, but the change was so decided and prompt that I am satisfactorily convinced that in *Mistletoe* we have an oxytocic that is superior to all remedies hitherto tried.

After the foregoing was compiled, Dr. George Black's exceedingly interesting brochure of 79 pages, *Viscum album, the Common Mistletoe*, etc., etc., appeared, and anyone wanting a complete history of the drug should procure a copy.

Dr. Black (Torquay, England) publishes all the known provings, and in addition some very thorough ones conducted by himself; from these we select the following striking symptoms:

Proll experienced a sensation as if a large spider were crawling over his hands; a glow rising from feet to head, and he seemed to be on fire, though his face was pale, this repeatedly; also violent aching pain in right foot recurring frequently. Proving with the tincture in increasing doses up to 40 drops.

Two women took the drug to produce abortion; every muscle of the body was paralyzed, including bowels, save those of the eye, and both died on the 8th and 9th day, starved to death.

The provings by Dr. Black. A well-built woman, aged twenty, took repeated doses of the drug from θ up to 30th. The most striking symptoms were: Sudden, severe thumps of the heart that then went on beating at a tremendous rate; it slowed down and was followed by trembling in the limbs; after this was very marked jerking of the limbs, and twitching; hot feeling, though not actually hot. "A feeling as if I should bite some one if I did not keep my teeth clenched. A wretched feeling as if I should do something awfully wrong if I did not keep myself under control." Several months later the effect of the drug was still strongly in evidence; "thinks she will go out of her mind, feels as if she would have an epileptic fit, says she would feel far happier in an asylum."

A second prover, Mrs.—— æt 37, experienced jerking and twitchings of the muscles, shooting pains in left ovarian region, and, on movement, lumbar pain and stiffness. Proving made with 3d dilution.

Third prover, æt 27, a woman. First marked symptom was a shooting pain in left ovary; then pain and twitching in leg, when aching stopped it felt very hot; aching repeated, and only relief was shifting the position of the leg to a cool place in the bed; again a dreadful pain in the region of the left ovary—"a fearful aching" "it was a pain you couldn't have put up with long without doing something;" later: "I have had no pain, but a great twitching in my hands and legs for a long time, just like a person with chorea—first my left hand jumped, then both legs, my heart seemed to beat very fast." "When hands were held it seemed to alleviate the jerking and twitching." The pain in ovaries, also in other parts of the body at times, the twitchings and jerkings, and the frequent hot feeling continued during all the proving. It was made with the 3d and θ.

The fourth proving was made by Dr. Black himself, chiefly with the 3x and θ.

This proving is quite long. From it we note the following symptoms: Severe pain in right shoulder joint. Muscular twitching in right leg. Dull pain under left false ribs. Neuralgic pain in sciatic nerve. Back, lumbar region, stiff and weak. Pain in right knee joint, painful to move and tender to the touch. Weight and oppression of the heart, with gripping feeling as if a hand were squeezing it; the load seemed to lift, with great relief, but came back again. A curious sensation of tickling about the heart. Twinges of pain in the great toes. The last record some days after ceasing the proving reads as follows: "I think it was the same night as the previously recorded symptoms that I went to bed between 12 and 1 o'clock, and after lying down experienced a curious general tremor through my body, as if all the muscles were in a state of fibrillary contraction; not a single involuntary jerk, nor the continued twitching of the muscle or a portion of one, but a general state affecting the whole body. It lasted until I fell asleep."

Therapeutically the drug has been used for palsy, "incompetency and tumultuous distressing cardiac action," mitral disease, chorea, epilepsy, retention of placenta, catarrhal deafness, menorrhagia, sciatica, rheumatism, periostitis, hydrothorax, and transient deafness.

The Druids sweepingly asserted that it would "heal all diseases."

WYETHIA HELENIOIDES.

NAT. ORD., Compositæ.
COMMON NAME, Californian compass plant.
PREPARATION.—One part of the fresh root is macerated in two parts by weight of alcohol.

(The following, by Dr. J. M. Selfridge, Oakland, Cal., was published in *Pacific Coast Journal of Homœopathy*, April, 1899:)

There is probably no State in the Union where there is a greater number of valuable remedies to be found than in the State of California. These remedies are waiting to be proved by those of us who have sufficient enthusiasm and who are willing to take the trouble and make what sacrifice is necessary to accomplish so desirable a result. I know it has been said that we have too many remedies which have not been properly proven. While this is doubtless true, it is equally true that many of the new remedies which have been introduced within the memory of some of us are absolutely indispensable in the treatment of certain forms of disease.

There is another reason why these California remedies should become a part of our armamentarium. It is claimed by Teste and others that where certain forms of disease prevail there, or in that vicinity, the curative remedy may be found.

Again, it has been said that there is a remedy somewhere in nature for every ill to which flesh is heir.

Whether this be true or not, we know there are certain diseases, which, so far as we are aware, are incurable, for the simple reason that we know of no remedy that will control the abnormal conditions. This being true, the incentive ought to be sufficiently great to urge us forward in the line of knowing more than we now know of the wealth of those remedies that lie at our very doors. All we know of these drugs, so far, are mere hints which have been given us by the older inhabitants of the Coast.

Thus, the *Eriodictyon Californicum* or "Yerba Santa," has been suggested for the cure of "poison oak" and for certain bronchial affections. A partial proving of it was made some years ago under the supervision of the late Dr. Pease, which can be found in "Allen's Encyclopædia," Vol. iv., page 218.

The *Micromeria Douglassi,* or "Yerba Bueno," is another plant which should be proved. Many years ago a friend of mine was suffering with a series of boils, when an old "Spanish woman" directed him to make a tea of this plant. This he did, and cured his boils; but, as the tea had an agreeable taste, he continued to drink it, believing, as some do, "that if little was good, more was better," until finally he became so weak he could not continue his work.

It was one of these hints that induced me some years ago to make a proving of *Wyethia Helenioides*, or "poison weed." Like many other provings, it was only partial. A schema of it was published in "Allen's Encyclopædia," Vol. x., page 168.

Two years ago an attempt was made to secure additional symptoms, which are given below in the language of the provers, who at that time were members of the "Organon and Materia Medica Club of the Bay Cities."

At the time of the proving, the potency and the drug were unknown to the provers.

I. "June 9th, 1896, began taking——, of which I took a drop in a teaspoonful of water before each meal. First dose 7:35 (did this for four days); 7:45, feels in nose as if about to sneeze; 7:50, sitting quietly, a momentary pain on inside of right foot from instep to the sole; 8:35, stretching and yawning, itching on the left side of the chin; 4:10 P.M., dry sensation in throat, although mucus is abundant; 5:30 P.M., sensation of dryness and tickling on the edges of eyelids, such as I felt when a sty was about to appear; sensation of dryness in throat; 5:35 P.M., a small itching spot on right side of neck; 8 P.M., dryness in throat with abundant mucus.

"June 7th.—7:30 A.M., throat sore; 8:35, tingling in right foot when standing; 11, while in church, sensations of formications in eyelids with lachrymations; 11:25, pain in the right testicle; 3 P.M., despondent; P.M., pain on top of right shoulder midway between neck and point of shoulder; motion does not affect it.

"June 8th.—Before breakfast, lips feel dry, back of throat (posterior wall of pharynx) sore, increased flow of tasteless saliva; 10:30, pain in left ear, itching in left external canthus; 1:30 P.M., mouth full of sweetish saliva; at lunch bit tongue severely; 9:30 P.M., mouth feels dry and as if scalded, with desire to drink frequently in order to moisten it.

"June 9th.—Scalded mouth continues.

"June 12th.—6 A.M., lips feel scalded and swollen.

"June 17th.—Itching in rectum.

"July 4th.—10 A.M., headache in left anterior part of brain, as if radiated from left inner canthus; 12:30, headache in left occipital protuberance.

"For several nights waken frequently and too early in the morning, without any disagreeable consequences.

"July 7th.—A sore hang-nail on third finger of right hand.

(Signed)
"A. McNEIL."

Dr. McNeil took the first decimal dilution. (S.)

II. "June 5th.—Began at 1 P.M., taking a drop before each meal.

"June 6th.—Depressed all forenoon, languid feeling of mind and body; despondent almost to desperation; irritable, cross, easily angered about trifles; melancholy about the future, with no reason for it; seemed that I was forsaken by all my friends and was on the verge of insanity; bodily uneasiness, unfitting me for any work; felt that I could 'fall all down in a heap;' muscles seemed to refuse to respond to the will.

"June 7th.—Entire incapacity for mental work; could not follow a line of thought twenty seconds; forehead cold to touch, with heavy feeling over the eyes as though the skin and flesh of forehead would come down over the eyes; intense drowsiness all day, worse after meals; irresistible sleepiness after lunch; accustomed cup of coffee was not relished.

"June 8th.—Dreams were vivid and real; was discovered talking in my sleep; the thoughts and work of previous day were on my mind on waking as though I had not gone to sleep.

"June 9th and 10th.—Aversion to company, did not wish to see anyone, not even intimate friends; great aversion to my work; had to punish myself to even visit a patient; quarrelsome, impatient, irritable.

"M. F. UNDERWOOD."

Dr. Underwood took the fifteenth decimal dilution. (S.)

III. "June 8th, 1896, commenced taking remedy given by Dr. Selfridge, one drop three times a day before meals.

"June 13th.—After a restless night, awakened at 7:30 A.M. with severe, sharp pain in the right tonsil; throat felt swollen and sore; tonsil red and inflamed; glands on right side of neck swollen and sore to touch.

"At 9:30, neuralgic pains commenced in left arm and hand, then in back, limbs and all over the body; skin felt sore to touch; was quite ill all day, with no appetite whatever.

"At 7:30 P.M. commenced to feel chilly; upon the slightest movement chills would creep up the back, with increase of pain; grew colder and colder; was very ill, and went to bed. At 9:30 fever commenced with desire for food; head very hot; cheeks very red and burning; temperature 102°, but still very chilly. Passed a very restless night, with chill, fever and sweat all at the same time, with constant twinges of pain all over the body, particularly in back and limbs; could not bear the slightest touch.

"June 14th.—Temperature 101-1/2° at 8 A.M. Right tonsil and glands of neck still very sore, in fact, worse; pains over body less, though back quite sore and lame; felt very weak and unable to remain out of bed.

"Still continued the remedy. All symptoms gradually improved, and was entirely well in a few days.

"June 20th.—Stopped taking the remedy on advice of Dr. Selfridge.

"June 21st.—Very depressed, both mentally and physically; menses commenced at 2:30 P.M., with slight uterine pain. Retired at 10 o'clock, when the pain became intense and burning. Suffered all night, the pain being constant, though increasing in paroxysms with sensation as if the uterus expanded in order to keep all the pain within its walls. Could distinctly outline the contour of the uterus. Never had such a pain before.

"June 22nd.—Pain much better, but still a paroxysm every little while. Felt very weak all day and mentally depressed.

"When menses ceased, observed no further symptoms.

"July 4th.—Commenced the remedy again.

"July 18th.—At 11 A.M. commenced to feel chilly, with aching pains all over the body, which gradually grew worse until 12 o'clock, when a most severe chill took place; shook all over; aching over body and headache intense. Took no more of the remedy; went to bed, and as I was growing worse, was given *Aconite* at 1 o'clock. There was great thirst for ice water during the entire chill, which lasted until 2:30 P.M., when fever came on; temperature, 101°; no thirst. In about fifteen minutes commenced to sweat. Temperature at 4 o'clock 100°; still sweating. At 10 P.M. menses commenced; no uterine pain, but still aching all over body which continued all night, preventing sleep; pains worse in limbs and back; at times jerking in character, making me start with every twinge; profuse sweating all night.

"July 19th.—Very weak; aching still continued, but less; cords of neck, right side, quite painful. Passed a restless night, still sweating profusely.

"July 20th.—Much better, but still very weak; some aching and sweating; did not go to sleep until 3 A.M.; was nervous and restless.

"July 21st.—Much improved in every way, and was all right in a day or two. Did not take any more of the remedy.

"July 26th.—At 1:30 P.M. commenced to feel chilly, with intense headache and aching all over the body. The chilliness rapidly increased until at 2 o'clock had a worse chill than ever, which lasted until 4 o'clock, when fever came on, temperature soon reaching 103°; sweating commenced almost simultaneously with the fever; headache was the most prominent symptom, which was terrific; intense, congestive headache; eyes extremely sensitive; bones of the face sensitive to touch; could not move the head a hair's breadth without intense agony; thought I should go mad from the intensity of the pain. This lasted until 10:30, when there was a sensation of faintness, due evidently to lack of food, and which passed away after eating some cream toast; the headache then also began to grow less, and I passed a fairly good night.

"July 27th.—Was much better, but was too nervous to remain in bed; felt very weak all day; retired early, but did not sleep a moment all night long.

"July 28th.—Arose at 6 A.M.; was weak and dizzy all day; had to lie down every little while. Slept well this night.

"Have been fairly well ever since. (August 7, 1896.)

"ELEANOR F.
MARTIN."

Dr. Martin took the thirtieth decimal dilution. (S.)

Lightning Source UK Ltd.
Milton Keynes UK
UKHW010943281222
414514UK00004B/239